Tāntric Hedonism of Mahānadī Valley
(Uḍḍīyāna Pīṭha)

Tantra in Contemporary Researches

1. Impact of Tantra on Religion and Art; by T.N. Mishra (ISBN 81-246-0073-2)
2. Lalitā-Sahasranāma — A Comprehensive Study of One Thousand Names of Lalitā Mahā-tripurasundarī; by M.L. Joshi (ISBN 81-246-0104-6)
3. Yoga-Tantra and Sensuousness in Art; by T.N. Mishra (ISBN 81-246-0239-5)
4. Tāntric Hedonism of Mahānadī Valley (Uḍḍiyāna Pīṭha); by Jitamitra Prasad Singh Deo (ISBN 81-246-0269-7)

Tantra in Contemporary Researches, no. 4

Tāntric Hedonism of Mahānadī Valley (Uḍḍīyāna Pīṭha)

by

Jitamitra Prasad Singh Deo

D.K. Printworld (P) Ltd.
New Delhi

Cataloging in Publication Data — DK
[Courtesy: D.K. Agencies (P) Ltd. <docinfo@dkagencies.com>]

Singh Deo, Jitamitra Prasad, 1946-
Tāntric Hedonism of Mahānadī Valley
(Uḍḍiyāna Pīṭha) / by Jitamitra Prasad Singh Deo.
p., 25 cm.
(Tantra in contemporary researches, no. 4).
Includes bibliographical references (p.)
Includes index.
ISBN 8124602697

1. Hedonism — India — Orissa — History.
2. Tantrism — India — Orissa — History. 3.
India — Civilization. I. Title. II. Series:
Tantra in contemporary researches, no. 4.

DDC 171.409 541 3 21

ISBN 81-246-0269-7
First Published in India in 2004

Published and printed by:
D.K. Printworld (P) Ltd.
Regd. office : *"Sri Kunj,"* F-52, Bali Nagar,
New Delhi - 110 015
Phones : (011) 2545-3975; 2546-6019; *Fax* : (011) 2546-5926
E-mail: dkprintworld@vsnl.net
Web: www.dkprintworld.com

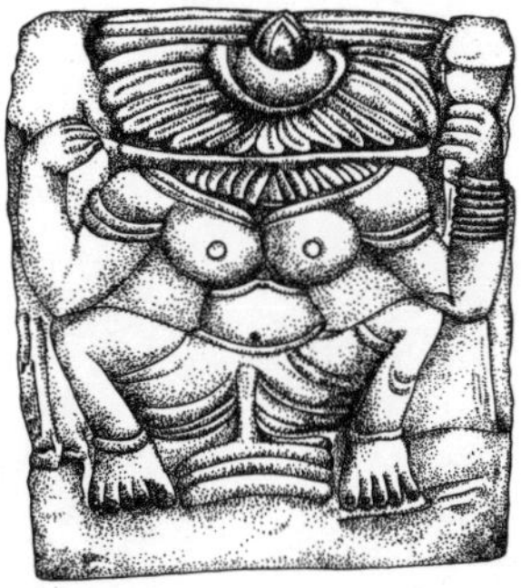

Preface

THE spiritual culture of India, i.e., Bhāratavarṣa, reached its topmost zenith through Vedic wisdom, which is meant for entire human beings of the earth. *Tantra* is a parallel cultivation of this Vedic wisdom which brought much refinement to the art of Vedic civilization. As overall development of Indian spirituality is based on truth, it brought about a synthesis of all aspects of life. It is for this reason that Indian civilization is eternal and a vibrant composite culture. As the Vedic civilization mostly developed in the Sarasvatī valley, Indians claim that though this river of north-west India has dried up now, Sarasvatī still flows on, i.e., Indian culture or civilization is perennial. This is Vedic culture.

The discussions of this book reveals that there was antediluvian culture in the Mahānadī valley and the nucleus of this culture, spirituality and civilization, developed from the central right of the valley which comprised the modern districts of Nuapāḍā, Kālāhāṇḍī, Bolaṅgīr and Sonepur in Orissa. It is difficult to confirm and appreciate antediluvian cultures. But with yogic intuitive knowledge, practical experiences, comparative study of archaeological findings, history and their synthesis, I have been able to trace the development of the *yoga* of sexual transformation, the genesis of the Lord Jagannātha deity and depiction of all *haṭha yogic* features latent or potential in the rare gigantic icon at Tala village situated in Bilāspur district of Chhattisgarh province in the upper hinterland of Mahānadī valley.

The development of the Kośali style of temple architecture has been studied with its *kāmakalā yantra* plan and its influences on the development of temple architecture in coastal Orissa, which came to be known as Kaliṅga Style of Temple Architecture, is also shown in this book.

Therefore, it can be claimed that the whole Mahānadī river valley is the land of *kāmakalā* where *uḍḍīyāna bandha* and *haṭha* yogic practices developed. Hence, it can be pointed out that the Mahānadī valley comprises the territories of South Kośala, Utkala and Kaliṅga, that is both the land of Kāmakalā and Uḍḍīyāna Pīṭha (Site). H.K. Mahatab[1] rightly states,

> Orissa as it is today consists of portions of three ancient regions, Kaliṅga, Utkala or Odra and Kośala which in course of centuries under political, social and economic pressure joined together in the twelfth century and developed to form the Oriya society as a distinct entity in the realm of India.

I appreciate my wife Srimati Rajshree Devi, Rani of Khariar, for providing me solitariness by taking up all worldly responsibilities and taking care of me as well. It is because of her sincere cooperation that I could devote myself to research and finally write this book. My wife is the cousin of the present Gajapati Maharaj Dibya Singh Deb IV of Purī and daughter of late Thatraj Raj Raj Deb of Purī. I am thankful to D.K. Printworld, for publishing the book, "Tāntric Hedonism of Mahānadī Valley (Uḍḍīyāna Pīṭha)."

29th August 2004
Khariar

Jitamitra Prasad Singh Deo
Raja Khariar, Palace Khariar,
P.O.: Khariar - 766 107,
Nuapada District
Orissa, India

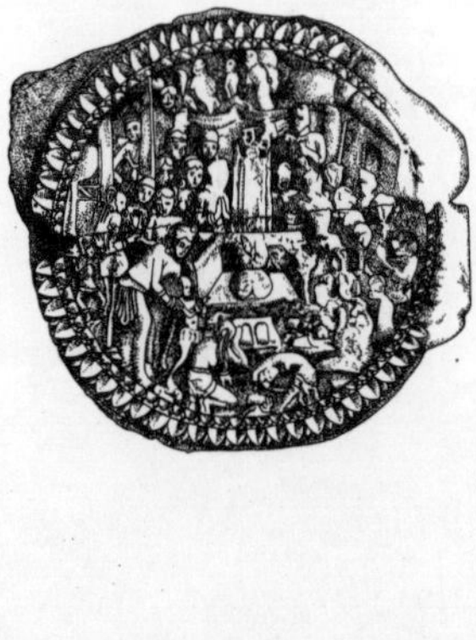

1. H.K. Mahatab, "Culture of Orissa," *OHRJ* (Golden Jubilee Volume), vol. xxx, nos. 2, 3 & 4, 1984, p. 1.

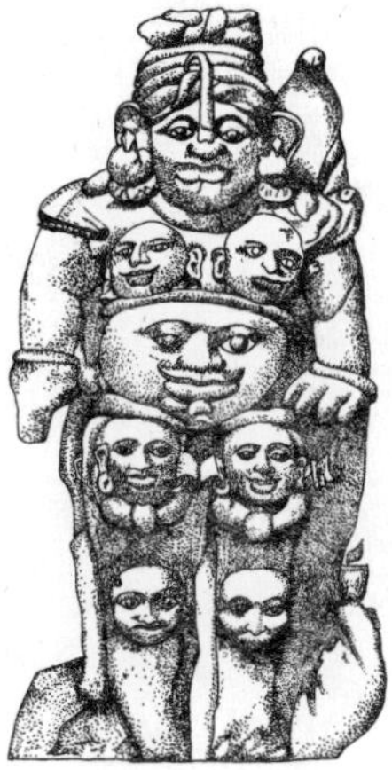

Contents

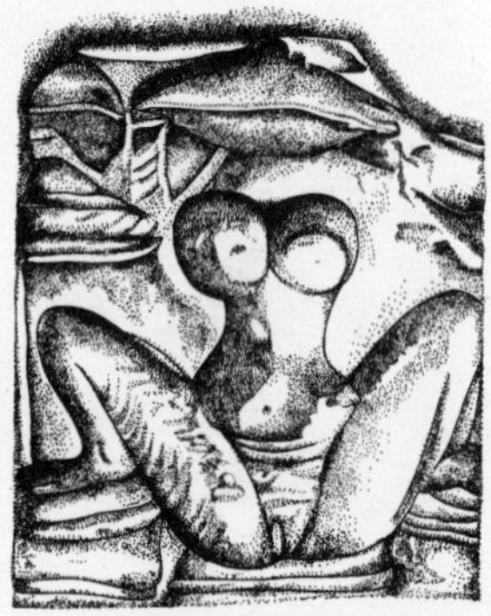

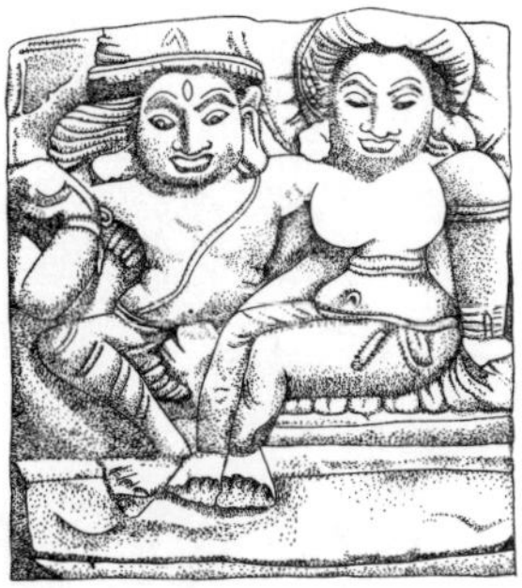

Abbreviations

BSOIHAC — *Bhishma's Study of Indian History and Culture*, General editor, S.D. Kulkarni, Shri Bhagavan Vedavyasa Itihasa Samshodhana Mandira, Mumbai, Thane.

EI — *Epigraphia Indica*.

HYPBS — *Haṭhayoga Pradīpikā* by Swatmarama, (Commentary) Sarasvatī, Swami Muktibodhananda, Bihar School of Yoga, Munger, Bihar, 1993.

JBORS — *Journal of Bihar and Orissa Research Society*.

NIATAL — *Naṭarāja in Art, Thought and Literature*, by C. Sivaramamurti, Publication Division, Govt. of India, New Delhi, 2nd edn., 1994.

NSS — National Service Scheme.

OHRJ — *The Orissa Historical Research Journal*.

ROII — *Riddle of Indian Iconography* (*Zetetic on Rare Icon from Tala*), ed. L.S. Nigam, Sharada Publishing House, Delhi, 2000.

SASWITW — *Sex and Sex Worship in the World* by O.A. Wall, Inter-India Publications, Delhi, 1979.

THACOTIP — *History and Culture of The Indian People*, General ed. R.C. Majumdar, Bharatiya Vidya Bhavan, Mumbai.

TSFO	*The Sarasvati Flows on* (*The Continuity of Indian Culture*), B.B. Lal, Aryan Books International, New Delhi, 2002.
TECOSA	*The Earliest Civilization of South Asia,* B.B. Lal, Aryan Books International, New Delhi, 1997.
TYATWG	*Tantric Yoga and the Wisdom Goddesses,* David Frawley, Motilal Banarsidass, Delhi, 1996.

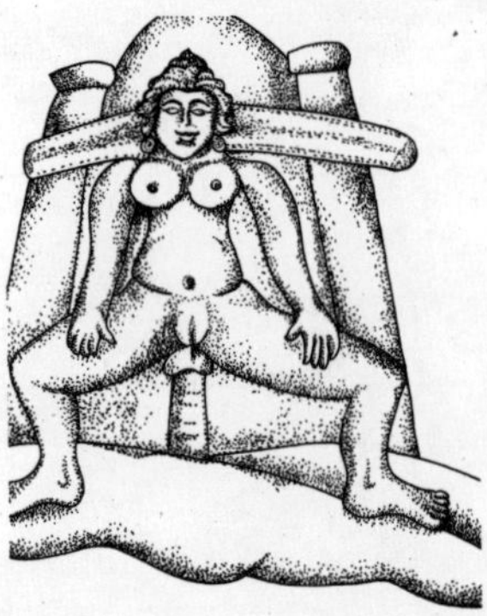

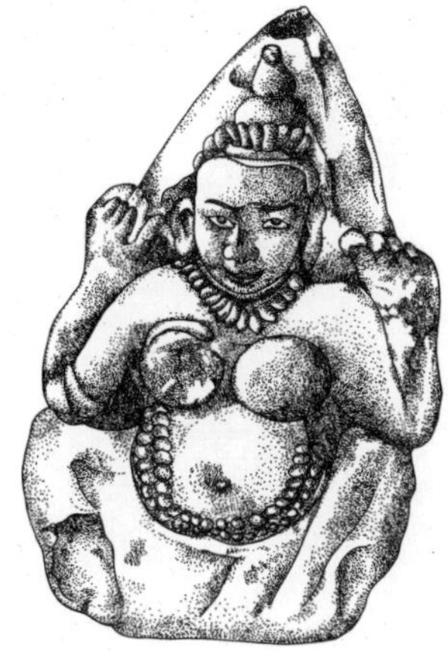

List of Plates and Figures

Plates

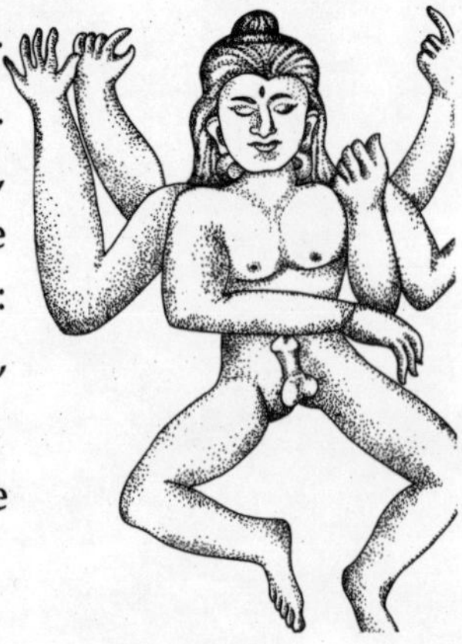

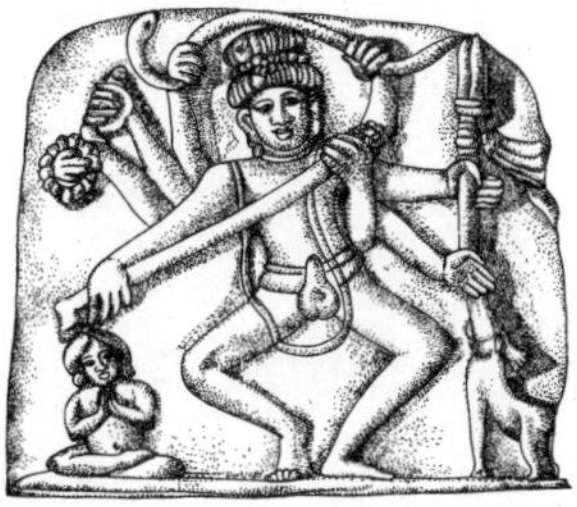

influence of the one on an image chiselled on the *Śivaliṅga* of Guḍimallam village, Andhra Pradesh, second century BC.

Pl. 29. Dakṣina Kālī as found in a northern niche of the Kedāreśvara Mahādeva temple at Ichhapur village of Kālāhaṇḍī district, Orissa. Modern construction within the eighteenth-nineteenth century AD.

Pl. 30. Nīlakaṇṭheśvara Śiva temple at Dadpur, Kālāhāṇḍī district. Kalacuri construction, within the twelfth-thirteenth century AD.

Pl. 31. Pātāleśvara Śiva temple of brick construction at Bodhi-Komnā, Nuāpāḍā district. Within the seventh-eighth century AD (before conservation).

Pls. 32. 33. & 34. The view of Pātāleśvara Śiva temple at Bodhi-Komnā (after conservation).

Pls. 35. to 42. Different views of the Citāberi Devī temple at Dhobni village, dist. Raipur, Chhattisgarh. Within seventh-eighth century AD.

Pl. 43. The Kapileśvara temple at Bauḍ, facing east. Ninth century AD.

Pl. 44. Three Tāntric temples at Bauḍ. Ninth century AD.

Pls. 45&46. The view of Tribidheśvar temple deity, Asika in Gañjam district, Orissa. The three *liṅga*s are sucked inside to the depth of 1½ ft, which shows the practice of the Vajroli *Haṭha* Yogic *mudrā*, i.e., the thunderbolt attitude in which the muscles of the male sexual organ and lower urinary tract are contracted, re-directing sexual energy upwards. A practice of the *Haṭha Yoga* and *Tantra*.

Figures

fig. 1. Pre-historic rock-shelter painting of Gurhandi, Kālāhāṇḍī district, Orissa.

fig. 2. Pre-historic rock-shelter painting of Yogīmaṭh Donger

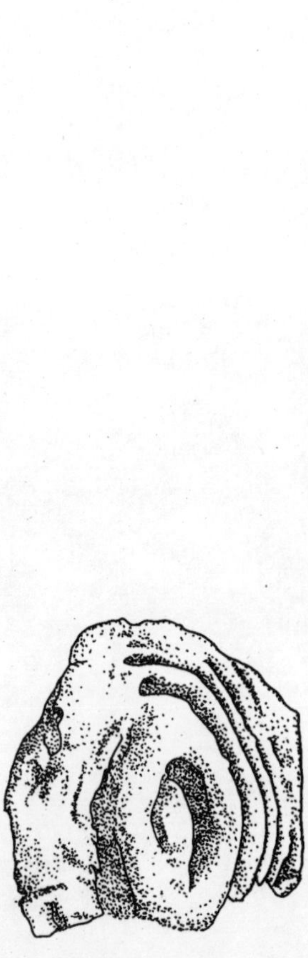

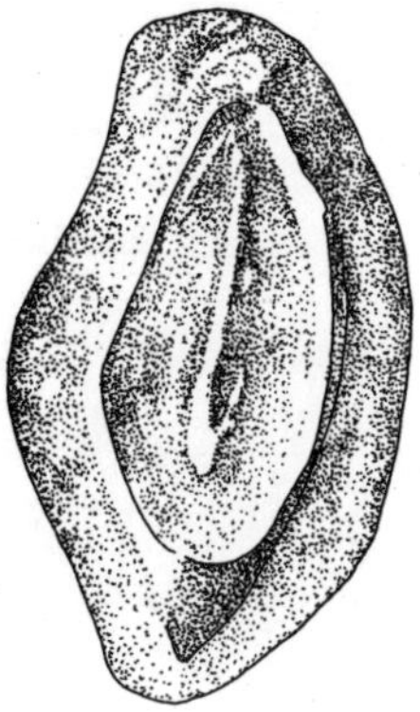

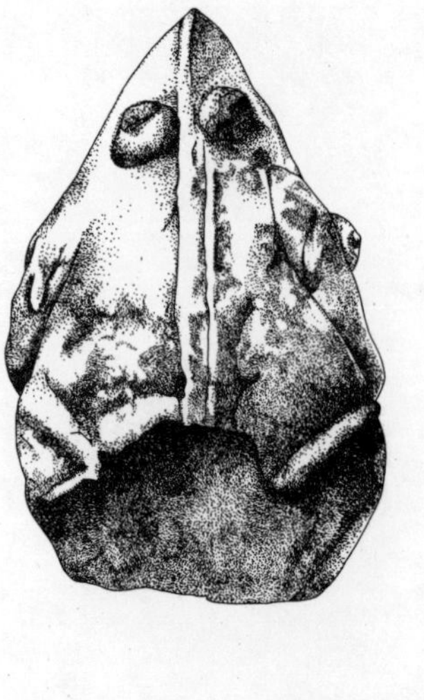

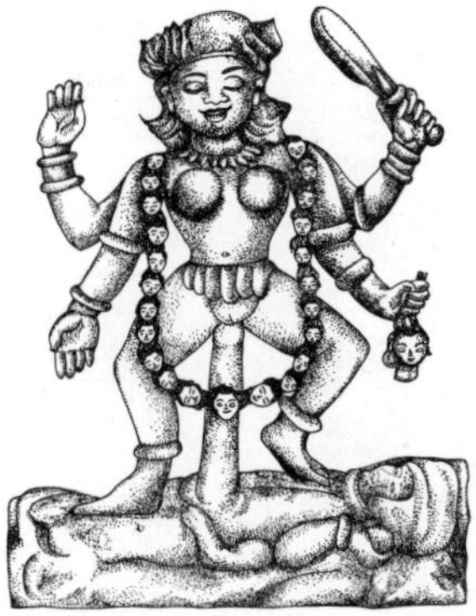

Transliteration Chart

अ *a* (but)

आ *ā* (palm)

इ *i* (it)

ई *ī* (beet)

उ *u* (put)

ऊ *ū* (pool)

ऋ *ṛ* (rhythm)

ए *e* (play)

ऐ *ai* (high)

ओ *o* (toe)

औ *au* (loud)

क *ka* (skate)[1]

ख* *kha* (blockhead)[1]

ग *ga* (gate)[1]

घ *gha* (loghut)[1]

ङ *ṅa* (sing)[1]

च *ca* (chunk)[2]

छ* *cha* (catch him)[2]

ज *ja* (john)[2]

झ *jha* (hedgehog)[2]

ञ *ña* (bunch)[2]

ट *ṭa* (start)[3]

ठ* *ṭha* (anthill)[3]

ड *ḍa* (dart)[3]

ढ* *ḍha* (godhead)[3]

ण* *ṇa* (under)[3]

त *ta* (path)[4]

थ *tha* (thunder)[4]

द *da* (that)[4]

ध* *dha* (breathe)[4]

न *na* (numb)[4]

प *pa* (spin)[5]

फ* *pha* (loophole)[5]

ब *ba* (bin)[5]

भ *bha* (abhor)[5]

म *ma* (much)[5]

य *ya* (young)

र *ra* (drama)

ल *la* (luck)

व *va* (vile)

श *śa* (shove)

ष *ṣa* (bushel)

स *sa* (so)

ह *ha* (hum)

ं *ṁ anusvāra* (nasalisation of preceding vowel)

: *ḥ visarga* (aspiration of preceding vowel)

* No exact English equivalents for these letters.

[1] guttural [2] palatal [3] lingual [4] dental [5] labial

Om Sri Sathya Sai Baba Saranam

Dedicated at the lotus feet
of
Sri Sathya Sai Baba
the living Purushottam Jagannath

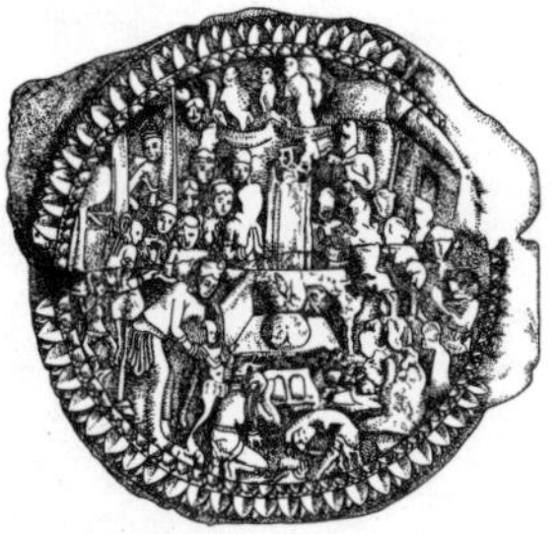

Introduction

HEDONISM is an ethic, whose doctrine is that pleasure is the highest good. There are four stages of happiness: pleasure, joy, bliss and beatitude. Beatitude is the happiness of the highest kind, it is heavenly happiness. Beatitude can be compared to *samādhi* in yogic conception. *Samādhi* is a particular type of consciousness whose practicality lies in the rise of *kuṇḍalinī*.

Kuṇḍalinī is a gift of *tantra* to mankind or human beings. In the words of Paramahansa Swami Satyananda Saraswati.[1]

> Since the dawn of creation, the *tāntrikas* and *yogīs* have realized that in this physical body there is a potential force. It is not psychological, philosophical or transcendental; it is a dynamic potential force in the material body and it is called *kuṇḍalinī*. This *kuṇḍalinī* is the greatest discovery of *tantra* and *Yoga*.

No definite period can be assigned to the beginning of *tantra*. It grew slowly throughout the ages. *Yoga* and *tantra* lay down systems for practical understanding of the human condition. The basic components of human beings are body, mind and spirit, i.e., *piṅgalā*, *iḍā* and *suṣumnā nāḍīs*. These flows of energy make up the entire human personality and are derived from the ultimate polarity of our macrocosmic universe into Śiva and Śakti, consciousness and energy.[2]

---

1. Paramahansa Swami S. Saraswati, *Kuṇḍalinī Tantra*, Bihar School of Yoga, Munger, 1992, vide introduction, passim.
2. *Ibid.*, p. 351.

Kuṇḍalinī is the subject-matter of *tantra.*[3] Paramahansa Swami Satyananda Saraswati states,

> *Kuṇḍalinī* does not belong either to the physical body, (though it has to be searched there), or in the mental body or even in the astral body. It exists in the unconscious causal body, in that particular state of awareness where the concept of time, space and object is completely lost. The seed of the unconscious in man is in the perineum, known in yogic terminology as *mooladhara.*[4] It is a gland, a muscle, a body in which all the unconscious powers and initiations of man are hidden.

Knowledge is of repetitive, derigative, educative and intuitive types. Intuitive knowledge is to be observed in different types of consciousness or *samādhis* acquired through the yogic process with the rise of *kuṇḍalinī.*[5]

The word *tantra* in *Kāśikāvṛtti* is derived from the root *tan*, to spread, i.e., to rise from the little awareness to greater awareness or knowledge. A tāntric text[6] called the *Vārāhī Tantra* gives an elaborate description of the main subjects of *tantra.* They are summarized as follows:

1. Consciousness.
2. The creation and destruction of the physical universe (*sṛṣṭi* and *pralaya*).
3. Worship of deities (*devī* or *deva pūjā*).

3. Paramahansa Swami S. Saraswati, *Kuṇḍalinī Tantra*, Bihar School of Yoga, Munger, 1992, p. 203.
4. Chela Buddhananda, *Moola Bandha The Master Key*, Bihar School of Yoga, Munger, 1984, passim.
5. (i) J.P. Singh Deo, "Preface," *Origin of Jagannath Deity*, Gyan Publishing House, New Delhi, 1991, pp. x-xi.

   (ii) J.P. Singh Deo, *Tāntric Art of Orissa*, Kalpaz Publication, Delhi, 2001, Appendix I, Knowledge and Reality, pp. 213-18.
6. Paramahansa Swami Satyananda Saraswati, *A Systematic Course in the Ancient Tāntric Techniques of Yoga and Kriyā*, Bihar School of Yoga, Munger, 1989, p. 322.

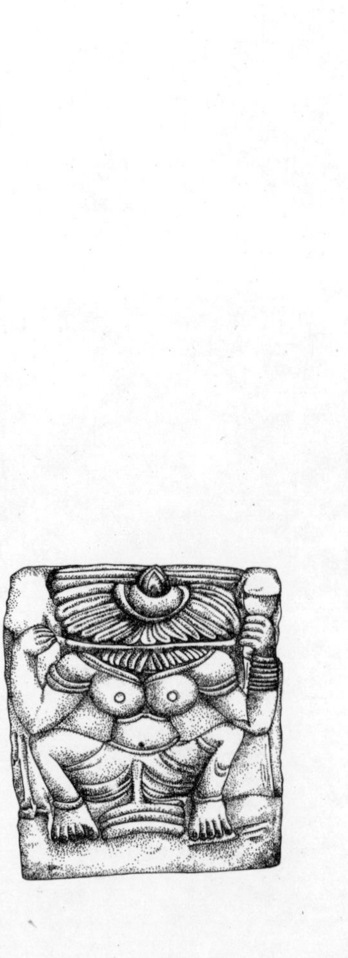

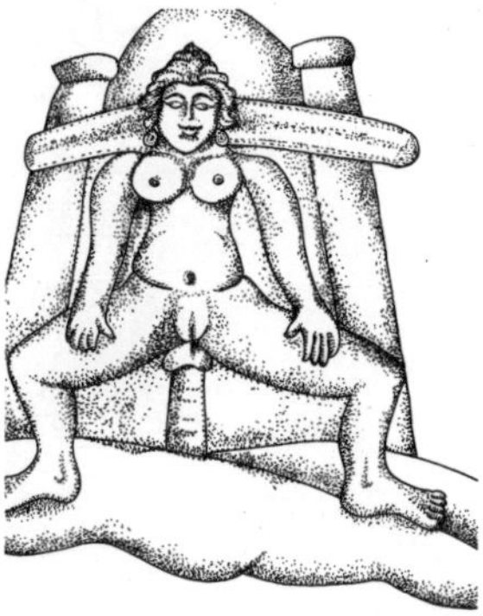

4. Classification of beings.
5. The heavenly bodies — astronomy and astrology.
6. The different levels of awareness (*lokas*).
7. The psychic pathways and centres in the human framework (*nāḍīs* and *cakras*).
8. Laws and duties in society.
9. Sacramental rites (*saṁskāras*).
10. Consecration of forms of deities (*mūrtis*).
11. Incantation (*mantras*).
12. Magic Circles (*maṇḍalas* and *yantras*).
13. Symbolic and invocative gestures (*mudrās*).
14. Spiritual practices (*sādhanā*).
15. Worship (*pūjā*), both internal and external.
16. Consecration of houses, wells, etc.
17. Description of holy shrines.
18. Magic (*yogamāyā sādhanā*).
19. Ceremonial rites and initiations (*dīkṣā*).
20. *Yoga* — including *āsanas*, *prāṇāyāma*, meditative methods, etc.
21. Medicines of many types, including *Āyurveda*, which is a herbal science combined with yogic practices.
22. Science.

To this list we would also add alchemy, the art of living a fruitful and blissful life, and the use of sexual energy as a means to unfold higher awareness.

According to Shree Swamiji Maharaj of Datia:[7]

> From the view of origin, *tantras* too have no beginning and are not man-made. *Bṛhad Dharma Purāṇa* says:
>
> *āgamasya bhavan kartā veda kartā hariḥ svayam.*
> *ādau āgama kartṛtve bhavan vai viniyojitaḥ.*
> *paścadvai veda kartṛtve hariḥ samyaṅg niyojitaḥ.*

---

7. Shree Swamiji Maharaj, *Lekha Saṁgraha*, Shri Pitambara Sanskrit Parishad, Datia, Madhya Pradesh, 1984, pp. 149-50.

āgamaścaiva vedaśca dvau baho mama puṣkalau dvabhyameva
dhṛtam sarvam traile kyam bhur bhuvadikam.

Shree Bhairavi says:

> O Sadāśiva, only on my instructions you evolved the Āgamas and Viṣṇu evolved the Vedas. The Āgamas and Vedas are my two heads. It is with these that I bear this universe. Thus the manifestation of Āgamas and Vedas through Śiva and Viṣṇu, are the twin inseparable forms of the Lord. Both the scriptures are eternal and are not man-made. Thus, any thought regarding the recent origin of the Āgamas is inappropriate.

Elsewhere Swamiji Maharaj of Pītāmbarapāṭh, Datia,[8] narrates,

> Lord Śiva is the propounder of *tantra* and *mantra*, which by glorifying *māyā* thus brings about the downfall of the evil-characters. The external manifes-tation of the Supreme Soul is Viṣṇu, and the inner manifestation is Mahādeva. Both these powers make guileful demons, victims of temptation and thus destroy them. To overcome them through sharp intelligence is typical of Viṣṇu. Evil-doers acquire pride and ignorance by *tantra* and *mantra* and perpetuate injustice unto others, and are thus led to destruction by Lord Śiva. Through the means of *tantra* and *mantra*, god destroying the ignorant and proud demons committing acts of injustice in their arrogance, is symbolic of Śiva, since in the genre of demons, there is no realization of non-dual monism. Its true realization is possible only in the case of virtuous devotees. The ultimate sermon of Śiva is the knowledge of all-pervading non-dual Supreme God.
>
> *Sat-karma*, the weapon of illusion, renders the message of benefaction to the righteous after destroying the wicked ones.

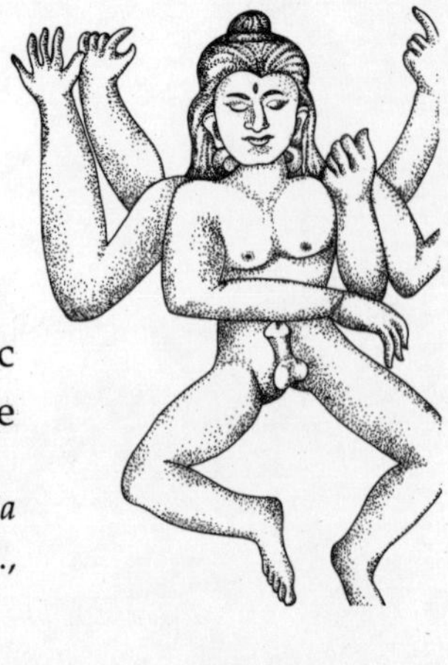

Learned Vedic Śāktas believe that the Śākta cult is both Vedic as well as tāntric. Had it not been so, *tantra*s would not have

8. His Holiness Rastraguru 1008 Swamiji Maharaj, *Vedic Upadeśa* (*Vedic Teachings*), Shri Pitambara Sanskrit Parishad, Datia, M.P., 1977, pp. 66-67.

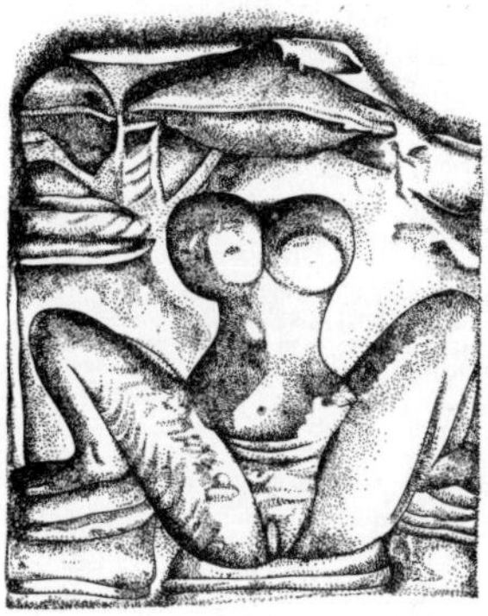

accepted the Vedic discipline. In the famous seven modes of *tantra* worship, the Vedic discipline occupies the foremost place. All the rituals of the *tantras*, have their base in Vedas completely.[9]

While dealing with the *Religion and Culture of the Sarasvati-Sindhu Civilization*, S.D. Kulkarni[10] states:

> Though no social sanction was received, the people continued to practise *tantra* in their rituals and continued to attach to it a philosophical content. *Tantra* was a parallel cultural current along with the philosophical one in the Indian culture.
>
> Expression of fertility rites is the other philosophy of *tantra* in India. Based on the dual conception of the creation phenomenon with the participation of "Śiva" and "Śakti," the germinator and the nurturer, respectively, it is a highly complex system of philo-sophical thought. The *tantra* practices, however, involved sexual intercourse and other abhorrent methods. In the *Ṛgveda* also the phallus worshippers are denounced. —*ṚV*, VII.21.5 & X.90.3

As dealt in this book, the *Yoga* of sexual transformation was finally included in *Bṛhadāraṇyaka Upaniṣad* of *Śukla Yajurveda*.

In chapter I, the original home of Ṛgvedic people has been dealt; the formation of peninsular India has been discussed; the origin of the *yoga* of sexual transformation and its eventual incorporation into Vedic culture has been shown. The first Vedic *ṛṣi* to cross the Vindhya mountain range was sage Agastya. Ratna Ma Navaratnam[11] states:

> The concept of Mother Śakti is enumerated in sage Agastya's

---

9. Shree Swamiji Maharaj, *Lekha Saṁgraha,* Shri Pitambara Sanskrit Parishad, Datia, M.P., 1984, p. 374.
10. *BSOIHAC,* vol. I (Beginnings of Life, Culture & History), 1988, p. 462.
11. Ratna Ma Navaratnam, *The Call of Mahāśakti Mother Divine,* Bharatiya Vidya Bhavan, Bombay, 1993, pp. 68-69 and 95.

Śakti Tantra, a treatise on power, which deals with an energy known as *Vidyut Śakti*, somewhat similar to electricity. It has a new theory of energy, not yet probed by modern science. Mind is considered a form of energy and also the vital life-force called *prāṇa*, which also embraces mental energy or conscious force.

Sage Agastya's *Śakti Tantra* depicts the magnetism of the mind power and describes the cosmic power of Śakti as a new dimension of energy. The powers of this prime Śakti are set forth by sage Agastya in the following order:

Rūpakarṣaṇī	Attracts form or image.
Rasakarṣaṇī	Attracts taste vibrations.
Gandhakarṣaṇī	Smell attracting.
Śabdakarṣaṇī	Attracts sound waves.
Sparśakarṣaṇī	Touch vibrations.
Prāṇakarṣaṇī	life-breath-vital magnetism.
Dhairyakarṣaṇī	Attracts strength vibrations.

Mother Śakti displays a form of energy like electricity. Therefore all properties of life can be separated into varied components by a form of magnetism. Visionary images can be attracted by photography. Similarly magnetic attractions of the mind and the vital life-current in the nervous system or *prāṇakarṣaṇī* are effected in *yoga* by the magnetic attraction of light or by focusing rays at one point or from a distance to proximity. Thus the component energies in a human being can be singled out and separated by a process based on the biological analysis of energy, and this results in decomposition into different energies till finally they merge into pure light.

The entire cosmos is endowed with Śiva's indivisible Śakti. Śiva and Śakti are united as fire and heat. When God is experienced as self-lumination He is Śiva, like the sun. When He becomes related with soul He is Śakti. The universe is His energy or Śakti. The supreme One appears manifold with different names, when Para-Śiva aspects *prakṛti* or Nature through His *kriyā*, *icchā* and *jñāna śaktis*.

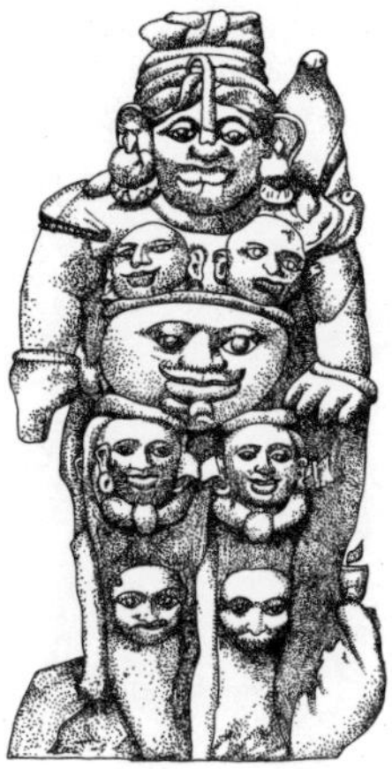

The glory of Śakti as "Paradevatā" or Supreme Goddess, is revealed to sage Agastya by Śrī Hayagrīva and elaborated by Agastya in his exposition of *pañca-dśākṣarī mantra* in *Śrī Vidyā Dīpikā*.

When the Vedic *ṛṣis* discovered the *yoga* of transforming sexual energy to raise the *kuṇḍalinī*, they included it in the *Bṛhadāraṇyaka Upaniṣad*,[12] which symbolizes woman as a medium of sacrifice, her lap as the sacrificial altar, her hair as sacrificial grass, her skin as Soma press and copulation as an act of sacrifice. It proclaims a series of rules and advises its followers to observe them unmistakably for a choicely progeny. The *Chāndogya Upaniṣad* portrays woman as a sacrificial fire and the generative organs as fuels.

With efflux of time, this *yoga* of sexual transformation was forgotten. In the earliest sculptural art of Śiva of Guḍimallam[13] of southern Andhra Pradesh dated second century BC, instead of the usual *ūrdhvaliṅga* (upward membrum virile), the phallus here is downcast as if it has shed its seed, so natural and dictated by the standing posture of the God, whereas the total concept of this ithyphallic *liṅga* form by synecdoche stands *ūrdhvareta*s, i.e., the drawn upseed — a pillar (*sthānu*) and symbol of chastity.

The *yoga* of sexual transformation was re-discovered or made popular again in the post-Gupta period, with the spread of Mattamayūra Śaivism and Nāthism in the Mahānadī valley.[14] Therefore the earliest and the second earliest eight-handed Naṭarāja sculptures with *ūrdhvaliṅga*s (*penis erectus*), dated fifth and sixth centuries AD are found at Sirpur and Āsanapaṭ sites,

---

12. R.P. Mishra, *Sahajayāna — A Study of Tāntric Buddhism*, Punthi Pustak, Kolkata, 1991, p. 4.

13. I.K. Sarma, *The Development of Early Śaiva Art and Architecture*, Sundeep Prakashan, Delhi, 1982, pp. 53-64.

14. R.P. Mishra, "Mattamayūra Śaivism in Orissa," *Culture and Collections*, ed. R.P. Mishra, Punthi Pustak, Kolkata, 1996, pp. 101-39.

in the Mahānadī valley.[15] The *ūrdhvaliṅga* (*penis erectus*) is also found on the rare icon discovered at Tala site of Bilāspur district, in the upper Mahānadī valley.[16] The *ūrdhvaliṅga* symbolizes the upflow of semen or the *yoga* of sexual transformation. For this act the *haṭha yoga* practice of *uḍḍīyāna bandha*, an abdominal retraction lock that involves drawing in of the abdomen and stomach towards the backbone after exhaling, is required. Therefore, it can be safely claimed that the Mahānadī river valley is tāntric Uḍḍīyāna *pīṭha* (site), as mentioned in *Pāg-Sām-Jon-Zaṅg*, with other tāntric *pīṭhas* (sites) such as Pūrṇagiri, Kamākhyā and Śrīhaṭṭa.[17] This chapter is divided into six sections and deals with the gradual development of tāntric hedonism in the Mahānadī valley, which developed *Yoginī* cult and erotic sculptural art in its final revelation.

The yogic development in the Mahānadī valley which evolved erotic mysticism is dealt with in chapter 2, which is divided into 15 sections. The existence of the *yoga* of sexual transformation in the Jagannātha cult has also been explained.

The existence of Lajjā Gaurī cult in the upper Mahānadī valley during the early medieval period has been discussed in chapter 3 which is divided into four sections. The identification of a terracotta art of a frog on one side and Lajjā Gaurī on its back, excavated at Mathurā and kept in the collections of Victoria and Albert Museum in Mumbai, has been discussed in this chapter and is nemed as "Lajjā Bīja Mātṛkā." Its identification had not been done so far. The explication of its identification proves that to understand Indian art, one should develop intuitive yogic knowledge and wisdom. Chapter 4 is divided into two sections. In section one, the yogic explanations of the composite tāntric figure discovered at Tala, in Bilāspur

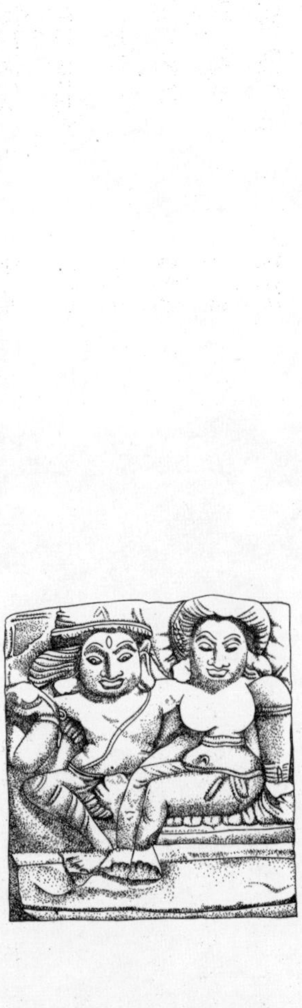

15. *NIATAL*, 2nd edn., 1994, pp. 159-60 & pp. 164-65.
16. J.P. Singh Deo, "Composite Tāntric Yogic figure of Mahākāla and Mahākālī," *ROII*, Delhi, 2000, pp. 127-34.
17. N.K. Sahu, *Buddhism in Orissa*, Utkal University, Cuttack, 1958, p. 142.

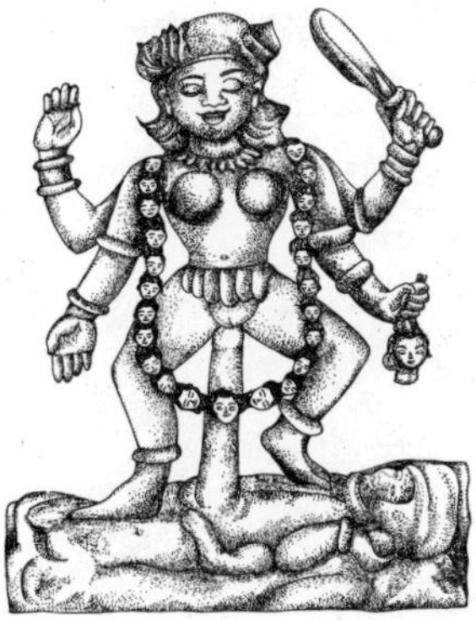

district of Chhattisgarh province, have been given. In section two, the Āgamic tradition of Mahānadī has been studied.

In Chapter 5, the *yoga* of sexual transformation, which can be named as "From Sex to Super Consciousness," has been described with details of intuitive knowledge.

The development of Kośali style of temple architecture has been studied in Chapter 6.

The influence of the Kośali style of *rekhā* temple on the development of the three tāntric temples at Bauḍ in the central right of the Mahānadī valley has been dealt with in Chapter 7.

The Kośali style of *rekhā* temple which developed in the upper Mahānadī valley with a tāntric background, influenced the development of fully matured Kaliṅga style of temple architecture in coastal Orissa. This tāntric influence on temple architecture of Mahānadī valley is shown in Chapter 8.

The book contains the first yogic interpretation of the archaeological remains of the Mahānadī valley, which is Uḍḍīyāna Pīṭha (site).

district of Chhattisgarh province, have been given. In section two, the Agamic tradition of Mahanadi has been studied.

In Chapter 5, the way of spiritual transformation, which can be named as "From Sex to Super Consciousness", has been described with details of intuitive knowledge.

The development of Kosala style of temple architecture has been studied in Chapter 6.

The influence of the Kosala style of rekha temple on the development of the three candi temples at Baud in the central region of the Mahanadi valley has been dealt with in Chapter 7.

The Kosala style of rekha temple which was developed in the upper Mahanadi valley with a Tantric background, influenced the development of fully matured Kalinga style of temple architecture in coastal Orissa. This tantric influence on temple architecture of Mahanadi valley is shown in Chapter 8.

The book contains the first vedic interpretation of the archaeological remains of the Mahanadi valley, which is Uddiyāna Pītha (sic!).

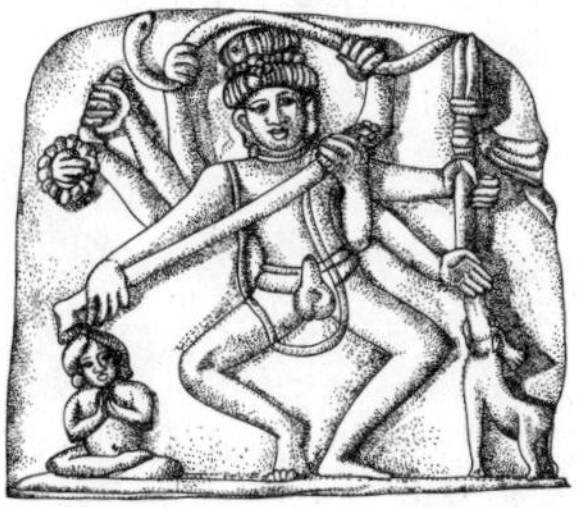

1

Tāntric Hedonism of Mahānadī Valley

THE Mahānadī is an important river in peninsular India. The valley of the Mahānadī forms a broad plain (Chhattisgarh) in the north-east, growing narrower as it passes through the hills of Orissa to the sea.[1] According to Bichitrananda Sinha,[2] river valleys are the net product of the action of rivers. They are fertile and at times present an undulating topography. The major river valleys of Orissa are associated with the Brahmāṇī, the Mahānadī and the Vaṁśadhārā rivers.

The pre-historic archaeology of the Mahānadī valley consists of the Stone age, which has sub-divisions of Palaeolithic, Mesolithic, Neolithic, Copper and Bronze and Iron ages, according to the established archaeological norms, which have been worked out by G.C. Mohapatra,[3] R.P. Pandey,[4] R.N. Dash,[5] K.C. Tripathy[6] and other scholars.[7]

---

1. R.C. Majumdar, "The Geographical background of Indian History," *THACOTIP*, vol. I, *The Vedic Age*, 1965, p. 97.
2. B. Sinha, "Land and People of Orissa," *Sidelights on History and Culture of Orissa*, ed., M.N. Das Vidyapuri, Cuttak, 1977, p. 4.
3. Gopal Chandra Mohapatra, *The Stone Age Cultures of Orissa*, Deccan College, Pune, 1962, passim.
4. R.P. Pandey, *Pre-historic Archaeology of Madhya Pradesh*, Sundeep Prakashan, Delhi, 1987, passim.
5. R.N. Dash, "Pre and Proto-history of Orissa," *OHRJ*, vol. XXX, nos. 2, 3 & 4 (Golden Jubliee Volume — Glimpses of Orissan Art and Culture), 1984, pp. 284-304.
6. K.C. Tripathy, *Lithic Industries in India* (*A Study of South-Western Orissa*), Leeladevi Publications, Delhi, 1980, passim.

→

The essence or the inner distinctive nature of the culture of the Mahānadī valley is that it is the land of *kāmakalā* (desire fulfilling) or tāntric hedonism.

I

The Vedic culture of India owes its origin to the *Ṛgveda* period. The river Sarasvatī of the *Ṛgveda*, according to S.D. Kulkarni's[8] research, is the modern river Syr Darya (Jexartes), which falls into the Aral Sea. The search for the Ṛgvedic Sarasvatī river in modern India is carried out by the Geological Society of India and by scholars like Bhagwan Singh, S.G. Talageri and B.B. Lal.[9] More archaeological discoveries are required to locate the Ṛgvedic Sarasvatī river.

By locating the home of the Vedic people, S.D. Kulkarni[10] shows that Vedic influence was all-pervasive and it spread right from modern Turkey and Egypt, covered the region between the Caucasus mountain and the Caspian sea down to Syria and Palestine and the Persian Gulf kingdoms of ancient Babylon, Asur, Sumer, Akkad, Ur, Kassite and included the modern Iran, Afghanistan, the Russian Azerbaizan and the southern regions of the Russian republics: Tadjikistan, Uzbek, Turkmen and Kirghis. It extended from the east to the Hindukush mountains and covered the region around the Varasakh river and included

---

7. K.K. Basa & P. Mohanty (eds.), *Archaeology of Orissa*, vol. I, Pratibha Prakashan, Delhi, 2000, passim.
8. S.D. Kulkarni (ed.), *BSOIHAC*, vol. I, 1997, pp. 119-20.
9. (i) B.P. Radhakrishna & S.S. Merh (eds.), *Vedic Sarasvatī* (*Evolutionary History of a Lost River of North Western India*), Geological Society of India, Bangalore 1999, passim.

   (ii) Bhagwan Singh, *The Vedic Harappans*, Aditya Prakashan, New Delhi, 1995, passim.

   (iii) Shrikant G. Talageri, *The Ṛgveda — A Historical Analysis*, Aditya Prakashan, New Delhi, 2000, pp. 94-97.

   (iv) B.B. Lal, *The Sarasvatī flows on* (*The Continuity of Indian Culture*), Aryan Books International, New Delhi, 2002, passim.
10. S.D. Kulkarni (ed.), *op. cit.*, vol. I, Thane, 1997, p. 147.

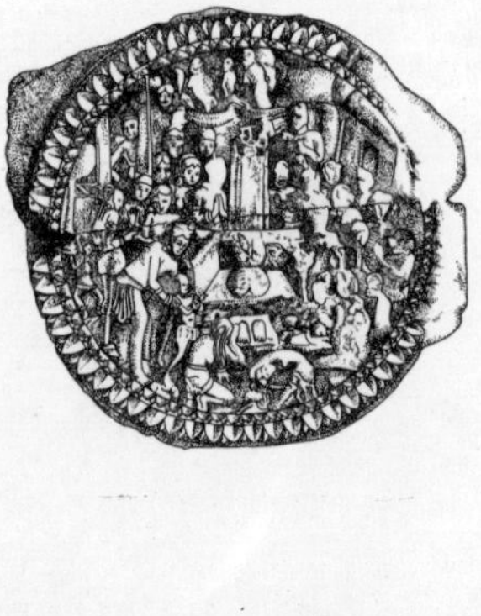

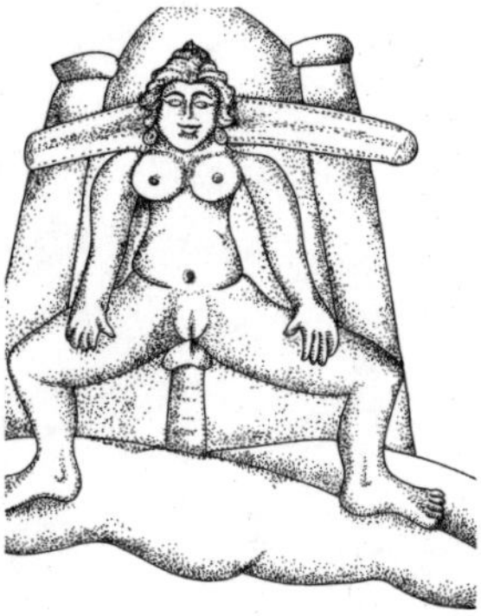

the Sindhu region of modern Sindh, Punjab and Kashmir. This was the position in about 5,000 BC. About 2,000 years or so earlier, the Daśarājanya battle was fought and the Vedics living together in this vast region, began to spread eastwards and southwards to present-day India, and towards west to Greece, Italy and to the North. The capital of the Emperor of Bhārata at the time of the Daśarājanya battle was Abhivasta, a place near Khorasan in eastern Iran and his sway spread over a vast region described in the preceding para. This region was then called Sapta-Sindu Pradesha.

During the Ṛgvedic period, the physical geography of Sapta Saindhava[11] or Sapta-Sindhu existed. J.P. Singhal[12] informs that in *Ṛgveda* there is no knowledge of the present provinces of Uttar Pradesh, Bihar or Mithilā, Bengal, Assam, Rājpūtānā, Gujarat and the Deccan, which clearly implies that *Ṛgveda* was compiled at the time when the Āryans were confined to Sapta-Sindhu and there existed the Tethys Sea below the half raised Himālayas binding the region on the east, south and south-west. This period is yet to be ascertained by the geologist. The time ascertained by the geologists is staggering. The geologists say that it was in the Miocene or the Pliocene period that a great upheavel occurred in the Himālayas which raised the bed of the Tethys Sea, causing a great flood in which the waters of this sea flowed down and joined the Indian Ocean submerging parts of the Lemuria continent. As the Deccan plateau was made up of very old and strong rocks it remained unaffected and the Bay of Bengal and the Arabian Sea were created separating the plateau from the other surviving parts of Lemuria continent. But there is no mention in the *Ṛgveda* of any such formation of the Bay of Bengal or of the Arabian Sea, or of any great flood.

---

11. Manohar Lal Bhargava, *The Geography of Rgvedic India (A Physical Geography of Sapta Saindhava)*, The Upper India Publishing House, Ltd., Lucknow, 1964, passim.

12. Jwala Prasad Singhal, *The Sphinx Speaks or the Story of the Pre-historic Nations*, Sadgyan Sadan, New Delhi, 1963, p. 9.

Thus, the *Ṛgveda* was evidently compiled before the occurrence of this upheaval.

There is no information about the formation of Peninsular India, because; as already observed, the Ṛgvedic people lived on the bank of Sarasvatī river, identified with modern Syr Darya (Zexartes).

Since the Geological Society of India has not yet laid any final period of the formation of peninsular India, a hypothetical study may be done from available sources. From the internal evidences furnished by the scattered descriptions of the "War of Ten Kings," it is established that the Ṛgvedic people initially inhabited in the regions of modern Iran, Afghanistan, Pakistan, Punjab, Sindh, Kashmir and spread eastwards later.[13]

The Ṛgvedic people, after the War of Ten Kings, seems to have migrated east and west from their original home in the Sarasvatī river valley. The final identification of location of the Sarasvatī river is not yet done and research at different level is still going on. The *Ṛgveda* does not mention any region east of the river Gaṅgā. When the Ṛgvedic people moved on to the plains of Punjab and spread out beyond them, they noticed this mighty stream similar to the one in their original habitat in the regions west of the river Sindhu and named it Sarasvatī. It is called "Prācī Sarasvatī" (Eastern Sarasvatī) in the Purāṇas. The Vedic civilization continued to flourish around this eastern Sarasvatī as it was so around the western one. The civilization known so far as "Indus" should therefore appropriately be called "the Sarasvatī Sindhu civilization."[14]

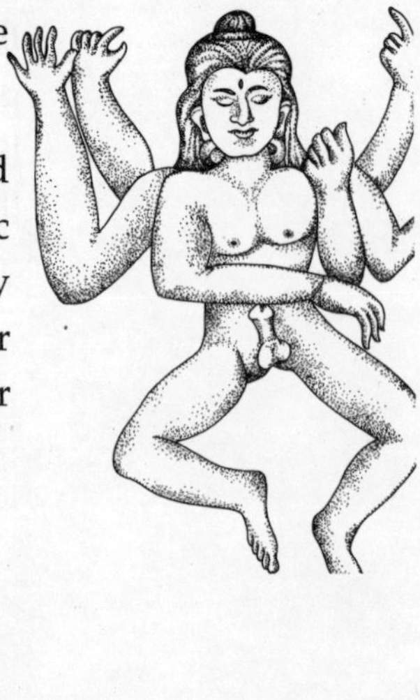

The time when this grand civilization evolved and flourished, most part of South Asia was still at the Neolithic stage. The most ancient civilization of South Asia, variously known as the Harappan or Indus-Sarasvatī civilization, far excelled its contemporaries in other parts of Asia in a number

13. S.D. Kulkarni (ed.), *op. cit.*, vol. I, Thane, 1997, p. 148.

14. *Ibid.*, vol. I, 1997, p. 427.

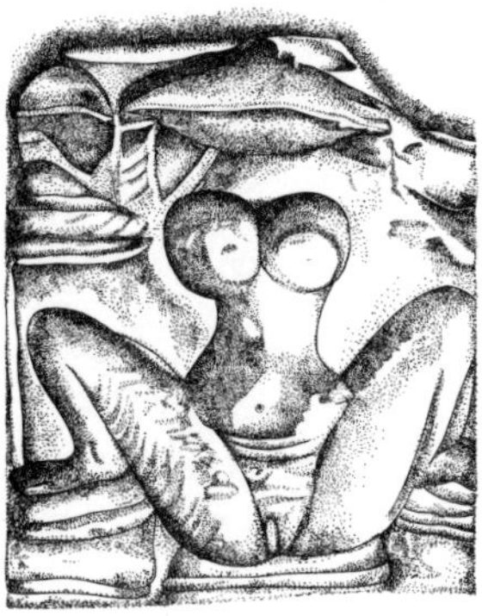

of ways. Not only did it cover a much greater area than any other civilization, but it also produced urban centres duly fortified and characterized by meticulous town planning, efficient drainage system, etc. Namazga-Depe and Altyn-Depe are two archaeological sites in the Syr Darya or Amu-Darya valley of the *Ṛgveda* period, identified as the Sarasvatī river, which has comparable artefacts from Harappan sites. The most noteworthy is the ithyphallic figure in terracotta found at Namazga-Depe, which recalls Mohenjo-Dāro examples.[15]

The Vedas are the heritage of mankind. It is for this reason that American scholars[16] in recent years have produced a work titled, *In Search of the Cradle of Civilization.* Even French and Italian scholars[17(A)] have shifted their vision of study and have produced a book named, *Crossings: Early Mediterranean Contacts with India.*

B.B. Lal[17(B)] examined the entire Ṛgvedic evidence and demonstrated that it goes counter to the aforesaid assumption. On the other hand, there are compelling geographical datas in the *Ṛgveda* itself which unambigously show that the Ṛgvedic Sarasvatī was none other than the present-day Sarasvatī-Ghaggar combine which flows through Haryana and Punjab. Though now it dries up near Sirsā, the dry bed, sometimes as much as 8 km in width as picked up with landsat imagery,

15. B.B. Lal, *The Earliest Civilization of South Asia,* Aryan Books International, New Delhi, 1997, pp. 4, 183, Fig. 87 and 189.

16. G. Feuersten, S. Kak & D. Frawley, *In Search of the Cradle of Civilization,* Motilal Banarsidass, Delhi, 1999, passim.

17(A). (i) F. De Romanis & A. Tchernia (eds.), *Crossings : Early Mediterranean Contacts with India,* Manohar, New Delhi, 1997, passim.

(ii) V.K. Verma, *Indo-Aryan Colonization of Greece and Middle East,* vol. I & vol. II, Pratibha Prakashan, Delhi, 2000, passim.

(iii) S.D. Kulkarni (ed.), *op. cit.,* vol. XVI, India Abroad, Thane, 1995, passim.

17(B). B.B. Lal, *TSFO,* New Delhi, 2002, passim.

shows that in ancient times it continued all the way down to the Rann of Kachchha.

The study of the institution of Vyāsas in Vedic culture, helps in knowing the probable period of the geological formation of peninsular India and spread of Vedic culture to the south of the Vindhya mountain ranges.

According to the institution of Vyāsas, the 19th Vyāsa was Bhāradvāja and his period is 6340 BC to 5980 BC. He was a contemporary of the famous Vaśiṣṭha, who was a priest of Sudāsa, the king on the eastern side of the Sindhu river.

About the personalities and events during Vyāsa Bhāradvāja's period, mention may be made of the sage Bhāradvāja who was the priest of Emperor Chayaman or Bhāratavarṣa, ruling from Khorāsān (Eastern Iran). He was also a priest of Divodāsa, the father of Sudāsa who led his armies in the Daśarājanya War.

After Daśarājanya War, Vaśiṣṭha's brother Agastya carried the Vedic civilization to south India.[18]

As observed, Vyāsa Bhāradvāja's period is within 6340 to 5980 BC. So, it can be claimed that the geological formation of peninsular India was formed during this period. But, according to Swami Prakashanand Sarasvati,[19] the Himālayas and India have been at their present locations for 1,972 million years. However, it is for geologists to make the final decision. Thus, *ṛṣi* (sage) Agastya was able to carry the Vedic civilization to south India by crossing the Vindhya ranges within the mentioned period.

Agastya was the elder brother of sage Vaśiṣṭha. One of the most significant achievements of Agastya referred to in the

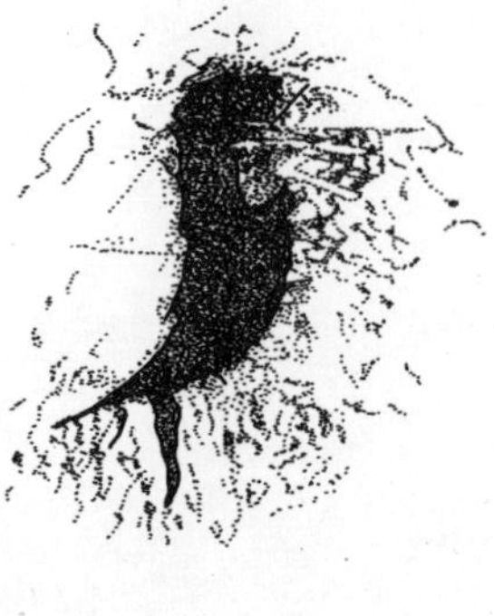

18. S.D. Kulkarni (ed.), *op. cit.*, vol. II (The Encyclopeadia of Indian History and Culture), Thane, 1993, p. 86.
19. Swami Prakashanand Sarasvati, *The True History and The Religion of India*, Motilal Banarsidass, Delhi, 2001, p. 451.

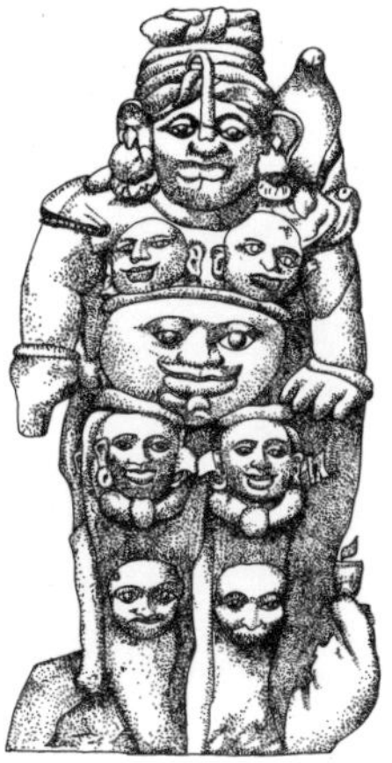

Ṛgveda is the reconciliation, which is said to have been brought about between Indra and the Maruts. The event is the subject-matter of three hymns in the *Ṛgveda* (1-165, 170, 171). The whole of this story, as has been suggested by Dandekar, appears to have been based on the historical fact of a causal estrangement between Indra, the heroic leader of the Vedic Indians and his trusted followers, the Maruts. It would appear that the seer Agastya played an important role in bridging the gulf between Indra and the Maruts and thus re-established the entente which proved most fruitful in connection with the victorious advance of the Vedics.

Agastya seems to have played a particularly prominent role in the *Mahābhārata*. He had to his credit three great achievements — victories over Indra, the Vindhyas and the ocean. In the *Rāmāyaṇa*, Agastya figures as an adviser and guide of Rāma and as the Head of the hermits who had settled in the south.

It must however be remembered that in the *Ṛgveda* itself there is no indication of the role of Agastya as the pioneer coloniser of the south. Indeed, there could not have been any such indications because the expansion of the Vedic Āryans towards the south of the Vindhyas took place in the latter Vedic and early post-Vedic periods. It must have been during these periods that the family of Agastya led the colonising Āryan missionaries to the south.

"Later literature, however, connects Agastya with the north as well as the south of India. He was the first Āryan explorer and originator of the art of colonisation. As great missionary, which he was, his influence can be traced across the seas to the distant lands of Cambodia, Borneo and Java. In the Indo-Javanese heirarchy of gods, the highest rank is given to Agastya. Agastya was indeed not only the Āryaniser of the south but also a Titanic architect — the great builder of a greater India beyond the seas. Agastya was an embodiment of the brāhmaṇa intelligence that brought about a liaison between the pre-Āryan and the Āryan cultures that supervend all over the regions in India and greater India beyond the seas."[20]

II

Before sage Agastya crossed the Vindhya ranges and came to south peninsular India, this land had passed through the pleistocene period in which there was rise of man.[21] Bovid tooth has been discovered at Mukramatia in Mayūrbhañj district[22] and a Habilines's (early human phase) tooth has been found in Churiagarh in Kālāhāṇḍī district, which is now preserved at Manikyapur Museum of Bhawanipatna.[23] So, there are palaeo-anthological evidences in the Mahānadī river valley also. *Palaeoanthropolity of Central Orissa*, worked out by P.K. Singh in 1985 is an unpublished Ph.D. thesis of Utkal University, Bhubaneshwar.[24]

The latest study in the Indian context shows that division of ages such as Paleolithic, Bronze and Iron appears to be too artificial. Along with the use of stone implements and articles, men used articles and implements made of metals as soon as he discovered these. And this period goes back to hoary antiquity. . . . Iron ore has been found in abundance in India and so the process of its smelting and getting rods and plates from iron ingots cannot lag far behind its initial discovery.[25] It thus shows

20. S.D. Kulkarni (ed.), *op. cit.*, vol. I, Thane, 1977, p. 218.
21. Amiya Kumar Roy Chowdhury, *Bhāratavarsha — An Evolutionary Synthesis of India* (*Dandakaranya & Mahakantara*) vol. I, Rupa & Co., Kolkata, 1975, pp. 90-122.
22. F.R. Alchin & D.K. Cakrabarti, *A Source Book of Indian Archaeology*, vol. I, Munshiram Manoharlal, New Delhi, 1979, p. 181.
23. (i) A.K.R. Chowdhury, *op cit.*, vol. I, 1975, p. 93.

    (ii) J.P. Singh Deo, "The Tell River Valley — Hati Valley Civilization," *Kalahandi Utsav — Souvenir 2000*, Bhawanipatna, 2000, pp. 63-64.
24. K.K. Basa & P. Mohanty (eds.), *op. cit.*, vol. I, Delhi, 2002, p. 59.
25. S.D. Kulkarni (ed.), *op. cit.*, vol. I, 1997, pp. 6-7.

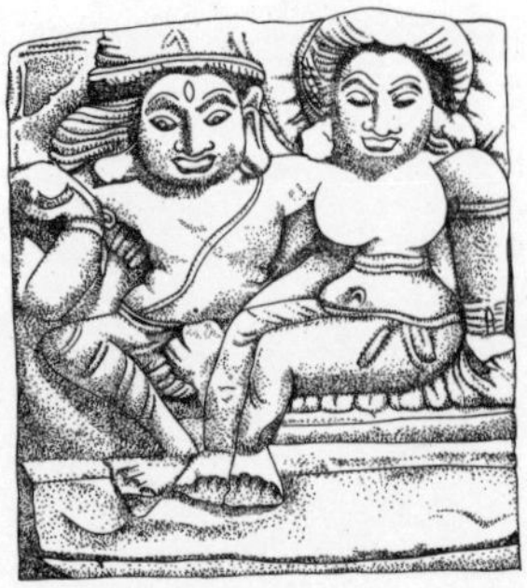

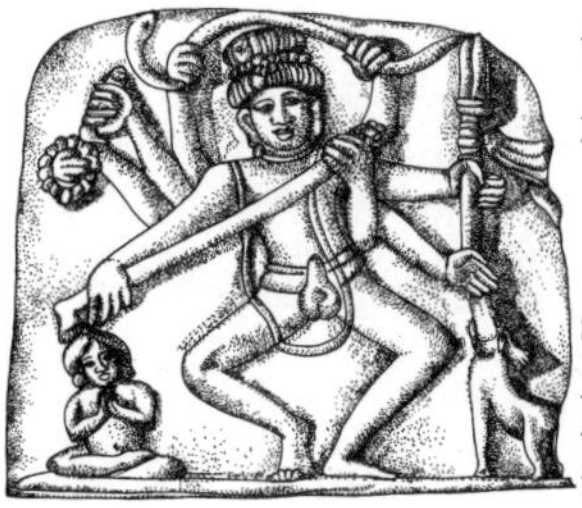

that iron smelting was well known throughout the Mahānadī river valley, because iron slags are found there in plenty.

The whole peninsular India is full of pre-historic rock-shelter paintings.[26] The Mahānadī valley also has many such paintings. The pre- and proto-historic paintings are found at the following sites in Chhattisgarh.

Raigarh District

1. Singhanpur, 2. Dharghora, 3. Ongana, 4. Karmagarh, 5. Kabra Pahad, 6. Basnajhor *alias* Tamnar, 7. Dotalada, 8. Kharsia, 9. Kherpal and 10. Kawagarh.

Rājnandagāon District

Chitva Dongari.

Bastar District

1. Alor and 2. Gupansar.

In Orissa, as stated by Sadashiv Pradhan,[27] the 28 rock art sites documented so far are (1) Guḍahāṇḍī in Kālāhāṇḍī district,

---

26. (i) M.D. Khare, *Painted Rock Shelters (100 Years of the Discovery of Painted Rock Shelters in India)*, Archaeology & Museums, Madhya Pradesh, Bhopal, 1981, passim.

    (ii) S.K. Pandey, *Indian Rock Art*, Aryan Books International, (?), passim.

    (iii) R.K. Sharma & K.K. Tripathi (eds.), *Recent Perspectives on Pre-historic Art in India and allied Subjects*, Aryan Books International, New Delhi, 1996, passim.

    (iv) Erwin Neumayer, *Lines on Stone (The Pre-historic Rock Art of India)*, Manohar, New Delhi, 1990, passim.

    (v) K.K. Cakravarty & F.G. Bednari (eds.), *Indian Rock Art and its Global Contest*, Motilal Banarsidass, New Delhi, (?), passim.

27. S. Pradhan, "Rock Art of Orissa," *Reference Orissa*, ed. A.N. Tiwari, Enterprising Publishers, Bhubaneswar, 1999, pp. 183-84. For the complete work vide S. Pradhan, *Rock Art in Orissa*, Aryan Books International, New Delhi, 2001, passim.

(2) Jogīmaṭh in Nuāpāḍā district, (3) Manikmada, Uṣākoṭi-I (near Rajpahal), Uṣākoṭi-II (near Candarpur), Uṣākūpa, Baurikūpa, Chormada, Jhinkamada, Jadabilmada, Imlimada-I, Imlimada-II, Tongo and a host of twelve rock-shelters bearing the name Lekhamada (Lekhamada group I to XII) in Sundargarh district, (4) Vikramkhol and Uṣākoṭi-III (near Ulap in Jharsuguḍa district and (5) Pakhnapathar near Jamala in Mayūrbhañj district. The district of Sundargarh alone accounts for more than three-fourth of the total rock art sites, i.e., 23 out of the 28 rock art sites (82 per cent) discovered so far. Though all these 28 rock art sites have got paintings, engravings have been documented only from thirteen (46 per cent) of them. They are Manikmada, Uṣākoṭi-I, Baurikūpa, Chormada, Jhinkamada, Jadabilmada, Imlimada-I, Imlimada-II, Tongo, Lekhamada-III, Lekhamada-VI in Sundargarh district and Vikramkhol and Uṣākoṭi-III in Jharsuguḍa district.

In recent years Sasanka Sekhar Panda has discovered five rock-shelter paintings around the forests of Railakhol in Sambalpur district. Rock art has also been found at Uṣākoṭi (Chandlipaṭ) in Srirampur Tahsil and Puja Ḍunguri in Sonepur district[28] and Pakhanpathar near Jamala in Mayūrbhañj district. The hill Pakhanpathar has three rock-shelters with paintings in monochrome of red.

The most interesting feature of rock art of Orissa is that it depicts female genitals or *yoni*s. S. Pradhan[29] informs that seven engravings of triangular forms resembling female genitals are found in Jhinkamoda rock-shelter, 21 in Jadabil, female genital patterns executed in oval, apsidal and triangular forms are in Imlimada-I, 24 specimen of engravings of triangular female genitals with traces of ochre in their grooves are in Imlimada-

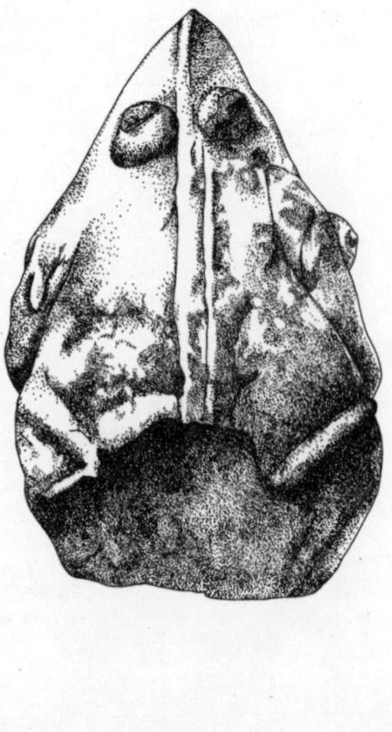

28. R.C. Das, "Puja Dunguri awaits your visit," *Souvenir* (Golden Jubliee Celebration of Independence — Sonepur district), District Council of Culture, Sonepur, 1998, pp. 18-19 (English section).

29. S. Pradhan, "Rock Art of Orissa," *Archaeology of Orissa*, vol. I, eds. K.K. Basa & P. Mohanty, Pratibha Prakashan, Delhi, 2000, pp. 640-47.

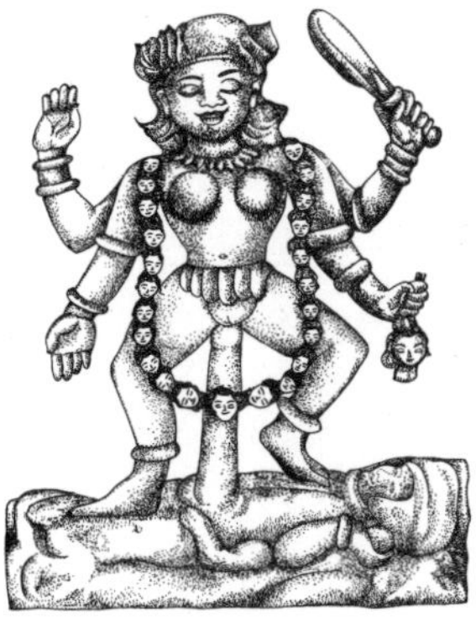

II, in Tongo rock-shelter serpentines at places take the shape of female genitals and in one case the shape of a scooped out female genital has been exquisitely engraved in yellow over red within the Lekhamada group nos. I to XII, engravings which include triangles, ovals, circles, entwined lines either with or without a slit and a hole resembling the female genitals, palm and footprints are found, 68 specimens of the usual triangular female genitals are found in Vikramkhol and the identifiable engraved forms in the midst of paintings of the Uṣākoṭi-III rock-shelter are palm and footprints, triangular female genital patterns, zig-zag lines, circles, brackets, dots, loops, hoops and cobrahood marks and many other forms that defy any geometric pattern or interpretation.

With this much informations of female genitals engraved and painted in the rock art shelters of Orissa, S. Pradhan[30] remarks that the other popular motifs and patterns in these rock engravings are female genitals, rhombic patterns, palm, foot brackets and cobrahood marks with dots. Some of the intricate patterns like the rhombic ones have a faint resemblance with the central Indian paintings of the mesolithic period. The carvings of the female genitals of varied shapes and sizes with natural or carved holes and slits that predominate the engraved forms in the rock-shelters baffle all interpretation. The carving of a female genital in a serpentine form at Tongo is not less intriguing. It is very difficult to say what do they mean? A Freudian interpretation of perversity or any association with fertility rites? Symbols of fertility rituals have always held a very important position in the religion of man.

Ranvir Singh[31] also remarks, "Occurrence of hundreds of female genitals in almost all the engraved rock-shelters is unique."

As stated, there was no Copper, Bronze and Iron ages in

30. S. Pradhan, "Rock Art of Orissa," *Archaeology of Orissa*, vol. I, eds. K.K. Basa & P. Mohanty, Pratibha Prakashan, Delhi, 2000, p. 648.

31. Ranvir Singh, *A Study of Decorative Motifs in the Rock Art of Orissa*, M. Phil Thesis, History Dept., Sambalpur University, 1996-97, p. 40, unpublished.

India. These metals were used in stone age itself, when they were discovered along with the use of Stone implements. Simultaneously, there is an apparent development of yogic concept in the people of Stone age. In peninsular India the earliest trace of *yoga* is found in the pre-historic rock-shelter painting at Guḍāhāṇḍī.[32] This painting of human — like figure has a head which symbolizes a lotus. In *kuṇḍalinī yoga*, the highest *cakra* of human being is described as a thousand-petalled lotus, i.e., *sahasrāra* (*Fig.* 1). So, it can be claimed that *sahasrāra cakra*, is a gift of Mahānadī river valley to mankind. In reality *cakra*s are within the realm of the psyche. Consciousness manifests at different levels, in accordance with the *cakra* that is predominantly active. *Sahasrāra* acts through nothing and yet again, it acts through everything. *Sahasrāra* is beyond the beyond (*parātparam*) and it is right here. *Sahasrāra* is the culmination of the progressive ascension through

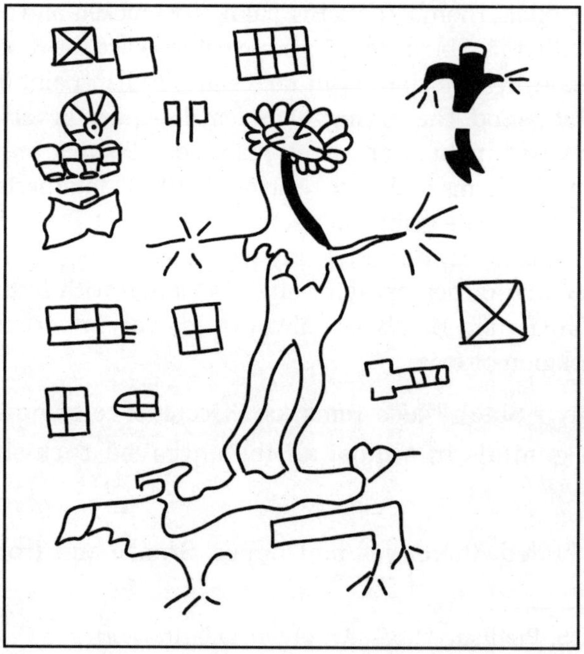

fig. 1. Pre-historic rock-shelter painting of Gurhandi, Kālāhāṇḍī district, Orissa.

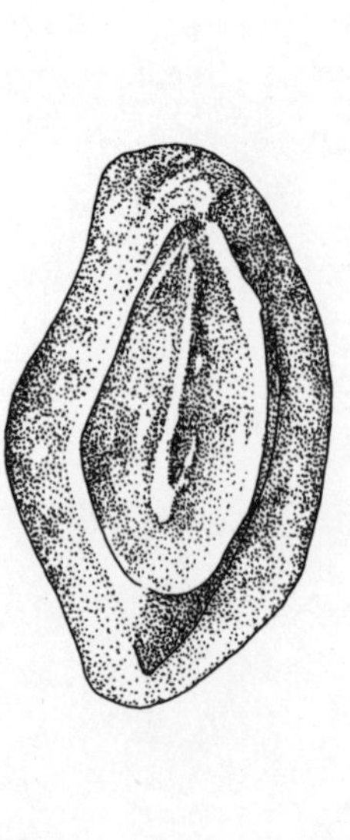

32. *The Journal of Kaliṅga Historical Research Society*, vol. II, p. 243.

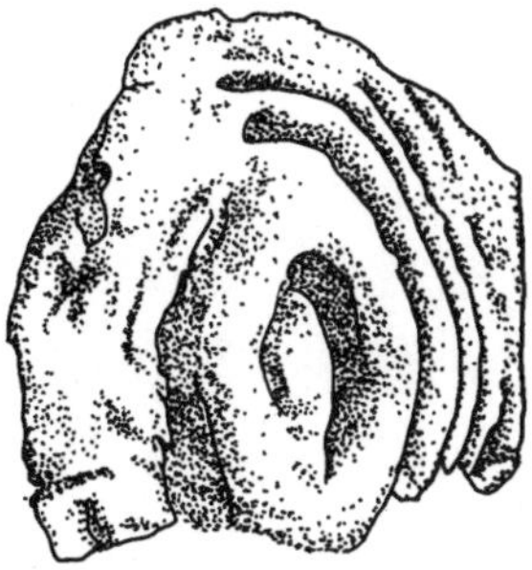

different *cakras*. It is the crown of expanded awareness. The power of the *cakras* does not reside within itself, but in *sahasrāra*. The *cakras* are only switches and all the potential lies in *sahasrāra*.[33]

The second earliest yogic conception of early men in the Mahānadī valley, was perhaps found in the paintings in the rock-shelter of Yogīmaṭh, discovered by the author on 21 December 1970, in Nuāpāḍā district of Orissa.[34] The line-drawn symbols painted in red-tint colour show the creation and run right to left. Paintings of bulls, rings and triple-strokes are yogic conceptions which speak of prevalence of phallism and the trinity functioning of god as the Creator, Organiser and Destroyer (*Fig.* 2).j

The rock art of the female genitals and serpentine forms shows the feminine conception of god and the serpent symbolizes the *kuṇḍalinī śākti*, which is a gift of *tantra*[35] to mankind. *Kuṇḍalinī*

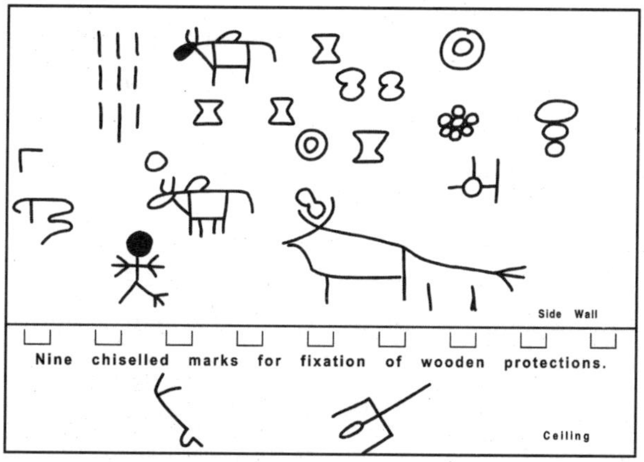

fig. 2. Pre-historic rock-shelter painting of Yogīmaṭh Donger (Hill) in red-tint colour. Nuāpāḍā district. Discovered by the author on 21st Dec., 1970.

33. Swami Satyananda Paramahansa Sarasvatī — *Kuṇḍalinī Tantra*, Bihar School of Yoga, Munger, 1992, p. 201.

34. J.P. Singh Deo, *Cultural Profile of South Kośala*, Gyan Publishing House, Delhi, 1987, p. 20.

35. *Kuṇḍalinī Tantra, op. cit.*, 1992, passim.

is a sleeping dormant potential force in the human organism which can be realized through intuitive knowledge. This view relates to the fact that in peninsular India, the practice of *yoga* and *tantra* prevailed in the bygone ages.

Valuable unpublished palm-leaf manuscripts named *Surisarvasva,* in seven volumes are preserved in the library of Mukti-Maṇḍapa of the Śrī Jagannātha temple at Purī. In its fifth *khaṇḍa,* details of 12 *jyotir-liṅga*s and 12 *jyotir-yoni*s are given. This is the earliest manuscript on *liṅga* and *yoni* worship and the publication of these seven volumes of *Surisarvasva,* will be very beneficial for knowing the details and beginning of *liṅga* and *yoni* worship by human beings.[36]

III

The origin of Śakti worship is shrouded in mystery. J.N. Banerjea[37] considers that the ring-stones, the female figurines along with the circular discs and the nude figurines of the historic period collectively establish the long continued existence of worship of the female principal in aniconic and iconic forms. Ring-stones are found in plenty throughout the Mahānadī river valley.

To know about the earliest Śakti conception, attention should be drawn to the period of geological formations. It is a truism that the course of human history in a region is in a considerable measure, shaped by its physical and geographical features, which in turn, in the ultimate, are determined by its geological history, through the dim vista of time.[38]

When the earth crust was under formation, at many places

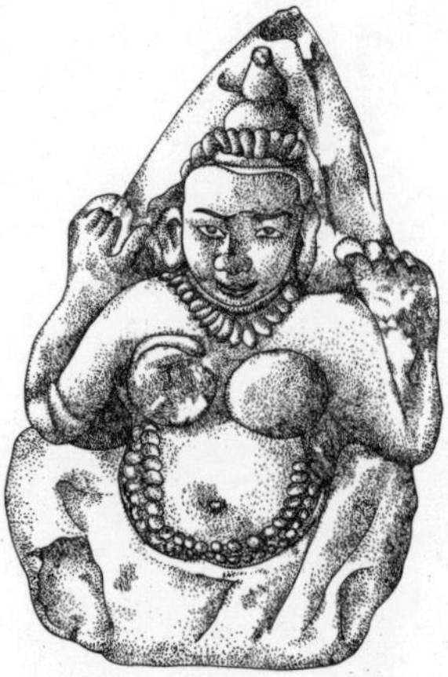

36. This information was supplied to the author by Pandit Banamali Ratha of Khariar on 26th December 2000 AD.

37. J.N. Banerjea, *Purāṇic and Tāntric Religion,* (?), p. 111.

38. D.N. Wadia, "The Geological Background of Indian History," *THACOTIP,* vol. I, The Vedic Age, 1965, p. 80.

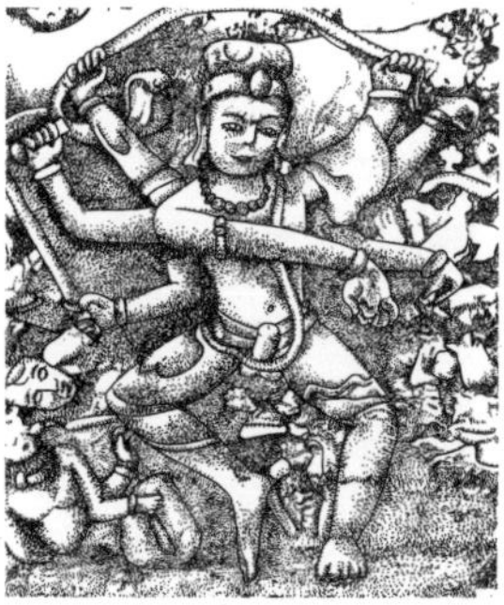

it took the shape of female vulva, the external organ of generation. In the words of O.A. Wall[39]

> The external feminine sexual parts, the vulva, is called *yoni* in India, it is still very widely worshipped in Asiatic religions and the worshippers of feminine attributes are called *yonicitas*. In subsequent reference to the vulva, we will speak of it as the *yoni*. The *yoni* in Sanskrit means vulva, uterus or origin, it is the female power in nature. The Supreme Being, wishing to begin creation, divided himself into two parts, Brahma and nature; from Brahma all males originated; from nature, all females, but the female is regarded as the real force in nature and most deserving of worship.

One such naturally formed female vulva or *yoni* of Mother Earth, is found under a bamboo thicket near Pātālgaṅgā the site in Nuāpāḍā district of Orissa. It is worshipped as "Dvārsani" and should be regarded as the earliest *śakti pīṭha* (site) of the Mahānadī river valley (*Pl.* 9). Such earthen vulva or *yoni* sites are found at Sindhekela village of Bolaṅgīr district and near Puruna Cuttack of Bauḍ district (*Pl.* 10) in Orissa.

Tantra gives prominence to the female energy or *śakti*. Śakti (Kālī) of the Śakti cult is the Mother or the Supreme Being. Similarly, Śiva of the Śiva cult is the father, or the Supreme Being and the master of *yoga*. The *tantra*s attempt to blend these two concepts, the motherhood and the fatherhood of god. *Tantra* gives importance to the Eternal Mother, for god's love for the creation is like a mother's love, deep and pure. So, the earliest *śakti* site of Mahānadī river valley is the "Dvārsani deity," situated in Nuāpāḍā district, Orissa.

One stone *yoni* is discovered in the Maraguḍā valley,[40] and is kept preserved with the author. It measures 8½ cm in

---

39. O.A. WALL, *Sex and Sex Worship in the World*, Inter-India Publication, Delhi, 1979, p. 464.

40. J.P. Singh Deo, "Yoni discovered at Maraguda valley, Orissa," *Essays on History, Education & Culture*, (*Comparatives Nos. 3 & 4*), Mayur Publication, Bhubaneswar, 1987, pp. 149-52.

circumference and is of quartzite stone and ferruginous in colour (*Pl.* 11). Another such *yoni* is discovered from Soseng village in the Sunabeda plateau of Nuāpāḍā district and is also preserved with author. Its middle portion is damaged because of human vandalism. One naturally formed stone *yoni* was found at Dhangrītāl village, both the sides of which have *yoni* formation (*Pl.* 13). This is also preserved with the author. Three such *yonis* are naturally formed on a flat rock belt, on the left bank of the Indra river within Nuāpāḍā district, in the vicinity of Chuipani village, on the foothills of the Sunabeda plateau.

One *yoni* with a triangle *yantra* and spot (*bindu*) in the centre is found with the help of Padma Dandasena. It is *Bhairavī-yantra* of quartzite stone, ferruginous colour and measures 6½ cm in circumference (*Pl.* 12). These findings have similarity with those found in the Sindhu valley. One broken stone *liṅga* in the actual human *liṅga* shape is collected from Bargāon village and preserved in author's private possession (*Pl.* 15). It has similarity with those found at Harappā and Mohenjo-Dāro (*Pl.* 14).[41]

B.B. Lal[42] gives a cultural Mosaic map within the period *circa* 2500-1800 BC of India and shows that during the developed and late Harappan civilization, the Mahānadī valley had neolithic culture (*Fig.* 3). As already observed, there was similarity between the *liṅga* findings of Harappā site and Khariar site of Orissa. A seated figurine or steatite has been discovered at Khariar and is preserved in author's private possession (*Pl.* 3). It proves the contact of Sindhu or Indus valley civilization with this area of upper Mahānadī valley, because new evidences of the Indus Valley civilization found in Pakistan, reveals that one seated figurine, with bent legs extending out in the front and having pinched applique facial features and

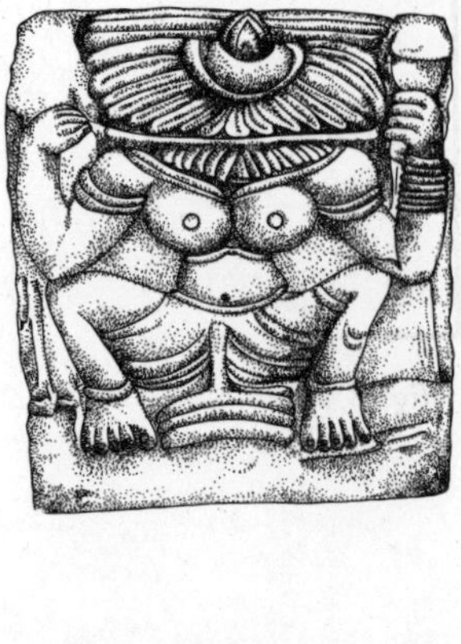

41. B.B. Lal, *TECOSA*, Plate. IC & D. Stone *liṅgas* from Harappā and Mohenjo-Dāro.

42. B.B. Lal, *TECOSA*, p. 16 & Fig. 31.

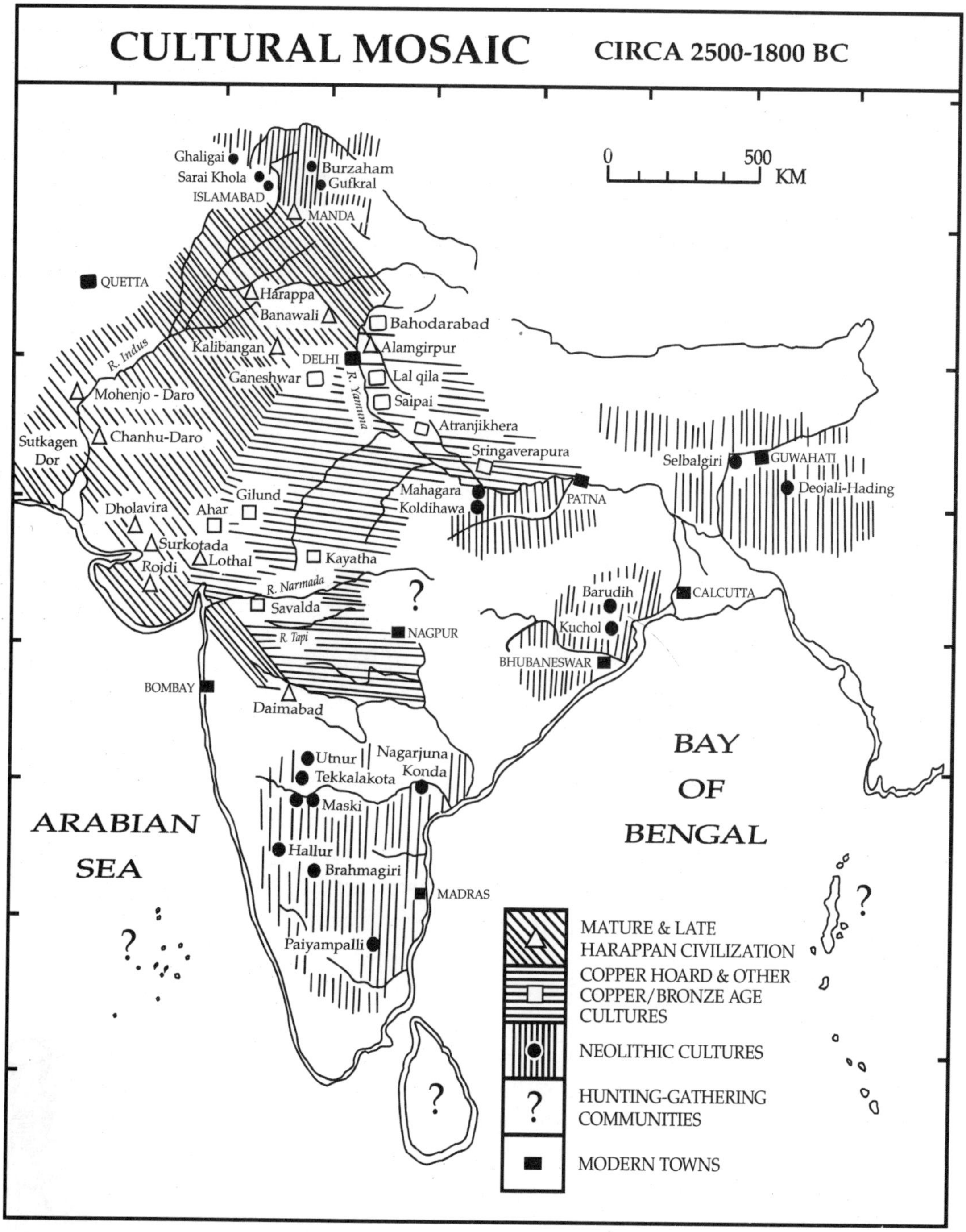

fig. 3. Cultural Mosaic Map of India. (Source: B.B. Lal, *The Earliest Civilization of South Asia*, Aryan Books International, New Delhi, 1997, *fig*. 3.1).

breasts has been found at Gumla. Seated figurines have also been discovered at Jalilpur in Pakistan.[43]

While searching archival records in the library of great scholar Prafulla Chandra Bhanja Deo, at Baripāḍā in November 1992, the author came across a copy of the English daily newspaper, *Hindusthan Standard*, dated 13th October 1953, published from Calcutta (present Kolkata). The newspaper mentioned:

> Babylonian Seal Unearthed.
>
> Baripada Oct. 11 — Śri Prafulla Chandra Bhanja Deo, M.P. yesterday communicated to the "Hindustan Standard," correspondent here over the phone that" an Ivory Babylonian Seal" has just been unearthed in the precincts of the Barunighat temple at Baripada.
>
> Śri Bhanja Deo told the "Hindustan Standard," that while excavation of a tank was in progress on the land on the northern side of the compound of the Barunighat temple an Ivory Babylonian Seal of the roller type was found underground at a depth of about seven feet. The temple and the grounds adjoining it belong to Lalsaheb Kumar Prafulla Chandra Bhanja Deo and are situated at a level of six feet below the level of Baripada town. Fortunately the proprietor who himself is an eminent archaeologist was present near the site of the excavation at the time of the discovery as labourers were about to throw this away as a piece of bone from the mass mud in which it was embedded. The labourers told the proprietor that on previous occasions several similar objects including strange skulls and skeletons had been unearthed on the same spot and that all such object had been thrown into the river as being inauspicious and undesirable objects after consultation with the temple authorities. Henceforth the proprietor gave strict orders that all finds

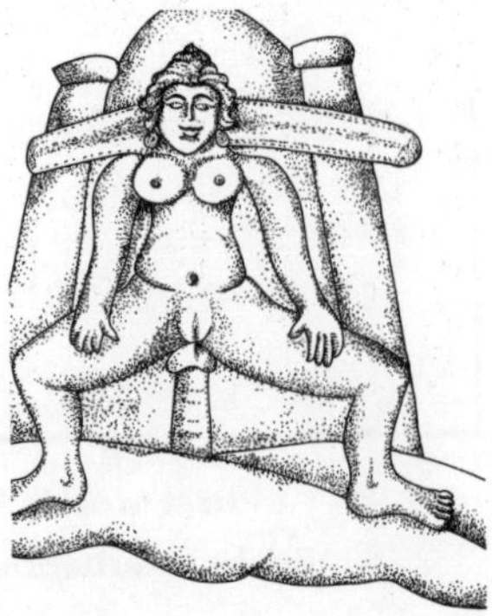

43. J.G. Shaffer, "The Indus Civilization: New Evidence from Pakistan," *Essays in Indian Proto-History*, ed. D.P. Agrawal & D.K. Cakrabarti, B.R. Publication Corporation, Delhi, 1979 pp. 18-22.

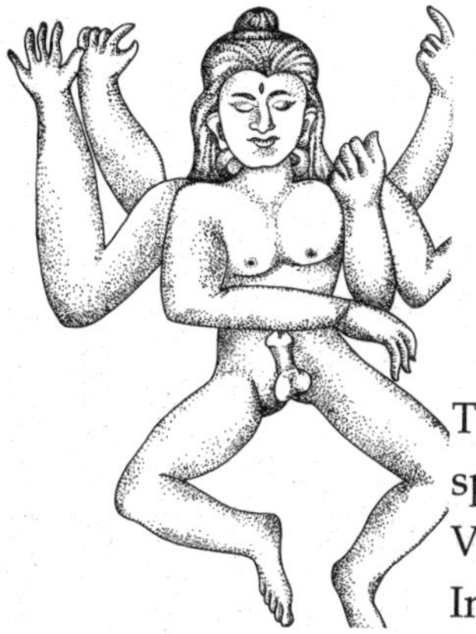

however seemingly insignificant or inauspicious should be kept apart for his personal scrutiny before their disposal in this manner by ignorant individuals. The seal is now in the possession of Śri Bhanja Deo who has preserved it for his new museum which contains many rare objects and discoveries.

This much information confirms that there was cultural, spiritual and trade and commerce link between the Mahānadī Valley and Sindhu/Indus valley civilization and Babylonia.[44] In recent years "Golabai," a proto-historic site, on the coast of Orissa has come to light.[45]

Regarding the concept of the *liṅga* and the *yoni*, D.C. Sircar[46] states that the worship of the *liṅga* of the Great God Śiva originated from the concept of the god as the father or procreator. But in the matter of the procreation of beings, the *yoni* (pudendum muliebre) of Mother Goddess should naturally be regarded as much important as the *liṅga* of Father God. Both the Father God and the Mother Goddess were worshipped by the pre-Āryan people of India. The objects discovered at Mohenjo-Dāro show that Śiva and Śakti were worshipped not only in the human form but also in the symbolic form of the *liṅga* and the *yoni*, the former representing procreation and virility and the latter motherhood and fertility (J. Marshall, *Mohenjodaro and Indus Civilization*, vol. I, London, 1931, p. 52 ff.).

About the religion and culture of the Sarasvatī-Sindhu civilization, S.D. Kulkarni[47] observes that the worship of Mother

---

44. J.P. Singh Deo, "Orissa's Contact with First Civilization of the World," *Reference Orissa*, ed. A.N. Tiwari, Enterprising Publishers, Bhubaneswar, 2nd edn., 2000, pp. 673-74.

45. B.K. Sinha, "Golabai: A Proto-historic site on the coast of Orissa," *Archaeology of Orissa*, vol. I, *op. cit.*, 2000, pp. 322-55.

46. D.C. Sircar, "The Śākta Pīṭhas," *Journal of the Royal Asiatic Society of Bengal, Letters*, vol. XIV, no. 1, 1948, p. 7.

47. S.D. Kulkarni (ed.), *op. cit.*, vol. I, 1997, pp. 461-62.

Goddess is a universal phenomenon. In fact, the earliest representation of the creative faculty in the universe was seen in the form of Mother Goddess with emphasis on worship of genital organs of both the female and the male. The cult constituted partly of the fertility rites and harvesting operations. In due course of time, replicas of the genital organs were worshipped. Many such articles, especially of terracotta were found at sites in the Sarasvatī-Sindhu region. With the advent of the male domination in society and organized social system in the West, the female deities were relegated to the background. But it was not so in India. Right from the Vedic times and continuing through the Sarasvatī-Sindhu culture phase, the Goddesses were worshipped along with male deities. With the rise of Upaniṣadic thoughts, rituals lost their prominence but they continued to play an active role in social life. It gave rise to the great tradition and little tradition of culture. While the great tradition involved abstract objects of worship, philosophical speculation was a part of elite culture. The little tradition was confined to the kitchen and mostly continued to be observed by women and was part of folk culture. The other expression of fertility rites is the philosophy of *tantra* in India. Based on the dual perception of the creation phenomenon with the participation of Śiva and Śakti, the germinator and the nurturer respectively, it is a highly complex system of philosophical thought. *Tantra* practices, however, involved sexual intercourse and other abhorrent methods.

In AD 2000 the author with the help of Padma Dandasena had come across a stone *yoni* (*yantra*) which is now worshipped as a household deity in her house in Mundapala village of Nuāpāḍā district. There is information of discovery of three more *yoni* with a *bindu* in the centre by Padma Dandasena, in the Mundapala village area on the left bank of the Udantī river. The *yantra* of *yoni* is a triangle facing down, which is *yantra* of Bhairavī. So the triangle *yonis* found from the sands of the Udantī river are *Bhairavī-yantras*, (*Pl.* 12).

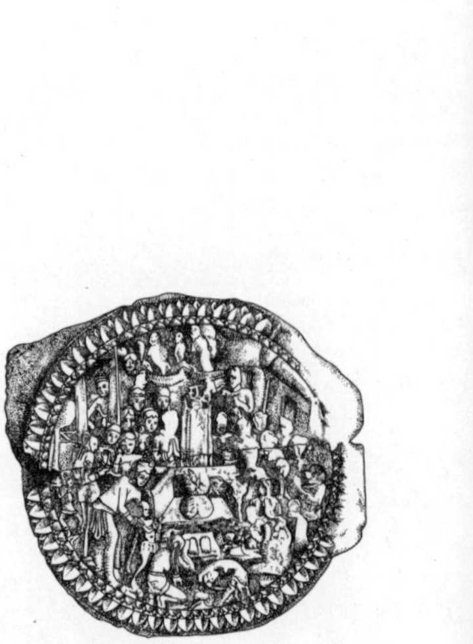

Technically speaking *yantra* means an instrument,

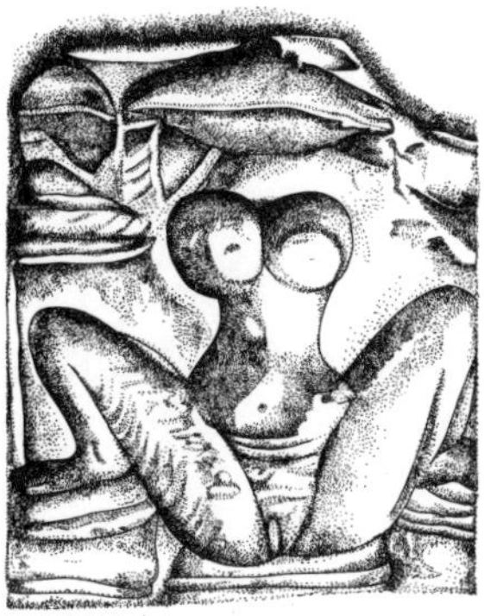

apparatus, a talisman or a mythical diagram. *Yantra* is not a magic but a shortest path or technique through which you can attain *siddhi* (endowned with supernatural power) and your desires provided they are followed with instructions and directions. *Yantra* Śakti is very wide, our *maharṣis* have practised and attained perfection in it. They have showed us the way. Now it is up to us in which manner we follow them. Do no wrong to anybody. Do good and reap good. In our various *śāstras*, *yantra* has been held in high esteem as it is the way of realization of God and desires. It is said that *devas* (gods) reside in *yantras* and without performing *pūjā* you cannot appease *devas* and neither can you attain the desired results of *yantras*.

> A man can express in three ways, through signs, speech and writings. *Yantra* includes signs and writings. *Mantras* and *tantras* are co-partners of *yantras* because they too are expressed through these mediuns.[48]

The finds prove that the *yoni yantra* of Goddess Bhairavī was well known to the spiritual heritage of the Mahānadī river valley in remote days or during early civilization.

The earliest conception of Śakti and Śiva in union has also been discovered in the Mahānadī valley in the form of stone sockets. These are in circular shape with a socket on the lower part and has components in the upper part which fits into the lower socket. The shape of this socket owes its origin to the rock-shelter painting of Yogīmaṭh Gonger (hill) (*Pl.* 1). Such a stone socket set was collected by the author from the Mohangiri site (*Pls.* 16, 17) and is preserved at the Manikyapur Museum of Bhawanipatna. It can be interpreted as the union of Śiva and Śakti, which represents the *yoga* of sexual transformation. Later it developed as *vajrolī* and *sahajolī* in the tāntric *haṭha yoga* practice. Such a socket set was jointly collected by Baba Mishra and Pradeep Mohanty from the Kharligarh site of Bolaṅgīr district in

48. L.R. Chawdhuri, *Practicals of Yantras*, Sagar Publications, New Delhi, 1984, pp. 1-2.

Orissa and exhibited at Manikyapur Museum of Bhawanipatna (*Pls.* 18, 19). Such an object had also been found from layer III (early historic phase), from Veerapuram in Andhra Pradesh, where it is interpreted as a votive *liṅga*.[49] The shape of such stone sockets had been utilized for the shape of Lord Buddha in the Amarāvatī Crossbar railing, which shows the presentation of Rāhula[50] (*Pl.* 20). Later this shape evolved to be the image of Lord Jagannātha at Purī and the composite tāntric figure of Mahākāla and Mahākālī at Tala in Bilāspur district of Chhattisgarh, depicting all *haṭha* yogic features throughout the body,[51] relating to the *yoga* of sexual transformation (*Pl. 27).*

T.N. Mishra[52] informs that no representation of the sexual art has been reported in the art and ritual objects of the Indus civilization. The earliest depiction of the sexual art among the objects excavated so far in India, is found on a pot of the Chalcolithic period at Dāimābād. Another early representation of sex has been noted in the Kupgallu cave in Mysore.

These prove that before the crossing of Vindhya mountains by Vedic *ṛṣi* Agastya and his coming to peninsular India, yogic conceptions had already developed in peninsular India and the Mahānadī valley in particular and the *yoga* of sexual transformation was popular.

While showing the Vedic origin of the tāntric tradition in

49. T.V.G. Sastri, K.N. Bai & J.V.P. Rao, *Veerapuram*, Bhavani Printers, Hyderabad, 1984, passim.
50. E.R. Sastri, *The Buddhist Art of Nāgārjuna Koṇḍa*, Motilal Banarsidass, Delhi, 1994, Illustration No. 32.
51. (i) J.P. Singh Deo, *Origin of Jagannāth Deity*, Gyan Publishing House, New Delhi, 1991, passim.

    (ii) J.P. Singh Deo, "Composite Tāntric Yogic figure of Mahākāla and Mahākālī," *Riddle of Indian Iconography* (*Zetetic on Rare Icon from Tala*), Sharada Publishing House, Delhi, 2000, pp. 127-34.
52. T.N. Mishra, *Impact of Tantra on Religion and Art*, D.K. Printworld (P.) Ltd., New Delhi, 1997, p. 101.

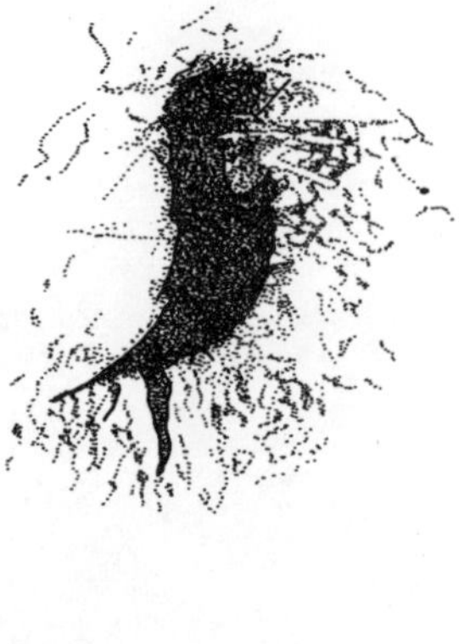

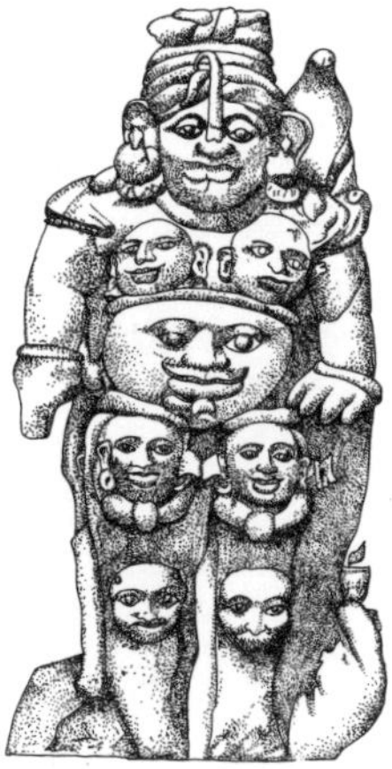

India, Sarbeswar Satpathy[53] informs, "The Vedas mostly deal with sacrifices which are divided into three classes, viz., *pāka yajña, homa yajña* and *soma* sacrifices. These sacrifices are based on the idea that *maithunīkaraṇa* leads to spiritual happiness."[54] *Maithunīkaraṇa* is consecration.[55] This *maithunīkaraṇa* is to be done secretly. The *Śatapatha Brāhmaṇa* (VI.5.3.5) also indicates that bricks are made for the *yajña* because the making of bricks causes generation. Even in the *Aitareya Brāhmaṇa* (II.5.3.) two *pāda*s or *caraṇa*s of an *anuṣṭubh* are raised in a manner to imitate sexual union. A female *devatā* is not worshipped unless she is coupled with a male *deva*.[56] They use a couple of *chandas*, one distinct as male from the other as female and the two taken together are believed to be the symbol of *maithuna* or sexual union and by such *maithuna* the desired result of ritual is achieved.[57] They believe that while the reading of the *ahanasya mantra*[58] confers bliss it is said that the highest and the best *maithuna* is *śraddhā* and *satya*, i.e., piety and truth[59] and this kind of *maithuna* in the abstract is directed for *agnihotrī*s who have purified themselves by observances of these acts in a religious spirit and every time when *maithuna* is performed *mantra*s are to be chanted.[60] Thus it is clear that one of the articles of faith of the Vedic people was that sexual union led the way to bliss and must be performed in true religious spirit to ensure spiritual welfare and wanton indulgence was severely deprecated.

After Vedic *ṛṣis*' contact with peninsular people, the *yoga* of sexual transformation was elaborately incorporated in the

53. S. Satpathy, *Śakti Iconography in Tāntric Mahāvidyās*, Punthi Pustak, Calcuta, 1991, pp. 4-5.

54. *Śatapatha Brāhamaṇa*, XI.6, 2, 10.

55. *Ibid.*, III.2, 1, 2.

56. *Aitareya Brāhamaṇa*, III.5, 4.

57. *Ibid.*, V.3, 1.

58. *Sāṅkhyāyana Śrauta-Sūtra*, XII.24, 1-10.

59. *Aitareya Brāhmaṇa*, VII.2, 9.

60. *Ibid.*, VII.2, 9.

Bṛhadāraṇyaka Upaniṣad of *Śukla Yajurveda*, as the Upaniṣads listed or classified under different Vedas in the *Muktikopaniṣad*.[61]

Vedic culture has strength to draw everything into its fold, because it is based on Cosmic Truth and its principles. Whenever and wherever any Truth is found, it can be assimilated into Vedic culture. As the earliest written records on the *yoga* of sexual transformation, variously known as *From Sex to Salvation*, *From Sex to Super Consciousness*, etc., are found in Vedic culture, it can be said that this *yoga* of sexual transformation has Vedic origin. Later, this *yoga* was elaborated in *Haṭha Yoga Prrdīpikā*, a *haṭha yoga* text of the early medieval period. Therefore, it is mentioned in the *Ṛgveda*, I-89 ni, "let noble thoughts come to us from every side."

IV

The whole Mahānadī river valley passed through a phase of megalithic culture and megalithic burial is still a living practice among the tribals of Baster district in Chhattisgarh and Malkangiri, Korapūṭ, Nabaraṅgpur, Kālāhāṇḍī and Nuāpāḍā districts of Orissa. Shyam Kumar Pandey[62] reports,

> About circa 1000 BC a new culture developed in this area. This has been known as Megalithic culture. This culture was widespread in south India, Bihar, central India and north India up to Kashmir. A large area full of megaliths especially menhirs and pit-circles has been found in Durg district. A few of them were excavated by M.G. Dixit in the fiftees. But no detailed information is known about these Megaliths.
>
> During the recent excavations at Malhar we have come across pottery akin to megalithic culture. The two periods viz., Chalcolithic and Megalithic are overlapping and there does not seem to be much change in material culture. The pottery

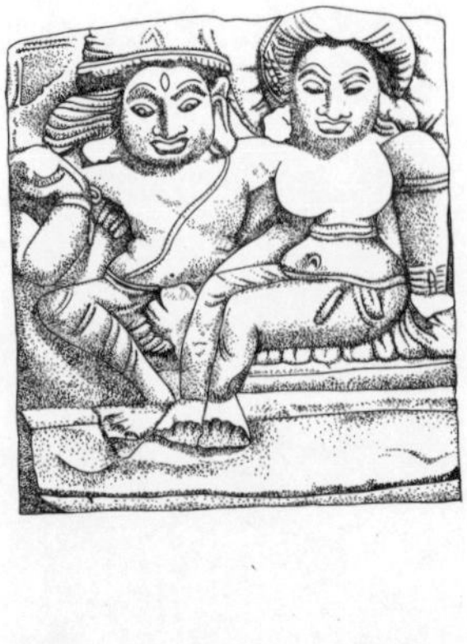

61. R.S. Nathan, *Our Heritage*, Book I, Central Chinmaya Mission Trust, Bombay, 1986. Appendix, p. 120.
62. S.K. Pandey "Archaeology of Chhattisgarh," *Prachya Pratibha* vol. V, no. 1, January 1977, Agam Kala Prakashan, Delhi, p. 100.

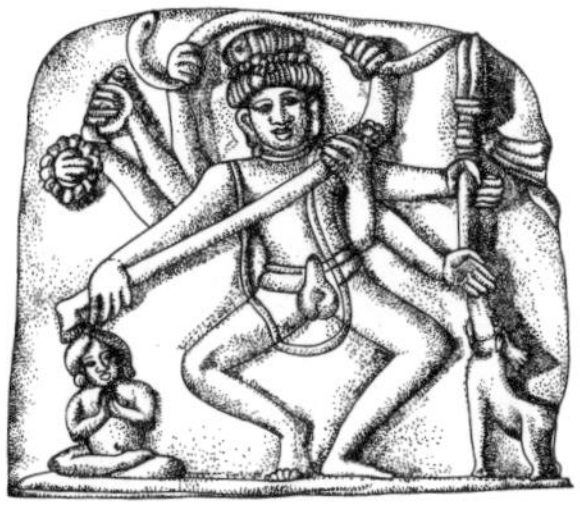

of this period is dominated by unpainted black and red ware, a few of them having graffitti marks. Other pottery includes black burnished ware, a piece of dish-on-stand in blackware, red slipped ware, coarse red ware and black polished wares. They were recovered from the lowest levels. A floor connected with this level was made of black cotton soil base covered with yellow Kankari. Dung was applied to this floor.

A.K. Sharma[63] has brought out the richness of cultural heritage, of Chhattisgarh during the megalithic period. He gives a detailed account of the results of the excavations conducted by him at Sorar-Karkabhat — a nucleus Megalithic site. He establishes the link between central Indian megaliths and those of north-east India and shows how during the first millennium BC the entire country extended its natural and geographical boundaries, right from Ladakh to Kanyā-Kumārī and Manipur to Kutch. A.K. Sharma has excavated one iron ploughshare at the Karkabhat site of Durg district.

While dealing with megaliths of Orissa, R.N. Dash[64] is of opinion that Megalithic culture is evident from Bhubaneswar, Gangahar M.I.P., Mayūrbhañj and at some places in Korapūṭ district. But the antiquity of Korapūṭ megalithic monuments is yet to be known though their living evidences are seen among the tribal residences. Stone circles are found in Mayūrbhañj and probably a buried urn is encircled by such circles. The urn recovered from Gangahar attests to this. A dolmenoid cist was discovered by the author close to the northen gate of Rajbhavan in Bhubaneswar. Dolmens were witnessed by the excavation branch of the Archaeological Survey of India near the western gate of Śiśupālgarh in 1948. Almost all major primitive tribes like Bonda, Gadaba, Kondh, Saora, Muṇḍa and Koyas practise this under various names. Furer Von Haimendorf, Verier Elwin, Dalton, Hutton and Gordon have thrown much light on the

63. A.K. Sharma, *Archaeo-Anthropology of Chhattisgarh,* Sundeep Prakashan, New Delhi, 2000, passim.

64. R.N. Dash, "Pre and Proto-History of Orissa," *OHRJ*, vol. XXX, nos. 2, 3 & 4 (Golden Jubilee Volume), 1984, p. 294.

same. It is not clearly known whether the Orissa's megalith is an extension of the south Indian megalithic practice.

Explorations by S. Pradhan[65] at Kurumpadar village, situated on the right bank of the Mahānadī, in the present Bauḍ district of Orissa has brought out a rich megalithic site, where menhirs, anthropomorphic stone circles, boulder settings and cairn were found.

P.K. Behera[66] explored a megalithic site about a kilometre east of the nearest National Highway (No. 6), where the bridge is constructed over the Mahānadī on its right bank in Sambalpur district. Eleven megalithic cairns were found there.

Nuāpāḍā district of Orissa is rich in Megalithic remains. Post-holes (*Pl.* 8) have been found at the top of the Rishipiti mountain with megalithic boulder piles and there seems to be an overlapping of neolithic and megalithic cultures. Post-holes have been found within Junen village area, which shows the habitation and dwellings of the megalithic people. The flat rocks on which pot-holes are found are being damaged because they are blown out for road-making chips.

Within Pendrapakhan village area of Nuāpāḍā district, a small hill named "Budharaja Donger (hill)," is found. It runs north to south. On its eastern slope a stone wall of megalithic construction is found, while on its top there is a star like megalithic stone formation. It seems to be the earliest trace of *yantra*, in the entire Mahānadī river valley.

Megalithic wall-like piles are common remains on hill tops of Candel donger of the Kudal protected forest, Manikgarh

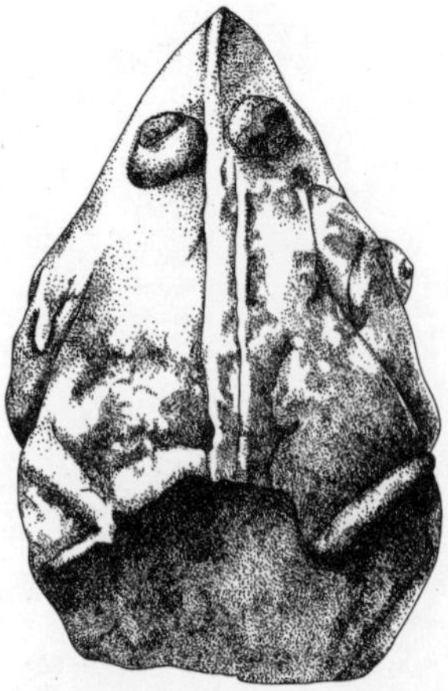

65. S. Pradhan, *Exploration in Phulbani District: A Preliminary Report*, P.G. Dept. of History, Sambalpur University, Jyoti Vihar, 1988, passim, unpublished.

66. P.K. Behera, "A Note on the recent discovery of Megalithic Cairns in the Middle Mahānadī Basin, at Burla, Orissa," *Prāgdhārā*, no. 6, Journal of the U.P. State Archaeological Organization, 1995-96, passim.

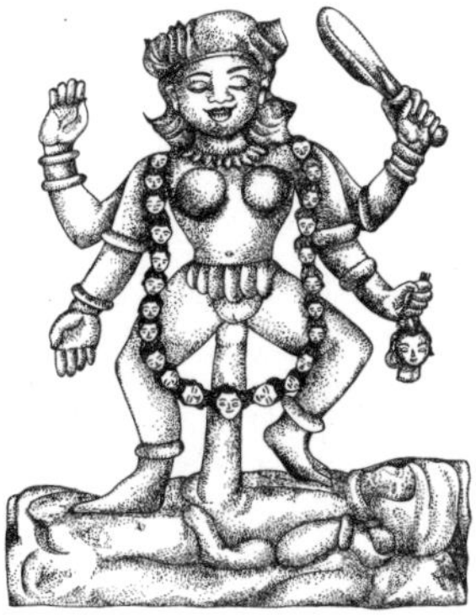

parbat, Ramgarh donger within Gandabahili village area, Tandel donger near Tikrapara village and boulder wall-like piles are found in Patdaraha area, the southern part of Sunabeda plateau, in Nuāpāḍā district.

Two megalithic stone circles or cairns have been discovered at Sandohel village on the left bank of the Sundar river.

On 28 December 1990, students of Khariar College held a National Service Scheme (N.S.S.) camp at Nehnā and on the advice of the author, excavated almost in the centre of one of the stone circles at Sandohel village. The stone circle measured 9 m in diameter. At the depth of 4 ft one twin-urn burial was found with thick black & red pottery, red pottery, iron objects and one huge iron spear. Human bone pieces were also found inside the two urns. The twin-urn burial associated with black and red ware and North Black Polish (NBP) was the characteristic of megalithic burials of south India and Maharashtra. The NBP shows the northern influence. One piece of black pottery with ring-like marks as decoration was found. The urn found in the northern portion of the pit was black outside and red inside, while the urn in the south was full red. Black and red ware is a kind of pottery which is usually black inside and red outside because of the inverted firing technique applied in baking pots. The technique involves double firing due to which probably the northern urn is black outside and red inside, which is very rare. One hook-like iron object was found during this digging. This hook-like iron object has similarity with one found during the excavation at Hashmantper by Birla Archaeological and Cultural Research Institute, Hyderabad, in 1971.[67] This proves that the megalithic twin-urn burial had a south Indian influence. Unfortunately, the iron hook like object excavated at Sandohel is now missing. The human bones found in these two urns, all the broken

---

67. M.L. Nigam, *Report of the Excavation of two Megalithic Burials at Hashmatpet*, Hyderabad, Andhra Pradesh, Birla Archaeological & Cultural Research Institute, Hyderabad, A.P. 1971, passim.

potteries, iron objects and the huge iron spear are now preserved in the Archaeology department of Khariar College. This megalithic twin-urn burial can be assigned to the first millennium BC.

One cairn is discovered inbetween Ghatmal and Citarama village area in Nuāpāḍā district, which is fast getting damaged, because the road passes over the cairn site.

On 28 March 1995, the author accompanied by Irfan Mohammad surveyed Podagarh site within the Chaura group of mountains in Nuāpāḍā district. A stream named "Badajharan" flows by the side of Podagarh, which has many wall-like megalithic boulder piles. At Podagarh was discovered one port stone, measuring 7½ inches in height and 10 inches in width, which is preserved with the author at Khariar. It is the first megalithic port stone discovered in Orissa so far (*Pls.* 5, 6). The discovery of second megalithic port stone in Orissa has been done by Ranvir Singh in the dense forest of Karlapat in Kālāhāṇḍī district. It measures more than 70 cm, in length, (*Pl.* 7).

On 1 March 1997, the author surveyed "Dengamacha," a megalithic rock shelter, on the mountains of the same name, situated at a distance of 3 km to the south of Kendumunda village, within the Singpali black area of Nuāpāḍā district. It is a megalithic dolmen facing west and measures 60 ft in length and 40 ft in width.

On 2 March 1997, the author discovered a stone plough near Citarama village (*Pl.* 2). It is worshipped by the local people. It is a wonder of its own type. It seems to be a stone model of a plough, created by the megalithic people, when iron was discovered and came to be used. Such wooden plough are still being used throughout India. The stone model plough is about 2 ft and 8 inches in height and is exposed to weather as it is kept in open space. One stone model plough was found on the left bank of the Jonk river in the Gatibeda village area on the Sunabeda plateau, situated in Nuāpāḍā district.

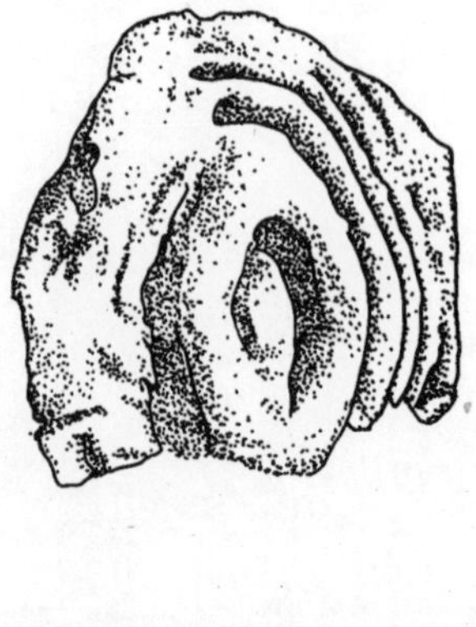

With the domestication of animals during the neolithic period, crude methods of farming were employed which

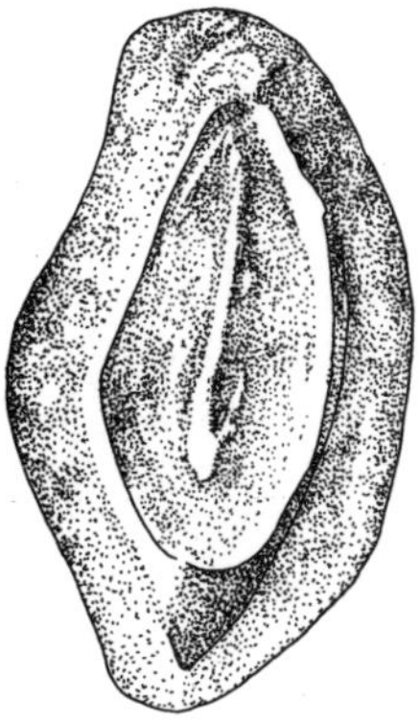

involved the use of celts and ring-stones, as mace heads or weights for digging sticks and slings.[68] But with the discovery of plough by megalithic people who succeeded the neolithic people in most parts of the Mahānadī valley, in 10000 BC, regular farming seems to have begun in the area according to the present archaeological dating norms established by the Western Indologists, which is accepted by the Archaeological Survey of India. The making of *The True History and Religion of India,* is now in progress, which dates back the Indian history to million years ago (vide Sarasvati, His Divinity Dharm Cakravarti Swami Prakashanand, *The True History and The Religion of India,* Motilal Banarsidass, Delhi, 2001, passim).

On the Gandhamardan hill ranges of Bargarh district, wall-like rock piles are found. The locals consider it a fort named "Bhojagarh," built by Cauhān King Bhojarāj Deo, the fifth Cauhān *rājā* of Patna. It seems they were megalithic wall-like rock piles similar to those found in nearby Nuāpāḍā district.

Two megalithic stone circles have been surveyed by Pradeep Mohanty and Baba Mishra[69] in Kālāhāṇḍī district, one near Dadpur village and another near Junagarh. The Dadpur site is locally known as "Rapanggudi," and the stone circle near Junagarh is locally called "Bhairavladia." Both these sites have yielded a large quantity of black and red ware. A menhir has been found in Sagada village, 15 km to the south of Bhawanipatna, on the way to Thuamul-Rampur. The site has revealed black and red ware and iron slags.

It is known from observations that in some sites, Neolithic

68. F.R. Allchin & D.K. Cakrabarti, *op. cit.,* vol. I, 1979, p. 256.

69. (i) B. Mishra & P. Mohanty, "Archaeological Heritage of Dadpur region, district Kalahandi, Orissa," *Journal of Bengal Art,* vol. 4, 1999, pp. 344-45.

(ii) P. Mohanty & B. Mishra, "From Stone Age to Early Historic: Recent Archaeological discoveries in Kalahandi district of Orissa," *River Valley Cultures of India,* ed. K.K. Cakravarti & G.L. Badam, Indira Gandhi, Rashtriya Manav Sangrahalaya, Bhopal, 2000, under print.

and Chalcolithic periods were succeeded by megalithic culture at different sites in the Mahānadī valley.

The technology and material life of the people of the Mahānadī valley can be known from antiquities discovered at Dhanora in Ḍurg district which is a megalithic site; Malhar in Bilāspur district which is a pre-Mauryan site and Sirpur in Raipur district which is a medieval site in Chhattisgarh.[70] Among the proto-historic sites, mention may be made of Khambeswaripali in Sonepur district, Kuanr in Keoñjhar district, Gopālpur in Nayāgarh district, Sankerjang in Aṅgul district and Golbaisasan in Khurda district of Orissa, while the early historic sites of Orissa are the Maraguda valley, Bodhi-Komnā, Komnā and Nehenā in Nuāpāḍā district, Asurgarh, Kharligarh in the foothills of the Gurhāṇḍī mountain, Churiagarh and Budhigarh in Kālāhāṇḍī district, Kharligarh in Bolaṅgīr district, Asurgarh in Sonepur district, Manamunda in Boudh district, Langudi, Rādhānagar, Śiśupālgarh, Jaugaḍa, Lalitagiri, Palur and Manikapatna.[71]

For a long time there has been a near unanimity among scholars about the non-existence of any written record between the Indus script and the Brāhmī script and the earliest positive evidence of the existence of the Brāhmī script does not go beyond the fourth century BC according to Upasak.[72] The most important proto-historic relic of the Mahānadī valley is the

70. R.A. Sharma, *Technology and Material Life of Central India*, Agamkala Prakashan, Delhi, 1991, p. 144.

71. (i) P. Mohanty & B. Tripathy, "The Pre-historic-Proto-historic and the Early Historic Culture of Orissa," *Prāgdhārā*, Journal of the U.P. State Archaeology Dept., no. 8, 1997-98, pp. 69-98.

(ii) K.K. Basa, "Neolithic and Post-Neolithic Cultures of Orissa: An Overview," and S. Pradhan "Chalcolithic Culture of Orissa." S. Pradhan (ed.), *Orissa — History Culture and Archaeology* (in felicitation of Prof. P.K. Mishra), D.K. Printworld, New Delhi, 1999, pp. 9-38.

72. C.S. Upasak, *The History and Palaeography of Mauryan Brahmi Script*, Nalanda, 1960, p. 183.

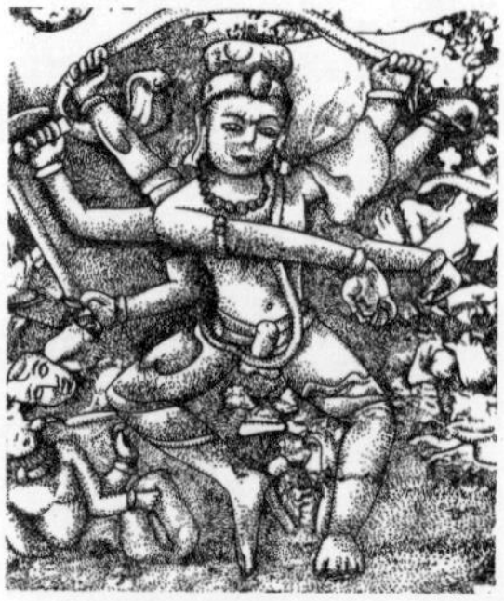

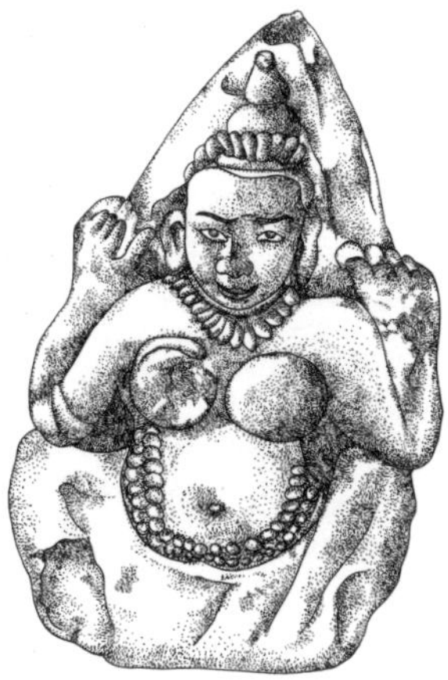

pictographic writing of Vikramkhol, situated in Sundargarh district of Orissa. This was discovered by an educated *sādhu* (*yogī*) Swami Jnanananda and being informed by him, K.P. Jayaswal[73] examined it thoroughly and published his treatise in 1933. He remarks:

> The characters in the Vikramkhol inscription belong to a period intermediary between the scripts of Mohen-zo-Daro and Brāhmī. Some letters still retain their original or proto-Brāhmī forms. This proves the origin of Brāhmī to be Indian and throws a flood of light on the history of writing, as from Brāhmī the Phoenician and European scripts are derived.

The letters of Vikramkhol were first painted and later developed to be engraved. They still remain undeciphered. Subrata Kumar Acharya[74] assigns the inscription to Vedic Āryans of the later Vedic period and *circa* 1,000 BC may be its approximate age. Thus, the Vikramkhol inscription is written in proto-Brāhmī script and in Sanskrit language, the language of Vedic Āryans. The script is in a stage of transition; a transition from the ideosyllabic to the alphabetic characters.

Satyanarayan Rajaguru had discovered a rock engraving within the hills of Naraj in Cuttack district of Orissa and had deciphered it, as hyroglyphic writing, but R.N. Das (vide *Samaj*, Oriya daily newspaper, 27 December 1987), identifies it, as a pre-historic engraving. The engraving depicts two men in a hunting mood, and a bird and a fish are engraved towards the left of the two hunters.

A large number of ring-plates discovered from the historical sites of Taxila to Pāṭaliputra, such as Mathurā, Rājghāṭ and Kauśāmbī signify the continuation of the tradition of symbolic worship of Mother Goddess. These ring-plates are of hard

73. *Indian Antiquary*, vol. LXII, 1933, pp. 58-60.

74. S.K. Acharya, "Vikramkhol Inscription and Origin of Brahmi Script," *Culture, Tribal History and Freedom Movement* (Dr. N.K. Sahu Commemoration Volume), ed. P.K. Mishra, Agamkala Prakashan, Delhi, 1989, pp. 5-14.

sandstone in black, violet or slate colours and are in a flat discoidal form, with or without a hole in the centre and showing the Mother Goddess in various combinations or only having plural geometrical patterns.[75] The author has discovered a broken piece of similar ring-plate from the Bikrampur site of Nuāpāḍā district which is kept in his personal museum.

V

Whatever may be the definition and nature of the Siddhānta Śaiva doctrine propounded by Maheśvara, it is possible that the Śaivāgamas continued to propel their evolution during the period beginning with the composition of the *Śvetāśvatara Upaniṣad* and ranging up to the rise of Madhvācārya in the fourteenth century AD. From the doctrinal shadow of the *Śvetāśvatara Upaniṣad* it appears plausible that these Siddhānta Śaivāgama doctrines began to evolve from the last part of the first century BC onward. Most probably the Siddhānta doctrine travelled from northern India to its southern part enroute the central province and South Kośala.[76]

Mattamayūra Śaivism originated in northern India, as it is a school of Śaiva Siddhānta, and it spread throughout the Mahānadī river valley. It had tāntric ideas and influenced the making of two Naṭarāja eight-handed sculptures with the *ūrdhvaliṅga* (erected penis) in the Mahānadī valley. The *ūrdhva-liṅga* symbolizes the upflow of semen, i.e., the practice of the *yoga* of sexual transformation.

The earliest Naṭarāja sculpture with *ūrdhvaliṅga*, dating to the fifth century AD is found at Sirpur in Raipur district, (*Pl.* 25). According to C. Sivaramamurti,[77]

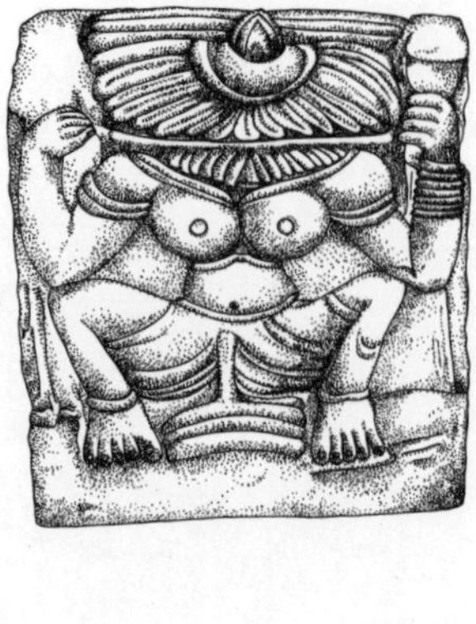

75. Balram Srivastava, *Iconography of Śakti* (A Study based on *Śrītattvanidhi*), Chaukhambha Orientalia, Varanasi, 1978, pp. 7-8.
76. R.P. Mishra, "Mattamayūra Śaivism in Orissa," *Culture and Collections*, ed. R.P. Mishra, Punthi Pustak, Calcutta, 1996, p. 117.
77. C. Sivaramamurti, *Naṭarāja in Art, Thought and Literature*, Publication Division, National Museum, New Delhi, 1994, pp. 159-60.

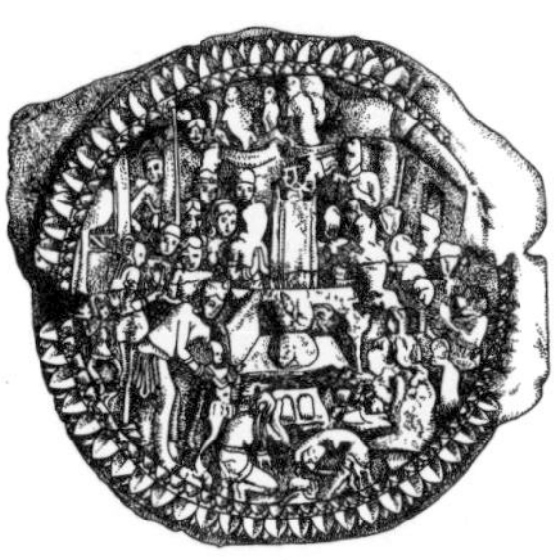

> All the grace and beauty of Gupta sculpture is seen in a late example of this school from Sirpur. Śiva dancing in the *lalita* pose, eight armed. He has a large pearl necklace, *jaṭās* arranged as usual in Gupta sculpture, with the crescent against it, the *ūrdhvaliṅga* recalls at once the tradition prevalent in this area of central India, as at Mandasor. While the topmost pair of hands holds up the snake, the other arms the *śūla, ḍamaru, kapāla,* while the last one fondles Devī, by caressing her chin. While the main right hand is in *gajahasta*, the main left, which should have been in *abhaya* or *saṁdaṁśa* brought nearer the ear; is broken. A drummer to the right plays the *ūrdhva* drum, while another beside him claps his hand to keep time. Gaṇeśa enjoys the dance, standing to Śiva's right, while Skanda, in juvenile fashion, dances exactly like his father, even while seated on the peacock. His left hand is in *gajahasta* and the right in *patākā*. Devī, seated to the left, watches her husband's dance with affection and emotion, and receives the caressing with joy. Between his legs peeps out a figure, dancing also in the *lalita* pose, exactly like Śiva. It is probably Tandu or Bharata imitating his Master. This is a great masterpiece. The jewellery is very sparse but the carving is every effective.

The second oldest eight-handed Naṭarāja sculpture with the *ūrdhvaliṅga* dates back to sixth century AD[78] and was found at Āsanapaṭ, in Keoñjhar district of Orissa and is now preserved at Orissa State Museum, (*Pl.* 26).

VI

The Nātha cult and 64 Yoginī cult were systematized and propounded in the Mahānadī river valley. About the Nātha cult, Ram Prasad Mishra[79] observes that entertaining Upaniṣadic influence in its prayer to Lord Śiva, this school most probably

78. C. Sivaramamurti, *Naṭarāja in Art, Thought and Literature*, Publication Division, National Museum, New Delhi, 1994, pp. 164-65.

79. R.P. Mishra, *Sahajayāna — A Study of Tāntric Buddhism*, Punthi Pustak, Calcutta, 1991, pp. 281-82.

followed the *yoga* of the Atharvavedic Upaniṣads of the later days which also influenced the *yoga* system of tāntric Buddhism. It appears that from the School of Śaivism, the cult of Nātha originated in Orissa and as the neighbourhood of Delhi was the primal seat of this School, the Nāthas treated Kurukṣetra as the seat of their primal Lord or Ādinātha Śiva. Candradvīpa where Matsyendra rescued the text of the sacred knowledge from the belly of a fish was most probably the Candrāvali-Dhāma regions of Orissa, which is even at present a popular citadel of the cult of Śaivism and the Nāthas. The Nātha cult as a school of Śaivism appears to have accultured much from different religious systems in the primary days of its genesis. It admitted the influence of the Upaniṣads, Śāktism, Vaiṣṇavism and tāntric Buddhism, although its adherents criticized a number of religious systems. Its supreme reality is called Saccidānanda, the Absolute Truth, the Real Truth transcending all dualism and non-dualism and this carries on the influence of the Upaniṣads. Śakti figures as inseparable from Śiva in this cult. The supreme reality in this cult is accompanied by Viṣṇu on the right and Śiva on the left. So Śiva as the supreme reality of this cult is quite different from the Śiva of other Śaiva school. He is *parama Brahman* and is beyond all thought constructions. The cult of Nātha most probably accultured the doctrine of *sahaja* both from the later Upaniṣadic culture and Sahajayāna. In *Akula Vira Tantra*, ascribed to Matyendranāth, *sahaja* is described as a state of supreme equilibrium which transcends all perceptual knowledge with positive and negative attributes. In this state, the *yogī* becomes one with the whole universe and realizes a non-dual existence.

In the words of H.K. Mahtab,[80] "Evidences of the Nātha *dharma* in Orissa can be traced to the last quarter of the eighth century." A statue of Matsyendranāth in the form of Padmapāṇi Avalokiteśvara in the forest of Rājnagar under Deravisi block

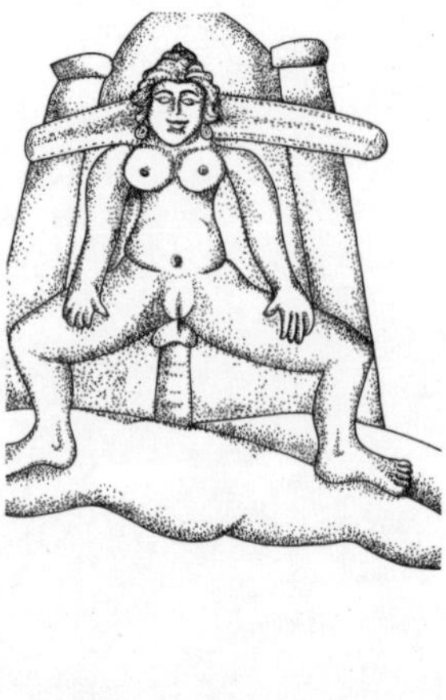

80. H.K. Mahatab, "Culture of Orissa," *OHRJ*, vol. XXX, nos. 2, 3 & 4, 1984, pp. 10-11 (Golden Jubilee Volume).

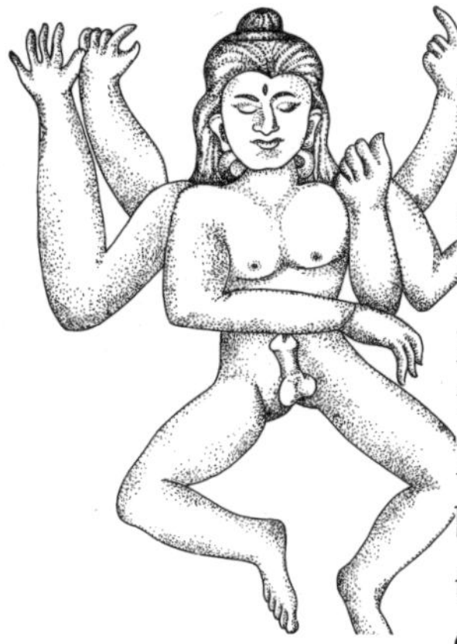

of Kendrapārā sub-division is still worshipped by the Nāthas of the surrounding villages. The inscription on both sides of the statue is in *kuṭila-lipi* or *proto-udralipi*. The present Oriyā script was not evolved by then and the period of that script is accepted to be in-between the sixth and eleventh centuries. The prototype of the same is seen at Kendrapārā bus stand with the same inscription and another at Trilocanpur village under Mahājājpur gram panchayat near Bahugrām is also worshipped by the Nāthas of surrounding villages. This proves that towards the last quarter of the ninth century Matsyendranātha and Gorakhanāth were worshipped in Orissa as incarnations of Viṣṇu and Śiva respectively. The most ancient specimens of Oriyā prose and poetry are ascribed to be the works of Gorakhanāth and other Nātha *siddhas*.

The theory of *piṇḍa-brahmāṇḍa* (cosmos in microcosm) of Gorakhanāth serves as the backbone Orissa's Vaiṣṇava philosophy of the *pañcaśākhā* literature as in the case of *nirguṇa santa kāvyas* of Hindī, Punjābī and Gujarātī literatures of the ancient and medieval period.

Since the dates of Sarala Das, the Nāthas of Orissa have been mentioned as Rudraja and Śiśuvedī brāhmaṇas. So far as social customs are concerned they observe most of the Vedic brāhmaṇical rites with some variations. According to Nāthas the sacred threads are ever pure, even during the period of uncleanliness due to birth or death. The dead body is buried in *yogāsana* posture in a compound specially preserved in the premises of *maṭhas* or homestead land. The *samādhis* are treated as sacred shrines. The *Śiśuveda* of the Nāthas is regarded as the fifth Veda. A person from any caste or religious sect can accept the Nātha *dharma*, but he must use the surname "Nātha" after due initiation. Hundreds of *nāthas*, *pīṭhas* and *gadīs* are scattered all over Orissa. Although idolatry is forbidden in the Nātha *dharma*, it came to be mixed up first with Buddhism and then with Hinduism. Buddhist and *Brahman* idols were accepted by the Nāthas. It is the Nātha *dharma* which made *yoga* popular in Orissa.

> One interesting fact is that Orissa is the state where in ancient times the *Atharvaveda* was the prevalent Veda. This was known when research was made on *Paipallala Sūtra* of *Atharvaveda* which was thought to have lost but manuscripts of which were found in many villages in Orissa. When the *Atharvaveda* was downgraded during ascendency of Brāhmaṇism many changed over to the *Yajurveda*, but they could not dispense with some rituals of the *Atharvaveda* during ceremonies such as marriage, etc.
>
> Thus the influence of this religious currents and cross-currents worked in Orissa cannot be gainsaid.

Two *mithuna-stambhas* have been found in Orissa so far. One *mithuna-stambha* is found in Goruāla village near Purī[81] and the other with an Oriyā inscription is fixed on the inner wall of the *jagamohana* or *maṇḍapa* of the Dadhibaban temple at Junagarh in Kālāhāṇḍī district.[82] These prove that Atharva-vedic practice was prevalent in Orissa, because the ritual of installing *mithuna-stambha*, is mentioned in the *Vāstusūtra Upaniṣad* of *Atharvaveda*.

As already mentioned, Nātha *dharma* made *yoga* popular in Orissa, i.e., in the whole of the Mahānadī river valley and India in general. Among the *yogas*, the *yoga* of sexual transformation was most popular, because, *Haṭha Yoga Pradīpikā*, a yogic text, composed by *yogī* Swatmarama, a disciple of *yogī* Gorakhnāth, has dealt with the *yoga* of sexual transformation and its *haṭha yogas* in detail.

About the origin of the yoginī cult, H.C. Das[83(A)] states:

> The cult of *yoginī* is a very important manifestation of the creative energy (*śakti*), who is the omnipresent, omniscient,

81. Boner-Sarma-Baumer, *Vāstusūtra Upaniṣad (The Essence of Form in Sacred Art)*, Motilal Banarsidass, Delhi, 1996, p. 84, Fig. 17.
82. J.P. Singh Deo, "Archaeological Remains of Junagarh," *OHRJ*, vol. XXXVII, nos. 1 to 4, pp. 61-71, vide Fig. VIII.

83(A). H.C. Das, *Tāntricism: A Study of Yoginī Cult*, Sterling Publishers, New Delhi, 1981, p. 3.

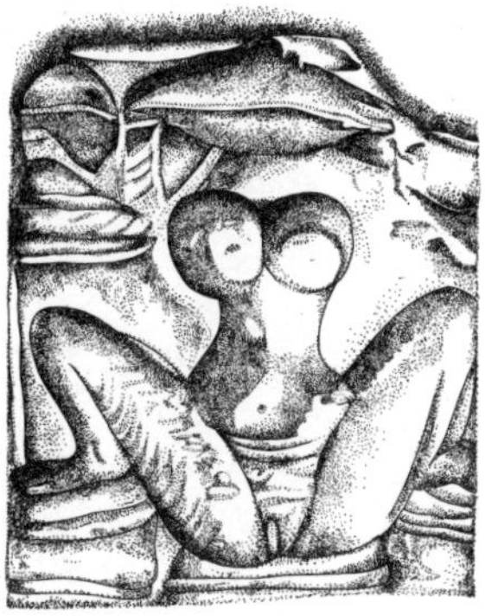

omnipotent, creator, preserver and destroyer of the universe. The origin of this cult is mysterious.

Archaeologists, historians, indologists and art historians have made serious attempt to carry on a systematic study of this obscure cult and advocated various theories to explain it satisfactorily. But no consensus has emerged yet to explain this all-pervasive and mythical cult. The main reason for this is non-availability of authentic texts.

The literature of the Vedic and post-Vedic period often mentions the name of *yoginī*s as manifestations of the female principal. But *yoginī*s in the shape of a cult known as Śākta Tāntric came into existence in the sixth-seventh century AD when efflorescences of Śāktism, Tāntricism and Śaivism either in individual form or in combination swayed the religious realm of India. Whatever might be the time of origin of the cult, it continued to flourish as an important manifestation of Śākta-Tāntricism and the propitiators acquired magical and super natural faculties through the help of *yoginī*s with a view of destroying enemies. Through the process of transformation over the ages the *yoginī*s finally multiplying into 64 gained supremacy particularly in the eastern zone of India. Matsyendranāth, in view of the popularity the cult had gained, systematized and expounded it in his famous work, *Kulajñānanirṇaya*, which has become its authoritative text of the cult.

This much of information by H.C. Das seems to be an expression of his educative mind, but he is ignorant of the *haṭha yoga* of sexual transformation, because he does not appear to have a yogic intuitive mind and its knowledge. Hence, he is bereft of this *yoga*. Therefore in a later work, *Śākta Pīṭha*s — *A Study*, while dealing of 64 *yoginī*s, H.C. Das[83(B)] mentions,

> The cult as well as its occult and secret practices and philosophy were systematized and expounded by Matsyendranāth in his work *Kaulajñānairṇaya*. He is described

83(B). H.C. Das, *Sākta Pīṭhas — A Study*, Bharati Prakashan, 1999, Bhubaneswar, pp. 71-72.

in his work as an incarnation of Bhairavaśiva, in the form of a fish who learnt the secret of *dhyāna-yoga*, and *yajña-yoga*, from Śiva when he disclosed it to Gaurī. The secret cult of Matsyendranāth was practised in the company of women in a circle known as *yoginī kaula*. But the new *kaula* expounded by Matsyendra is called *Matsyendra kaula*. This particular cult was revealed by Bhairava in Candradvīpa in general and in the Kāmarūpa in particular to Bhairava who is none other than Matsyendra himself. Hence perhaps, it is called *Matsyendra kaula* (got from the belly of the fish, i.e., Matsyendra). Since it was practised in the company of women, it was disliked by Kārttikeya, who being a *brahmacārī* and purist tried twice to destroy it by submerging into the sea. For the same reason Gorakhanāth also disliked it and he is well-known for his staunch yogic Śaivism. It is reported that this peculiar secret knowledge was known as *mahat kaula* and *siddhāmṛta*, in earlier ages. Matsyendranāth is stated to have expounded his secret *yoginī kaula* in Kāmarūpa where every woman was a *yoginī* in the company of whom he discovered his new cult. According to *Kaulajñānaniṇaya*, the ultimate aim of the *kaula* is to attain a state in which the mind and the sight merged into the object to be visualized. The *Saubhāgya Bhāskar* describes *kaula* as Śakti and *akula* as Śiva; the union of the two is *kaula* and the process of establishing this relationship is the *kaulamārga*. Śiva, the *akula* is represented in the *yoginī* temples of Orissa and Khajurāho in supreme poise and beatitude with uplifted male organ symbolizing the complete cessation of the triple stirrings of consciousness, breath and semen. The image echoes the reconciliation of the impressiveness of *yoga* with the lyricism of sex. The mystic and esoteric *kaula* rites that prevailed in India were systematized by Matsyendranāth, the author of *Kaulajñānanirṇaya*, who preached the doctrine of *yoginī kaula*. The Bhaumakaras and Somavaṁśīs in Orissa, Candelās and Kalacuris in Madhya Pradesh, erected the *yoginī* temples in honour of the cult associated with the *kaula kāpālika* practice.

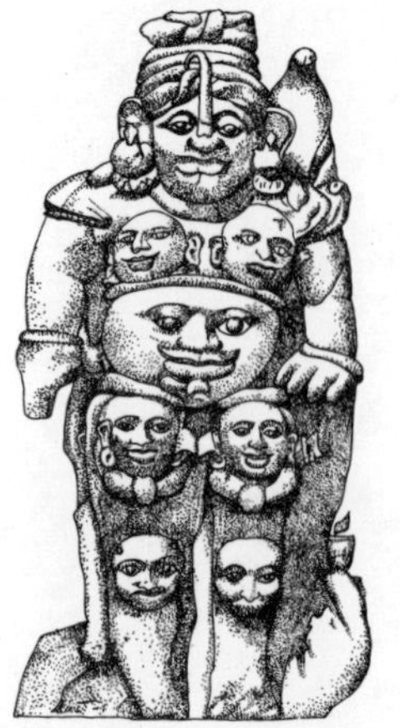

This opinion of H.C. Das by quoting earlier scholars, who were ignorant of the *haṭha yoga* of India, is absolutely blasphemy. Without delving deep into its yogic intuitive knowledge, the

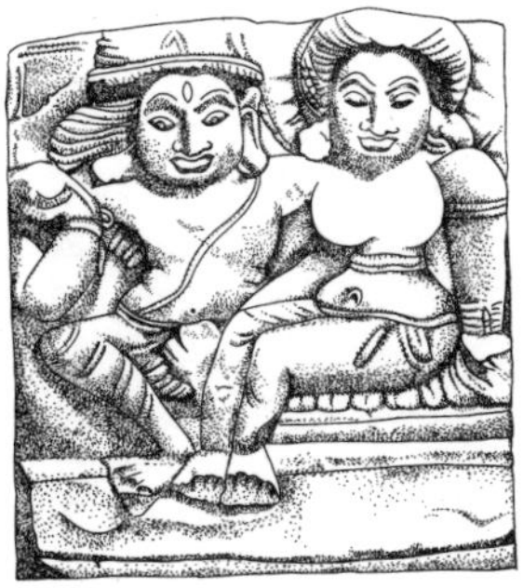

scholar has given such an erroneous view. For example, H.C. Das speaks of "uplifted male organ," as symbolizing the complete cessation of the triple stirrings of consciousness, breath and semen. It is completely wrong. The uplifted male organ of Śiva is *ūrdhva-liṅga* (penis erectus) which symbolizes the upflow of semen through *iḍā* and *piṅgalā nāḍīs* to the *suṣumnā nāḍī* (main *nāḍī* in the centre of the spinal cord which conducts *kuṇḍalinī śakti*), i.e., the practice of the *yoga* of sexual transformation and Lord Śiva is regarded as the master of *yoga* in tāntric-yogic literatures of India. All details of the *yoga* of sexual transformation are found in the *Haṭha Yoga Pradīpikā*, text. According to Paramahamsa Swami Satyananda Sarasvatī,[83(C)] out of many authorities on *haṭha yoga*, one outstanding personality is Swatmarama who compiled *Haṭha Yoga Pradīpikā*. It can also be translated as "Light on Haṭha Yoga." However, the term *pradīpikā* actually means "self-illumi-nating" or "that which illumines." It is the text which illumines a multitude of physical, mental and spiritual problems for the aspirants. Gorakhnāth, the chief disciple of Matsyendranāth, had earlier written books, poems and prose on the *haṭha yoga* system in the local dialect, but Swatmarama compiled the entire wisdom of *haṭha yoga* in Sanskrit. In common with other texts, he has expounded techniques such as *āsana*, *prāṇāyāma* and *ṣaṭkarma*.

> The beauty of the *Haṭha Yoga Pradīpikā* is that it solves a very great problem of every aspirant. Swatmarama has completely eliminated the *yama* (moral codes) and *niyama* (self-restraints) which are the starting points in the Buddhist and Jain systems and also in Patañjali's *rāja yoga*.

The *Yoginī Tantra*, being a tāntric text of the eleventh century AD states that the *ādi-pīṭha* (first site) of the *yoginī* cult is at a

---

83(C). Swami Muktibodhananda Sarasvati, *Haṭha Yoga Pradīpikā* (*Light on Haṭha Yoga*), under the guidence of Paramahamsa Swami Satyananda Sarasvati, Bihar School of Yoga, Munger, 2nd edn., 1993, pp. 3-4.

place where Someśvara-*liṅga* is worshipped.[84] Someśvara-*liṅga* is worshipped in the Someśvara Śiva temple,[85] which stands at the Rānīpur-Jharial site of Bolaṅgīr district of Orissa. Therefore, it can be stated that Rānīpur-Jharial is the *ādi-piṭha* of the 64 *yoginī* cult, where this cult evolved at the right middle of the Mahānadī valley and spread to different parts of the country and abroad. Therefore the opinion of H.C. Das[86] "The Hirapur village was established by Hiradevi, one of the Queens of Bhaumakara, family in *circa* ninth century AD when the wave of tantrism was at the zenith. Most of the śākta-tāntric temples of Orissa are assignable to the Bhaumakaras. . . . The hypaethral *yoginī* temple at Hirapur is the earliest of all," is completely wrong on the basics of the tāntric-yogic text proof. K.C. Panigrahi,[87] a seasoned archaeologist, while dealing with the 64 *yoginī* cult of Hīrāpur states, "It seems that the Sōmavaṁśī rulers, when they lived in Orissa, created this shrine or helped the creation of it in the model of the Rānīpur-Jharial shrine, which lay in their original seat of power." This opinion seems to be fully correct.

Nine temples of the 64 *yoginī* cult have been discovered in India so far. Two are located in the Mahānadī valley at Rānīpur-Jharial and Hīrāpur in Orissa, three at Bherāghāṭ, Khajurāho and Shahdol in Madhya Pradesh. The Shahdol images are now preserved in Dhubela Museum in Chhatrapur district, at Mitauli and Dudahi in Lalitpur district and Lokhari in the Bāndā district of Uttar Pradesh and in Coimbatore district of Tamil Nadu. Such temple at Suruda in Kālāhāṇḍī district of Orissa, as mentioned by A. Cunningham,[88] is not yet located.

84. R.P. Mishra, *Fragments of Indian Culture* (*Ranipur-Jharial*), Punthi Pustak, Calcutta, 1995, p. 207.

85. Dipakranjan Das, *Temples of Orissa — The Study of a Sub-style* Agamkala Prakashan, Delhi, 1982, pp. 26-29.

86. H.C. Das, *op. cit.*, Bhubaneswar, 1999, pp. 69-70.

87. K.C. Panigrahi, *History of Orissa*, Kitab Mahal, Cuttak, 1981, p. 454.

88. Alexander Cunningham, *Archaeological Survey of India Report*, vol. IX, p. 74.

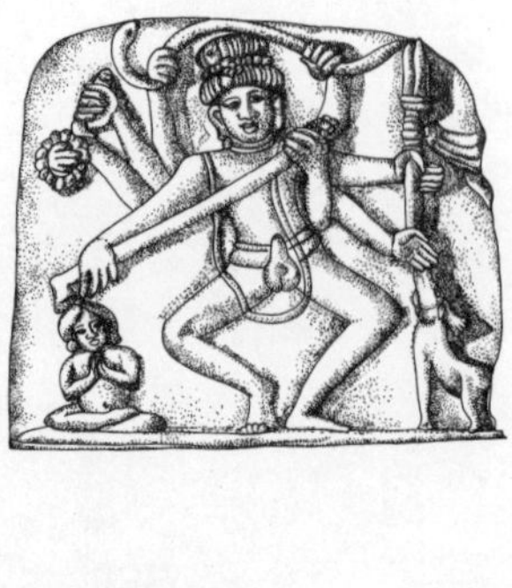

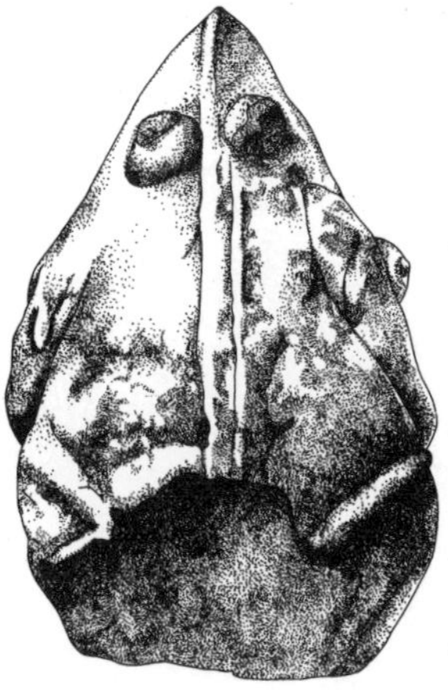

According to *Haṭha Yoga Pradīpikā*,[89] which is an authoritative book on *haṭha yoga*, "a *yoginī* is one who practises *vajrolī*." The *vajrolī-mudrā* is a *haṭha yoga* practice. It is a thunderbolt attitude in which the muscles of the sexual organ and lower urinary tract contract to redirect sexual energy upwards. It is a practice of *haṭha yoga* and *tantra*. The *sahajolī-mudrā* is a practice of *vajrolī* by a woman that involves contraction of the lower urinary muscles. Verse 99 of Chapter 3, of the same text mentions:

> If a woman practises *vajrolī* and saves her *rajas* and the man's *bindu* by thorough contraction, she is a *yoginī*.

This proves that the *yoga* of sexual transformation was very popular throughout India, between the eigth century AD to twelfth century AD as 64 *yoginī* temples are assigned within this period.[90]

All standing temples of the Mahānadī river valley are not older than the fifth century AD. The post-Gupta period was the juvenile period of the revival of Vedic culture with tāntric influence. Prof. Satyavrata R. Patel[91] quotes Sri Aurobindo Ghosh in this context,

> Indian art portrays all human activities, sacred and profane, secular and religious, from sex to salvation. It embraces all life, even the cosmos in its vast existence.

While dealing with *tantra* (Āgama), Swami Sivananda[92(A)] states,

> Sanskrit literature can be classified under six orthodox heads and four secular heads. They are (1) Śruti, (ii) Smṛti, (iii)

89. Swami Muktibodhananda Sarasvati (Commentator), *Haṭha Yoga Pradīpikā*, Bihar School of Yoga, Munger, 1993, p. 362.

90. H.C. Das, *op. cit.*, 1981, p. 3.

91. Prof. S.R. Patel, *East and West — A Cultural Dialogue*, Bharatiya Vidya Bhavan, Bombay, 1992, p. 74.

92(A). Swami Sivananda, *Bliss Divine*, The Divine Life Society, Shivanandanagar, 1974, p. 578.

Itihāsa, (iv) Purāṇa, (v) Āgama (vi) Darśana; and (i) Subhāṣita, (ii) Kāvya, (iii) Nāṭaka and (iv) Alaṅkāra.

The Āgamas are theological treatises and practical manuals of divine worship. The Āgamas include *tantras*, *mantras* and *yantras*. These are treatises explaining the external worship of God in the form of idols, temples, etc. All the Āgamas are treatises on (i) *jñāna* or knowledge, (ii) *yoga* or concentration, (iii) *kriyā* or making and (iv) *caryā* or doing. They also give elaborate details about the ontology, cosmology, liberation, devotion, meditation, philosophy of *mantras*, mystic diagrams, charms and spells, temple-building, image-making, domestic observances, social rules and public festivals.

Śiva-Śakti in Āgamic principle are found at Ranipur-Jharial Site (*Pl.* 4 & *Fig.* 4)

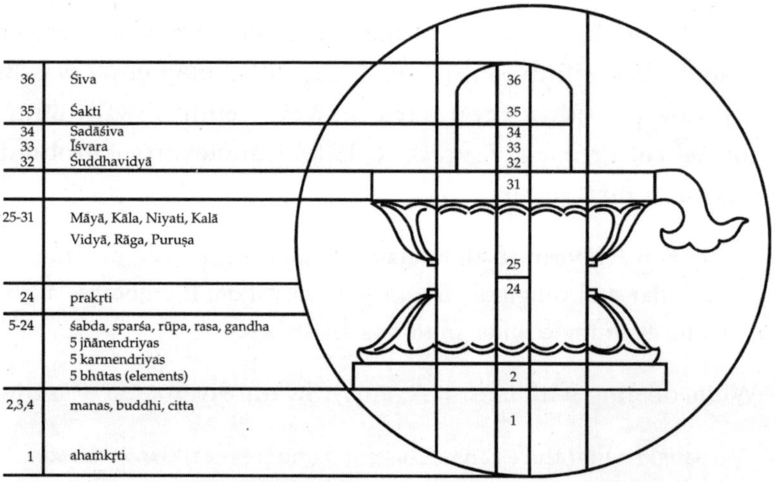

fig. 4. *Tattvas in Śivaliṅga*, according to Āgama literature. (Source: S.S. Janaki, "Pañcabhūtas in Śaiva ritual: with special reference to Bhūta-śuddhi," in *Prakṛti*, vol. 3. (*The Āgamic Tradition and the Arts*), General ed. Kapila Vatsyayan, D.K. Printworld (P) Ltd., New Delhi, 1995, *fig.* IV, p. 46.

According to Swami Satyananda Sarasvatī,[92(B)] *tantra* aims

92(B). Swami Satyananda Sarasvati, *A Systematic Course in the Ancient Tāntric Technique of Yoga and Kriyā*, Bihar School of Yoga, Munger,

→

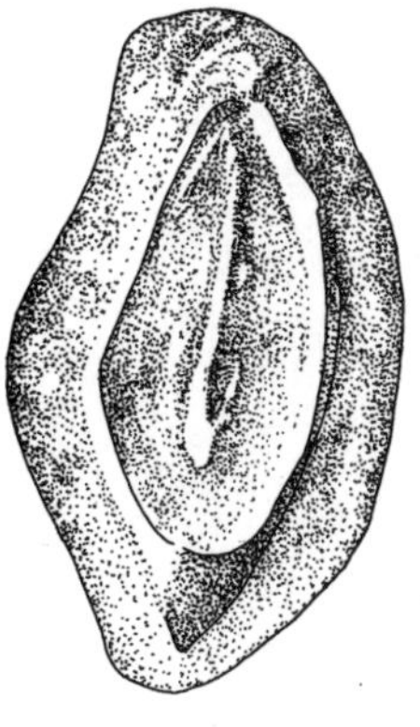

at transforming every action of life into a ritual so that the individual performs every action and thought with a feeling of worship and awareness. The action of bathing, dressing, sitting for worship, offering various symbolic sacrifices, sexual relations, stages of development from inception in the womb, birth to marriage, etc., are transformed into worship.

> The aim of *tantra* is to unfresh the cosmic energy in man so that he rises to higher levels of awareness.

These observations shows that Swami Harshananda[93] is very correct when he mentions thus:

> Again, the temple represents this world in all its aspects, the actual and the ideal. The imposing *gopuramas* at the entrance reflect the awesome grandeur of the external world. The friezes and sculptures on the external walls of the temple proper depict the animal world and the mundane life of ordinary human beings including the ridiculous side and the aberrations. Criticism is often voiced against the *mithuna* figures (figures of amorous couples) that adorn most of the temples on their exterior walls. These figures, obviously connected with fertility rites, are considered to be auspicious. More often, they are iconographical representations of creation and of the bipolar nature of this created world, which is described in philosophical treatises as arising out of the union of *prakṛti* and *puruṣa* (Nature and Spirit). Uninhibited eroticism as found in the temples at Konarak (Orissa) and Khajuraho (Madhya Pradesh) is perhaps the outcome of Tāntricism.

K.S. Behera,[94] has failed to give a convincing argument, on the erotic art of world fame Koṇārk temple of Orissa because he seems to be ignorant of intuitive knowledge which is revealed,

→ 2nd edn., 1989, p. 335.

93. Swami Harshananda, *All About Hindu Temple*, Sri Ramakrishna Ashrama, Mysore, 2nd edn., 1981, pp. 12-13.

94. K.S. Behra, *Konark The Heritage of Mankind*, Aryan Books International, New Delhi, 1996, pp. 229-49.

achieved and got through *yoga* and the *yoga* of sexual transformation.

Prithvi K. Agrawala[95] and G.V. Bhaskara Reddy[96] though have made a passing reference to *vajrolī, amarolī* and *sahajolī*, are in fact ignorant of the yogic life and they have discussed it only academically within the pursuit of educative knowledge.

Even N.N. Bhattacharyya[97] and Devangana Desai[98] have done religious, social and cultural studies but seem to be ignorant of the tāntric-yogic conception of the erotic sculptural arts. Only recently D. Desai[99] mentions,

> Going beyond the erotic, the head-down pose, the south juncture wall of the Kandarīya Mahādeva temple, the *kāmakalā yantra* is superimposed here to show the possibility of this sculpture to be composed on the lines of the *yantra*. The *Śilpa Prakāśa*, enjoins the sculpturing of erotic figures on the lines of the *kāmakalā yantra* in order to hide the actual *yantra* from the gaze of the uninitiated and to give delight to layman.

No manuscripts on temple architecture has been found at Khajurāho or in its vicinity so far. It seems Khajurāho was dependent on the Manuals of Temple Architecture of Orissa.

---

95. Prithvi K. Agrawala, *Mithuna — The Male-Female Symbol in Indian Art and Thought*, Munshiram Manoharlal, New Delhi, 1983, passim.
96. G.V. Bhaskara Reddy, *Erotic Sculptures of Ancient India*, Inter-India Publications, New Delhi, 1991, passim and special reference p. 100.
97. N.N. Bhattacharyya, *History of the Tāntric Religion*, Manohar, New Delhi, 1987, pp. 370-98.
98. Devangana Desai, *Erotic Sculpture of India — A Socio-Cultural Study*, Tata McGraw-Hill Publishing Co., New Delhi, 1975, passim.
99. Devangana Desai, *The Religious Imagery of Khajuraho*, Project for Indian Cultural Studies Publication IV, Mumbai, 1996, p. 195.

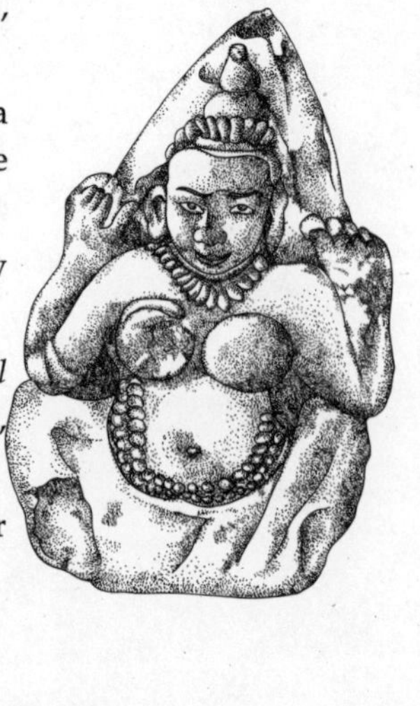

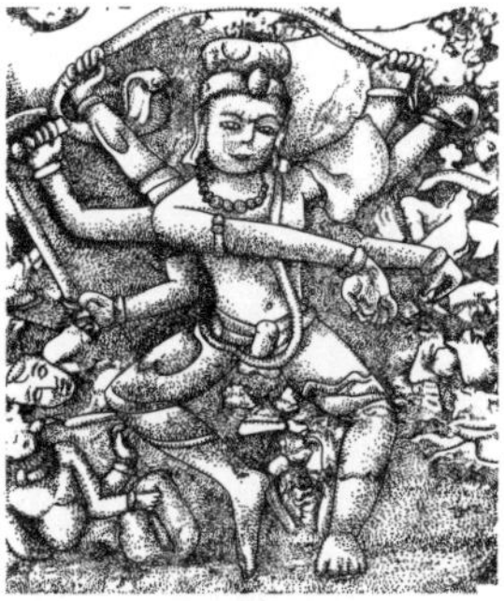

So far, the following *śilpa śāstra*s have been discovered in Orissa. They are:[100] 1. *Bhuvana Pradīpa*, 2. *Śilpa Prakāśa*, 3. *Saudhikāgama*, 4. *Baya Cakada* (A Book of accounts and building chronicle of the sun temple of Koṇārka), 5. *Śilpa Sāriṇī*, 6. *Vāstusūtra Upaniṣad* and 7. *Śilpa Ratnakośa*.

100. R.P. Das, "The Study of Śilpa Śastras," *Reference Orissa*, ed. A.N. Tiwari, Enterprising Publishers, Bhubaneswar, 1999, pp. 174-81.

2

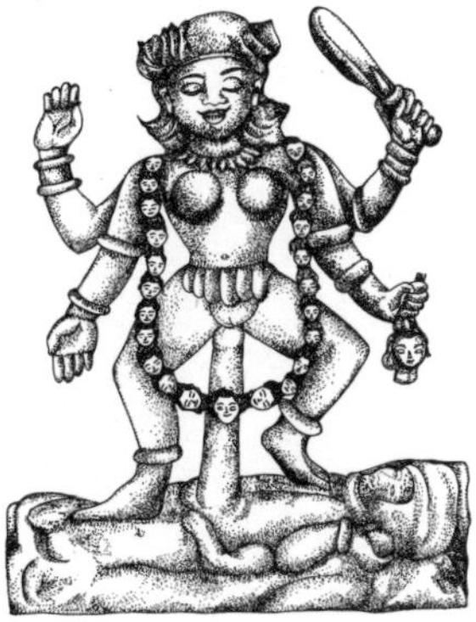

Yogic Development in Mahānadī Valley, Evolved Erotic Mysticism

A STUDY of yogic development which evolved Uḍḍīyāna-*Pīṭha* (site) has been done in this chapter and it shows the natural unfoldment of erotic mysticism, which is a silent expression of the antiquities of Mahānadī valley, so eagerly awaiting to be exposed and expounded for guidance to the modern *kali-yuga* (age) people. Great discoveries have been done, but human beings have forgotten to delve into the self. The self-indulgence of the author in discovering the secrets of Mahānadī valley has spotlighted the evolution of yogic erotic mysticism.

I

The Early Upland Dwellers of Mahānadī River Valley

While dealing with the early upland dwellers, Nupur Dasgupta[1] states,

> The involvement of nature and the elements in the growth of human societies can't be overemphasized. Nowhere is this symbiosis more obvious as when we look into the earliest days of human society's evolution, when man first began to explore and adjust with nature. In these early days the ancients, in their search for natural shelters and life sustaining resources, chose the likely places for habitation.

1. Nupur Dasgupta, "The Early Upland Dwellers: Evidences for Evolution of Human Societies in the Mountains and Hills," *The Quarterly Review of Historical Studies,* Institute of Historical Studies, Kolkata, vol. XI, nos. 1 & 2, April to September, 2000, p. 32.

> The middle reaches of mountains offered them with many amenities. The rock caverns provided shelter as well as some element of invincibility. The mountain woods, rich in timber and plant value and animal life, provided resources for hunting and gathering. The mountain streams offered the most, precious of all natural boons — clear drinking water.
>
> Thus we find some of the earliest evidences of settlement in the temperate forests of the northern mountain ranges in India, Afghanistan, Baluchistan, Kashmir, Punjab and Himachal Pradesh and in north-east Himalayan belt, as well as in lesser ranges in Central India and Deccan.

Dasgupta[2] concludes thus,

> But our studies[3] of the early Indus cultures in the Afghanistan and Baluchistan highlands and their links with the sedentary high farming cultures evolved in the valleys of Indus and other southern rivers lead us to similar conclusions.

In this background, let us acquaint ourselves with the history of India in the Ṛgvedic period. According to David Frawley,[4]

> There were two main Vedic cultures in ancient India. The first was a northern kingdom centred on the Sarasvatī-Dṛshadvatī river region dominated by the Purus and the Ikṣvākus that produced the existent Veda texts that we have. The second was a southern culture along the coast of the Arabian Sea and into the Vindhya mountains, dominated by the Turvaśas and Yadus and extending into groups yet further south. These northern and southern groups vied for supremacy and influenced each other in various ways as the Vedas and Purāṇas indicate. The northern or Bharata culture

2. *The Quarterly Review of Historical Studies*, Institute of Historical Studies, Kolkata, p. 39.

3. Nupur Dasgupta, "Pastoral Economy in the formative stage of Indian History, *Journal of History*, Department of History, Jadavpur University, vol. XIII, 1994-95, Kolkata, pp. 1-2.

4. David Frawley, *The Ṛgveda and the History of India*, Aditya Prakashan, New Delhi, 2001, cover flaps.

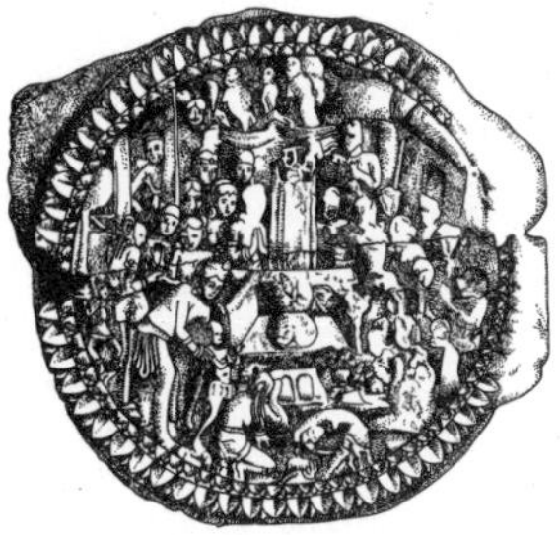

> ultimately prevailed, making India the land of Bharata or Bharatavarṣa and its main ancient literary record the Vedas, though militarily the Yadus remained strong throughout history. The southern culture was the older of the two, with the Vedic people coming originally from the south, not the north-west. This was the basis of the maritime symbolism at the core of Vedic thought, which reflects an ancient heritage.
>
> In addition, there was a third Vedic culture that prevailed in Punjab and Afghanistan, that of the Anus and Druhyus, which was at first part of the northern kingdom but gradually developed its own identity. It was partly assimilated by the Bharatas who became the dominant northern people. Another portion of it extended to north and west outside the Indian subcontinent. Its influence was secondary to that of the northern and southern kingdoms and much of it passed out of the Indic sphere of culture. However, it was the basis of most of the Indo-European and Iranian peoples and culture that we find in Europe, Central Asia and the Middle East.
>
> Therefore, we must look at the south and east connections to understand not only the Indic civilization and Hinduism, but also the Vedas. The western connections to the Europeans and Iranians were more an outflow, while the southern connections were more original and endu-ring. Western scholars, dominated by a European mind-set, only traced the Indo-European culture from Europe and the Middle East to India as its eastern border. They failed to see that the boundary was only in their minds.

With this knowledge and background, let us examine the developments of early upland dwellers of Mahānadī valley. This is the major river of the two provinces — Chhattisgarh and Orissa, an area which is no more *terra incognito* to the historical world. The stone age culture and megalithic culture of the whole valley are being studied by the scholars[5] and its explorations

---

5. (i) Gopal Chandra Mohapatra, *The Stone Age Cultures of Orissa*, Deccan College, Poona, 1962, passim.

→

are still continuing. Mahānadī river valley is situated at the centre of India, which received cultural and spiritual waves, both from the north and the south. Therefore cultural, religious and spiritual synthesis developed, but the early upland dwellers of the whole Mahānadī valley had developed their own antediluvian culture. Though technologically the antediluvian culture was not much developed, but spiritually it was much refined, pure advanced. This is known from the archaeological findings.

The most important antediluvian finding is the Dvarsanī deity, worshipped near Pātālgaṅgā site in Nuāpāḍā district in Orissa (*Pl.* 9). When the crust of the earth was under formation, it took the shape of female vulva at many places. In the words of O.A. Wall,[6]

> The external feminine sexual parts, the vulva, is called *yoni*, in India; it is still very widely worshipped in Asiatic religions and the worshippers of feminine attributes are called

---

→ (ii) R.P. Pandey, *Pre-historic Archaeology of Madhya Pradesh*, Sundeep Prakashan, Delhi, 1987, passim.

(iii) R.N. Dash, "Pre and Proto history of Orissa," *OHRJ*, vol. XXX, nos. 2, 3 & 4, pp. 284-304.

(iv) K.C. Tripathy, *Lithic Industries in India* (*A Study of South-Western Orissa*), Leeladevi Publications, Delhi, 1980, passim.

(v) K.K. Basa & P. Mohanty (eds.), *Archaeology* of *Orissa*, vol. I, Pratibha Prakashan, Delhi, 2000, passim.

(vi) S. Pradhan, *Exploration in Phulbani District: A Preliminary Report*, P.G. Department of History, Sambalpur University, Jyoti Vihar, 1988, passim, unpublished.

(vii) P.K. Behera, "A Note on the recent discovery of Megalithic Cairns in the Middle Mahānadī basin, at Burla, Orissa," *Prāgdhārā*, no. 6, Journal of the U.P. State Archaeological Organization, 1995-96, passim.

(viii) A.K. Sharma, *Archaeo-Anthropology of Chhattisgarh*, Sundeep Prakashan, New Delhi, 2000, passim.

6. *SASWITW*, p. 464.

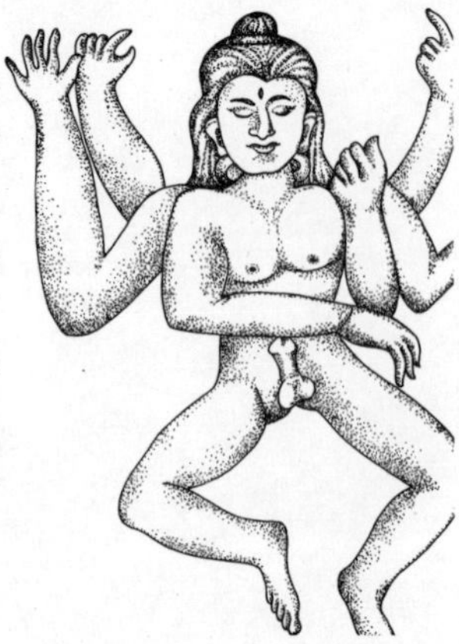

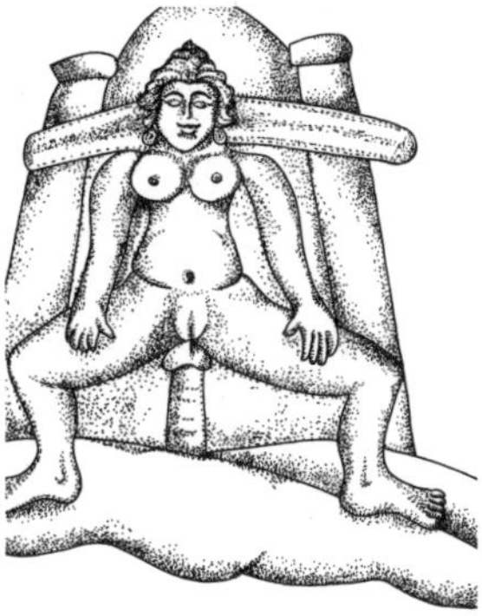

yonicitas. In subsequent reference to the vulva we will speak of it as the *yoni*.

Eight *yoni*s are discovered in Nuāpāḍā district so far. They are:

1. A land mass in a shape of *yoni*, near Pātālgaṅgā site is worshipped as Dvarsanī.
2. One naturally formed stone *yoni* was found in Dhangrital village which is now in the author's private possession at Khariar.
3. Three *yoni*s have been found on the rock belt, on the left bank of the Indra river, at a distance of 2 km from Chuipain village, on the foothills of the eastern slope of the Sunabeda plateau. This finding was first reported by Syamlal Purohit.
4. One stone *yoni* has been found at Soseng village area, on top of the Sunabeda plateau. Its middle portion is damaged because of human vandalism. It is now kept in the author's private museum at Khariar.
5. One beautifully chiselled *yoni* was discovered while digging for the foundation of the spill way of the Jonk Irrigation Dam in the Maraguda valley in 1982. It is also kept in the author's private museum.
6. One stone *yoni* was discovered from the sands of the Udanti river, with the help of Padma Danḍasena. There is a triangle with a spot (*bindu*) in the centre, which signifies the Bhairavī *yantra*. It measures 6½ cm in circumference and is worshipped in the house of Brusabhanu Naik of Mundapada village on the left bank of the Udanti river in Sinapali block area of Nuāpāḍā district.

Yoni symbolizes *yantra* in the form of a triangle pointed downwards. It is the *yantra* of Goddess Bhairavī, the fifth Goddess of *Daśamahāvidyā*. So, all these eight *yoni*s are the manifestation of Śakti in its *Bhairavī* form.

According to the tāntric literature *Śākta Pramoda*,[7] Bhairavī is a benign manifestation of Śakti and is considered as the giver of knowledge. The earliest archaeological remain of *Kuṇḍalinī Tantra*'s, *sahasrāra cakra*,[8] is found in the pre-historic rock-shelter paintings of Gurhāṇḍī in Kālāhāṇḍī district. The remain proves that knowledge originated and spread from this area and developed into imitative, repetitive, derigative, educative and intuitive forms.

The *yoni yantra*, developed the *śrīyantra* or *śrīvidyā*, which is a diagrammatic embodiment of the creative sexual activity of the universe.[9] Teun Goudriaan[10] says,

> In the *śrīvidyā* theory, Uḍḍīyāna is located within the central triangle of the *śrīcakra* (*Kāmakalāvilāsa*, 51), an indication of the ever increasing tendency towards interiorrization and symbolization of outside realities.

On the circular *yoni* discovered from the sands of the Udanti river, there is a triangle with a dot in the centre which is the *mahābindu* signifying *uḍḍīyāna*, which finally developed into *śrīvidyā*. So, it can be claimed that the *uḍḍīyāna* thought developed in the Nuāpāḍā area first, and then developed into *uḍḍīyāna-bandha* in the *haṭha yoga*. *Uḍḍīyāna-bandha* means abdominal retraction lock, the drawing in of the abdomen and stomach towards the backbone after exhaling.[11]

Like the *uḍḍīyāna-bandha*, the *haṭha yoga* practice is also essential for the *yoga* of sexual transformation. The area in which this *yoga* was disovered and became popular, came to be known as Uḍḍīyāna *pīṭha* (site).

7. *Śākta Pramoda*, ed. Sri Venkatesvara Press, Bombay, 1951, p. 262.
8. *Kuṇḍalinī Tantra*, Bihar School of Yoga, Munger, 1992, p. 201.
9. Pranab Bandyopadhyay, *The Goddess of Tantra*, Punthi Pustak, Kolkata, 1987, p. 48.
10. Teun Goudriaan, "Tantrism in History," *Hindu Tantrism*, Handbuch Der Orientalistek, II, ABT, IV, Band. 2, ABSCH, No., Leiden/Koln, E.J. Brill, Belgium, 1979, p. 38.
11. *HYPBS*, Munger, 1993, p. 563.

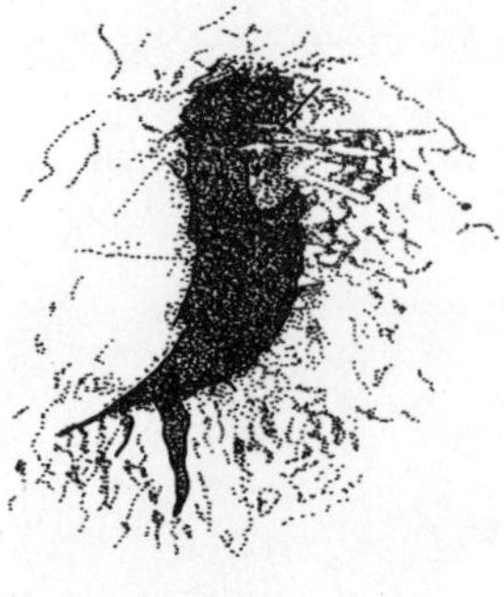

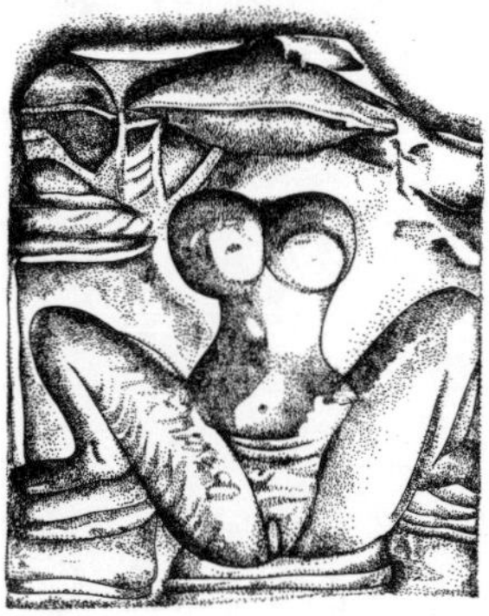

Shri Svāmījī Mahārāj of Datiā,[12] mentions that according to the Śākta scriptures the *mahābindu* is the origin of all creations. This *mahābindu* or the supreme point contains the two principals, Śiva and Śakti. On it are the red, white and mixed spots. The white spot or *bindu* symbolizes the Śiva and the red spot the Śakti principals. The spot of mixed colours symbolizes both. From the white spot springs the *nāda* or sound. This *nāda* produces multitude of words. The red spot is the matrix which gives meanings to words. This world of words and meanings is dissolved for the *yogī*. The *yogī* too loses his identity and merges into the *mahābindu* or the supreme point. Thus does the *yogī* realizes his *laya yoga*. The world of meanings comprises the entire material creation which dissolves and merges into the *yogī*. The *Īśāvāśya Upaniṣad* says,

> The *yogī* sees all creatures within his own self or *ātman*. . . .
> The *mahābindu* and the *mahāśūnya* or the great cypher are one.

Earliest model stone ploughs are found between Ghatmal and Citarama villages (*Pl.* 2) and also within the Gatibeda village area, on the left bank of the Jonk river on the Sunabeda plateau, in Nuāpāḍā district. These prove the agricultural practice of upland dwellers. Domestication of animals finds expression in the pre-historic rock-shelter art of Yogīmaṭh donger (hill), discovered by the author,[13] in Nuāpāḍā district on 21 December 1970. In Yogīmaṭh donger three lines are painted thrice. This proves that the conception of Trinity was well developed in those early days, in this region. The *yoni yantra* and many such female genitals have been painted in pre-historic rock art of Chhattisgarh and Orissa, which are well documented by

12. Śrī Svāmījī Mahārāja, *Siddhānta Rahasya* (Secrets of Spiritual Living), Śrī Pitambarapeeth Sanskrit Parishad, Datia (Madhya Pradesh), Chaitra Purnima, Samvat 2040, pp. 65-68.

13. (i) J.P. Singh Deo, "Pre-historic Cave Painting of Jogimath Donger," *OHRJ*, vol. XXII, no. 2, pp. 21-22.

    (ii) J.P. Singh Deo, *Cultural Profile of South Kośala*, Gyan Publishing House, New Delhi, 1987, p. 20.

Sadasiba Pradhan[14] and others. Sadasiba Pradhan has documented 55 rock-shelter paintings of Orissa. There might be more.

While dealing with the later development of *mantra* and other aspects of tāntric practice, Dirk Jan Heens[15] states that triangle (*trikoṇa*) consists of the *icchā*, *jñāna* and *kriyā-śaktis*. Even (*Śāradātilaka*, I, 78)[16] records that from the *saguṇa* Śiva rise *śakti*, *nāda* and *bindu*. This *bindu* is threefold: (a) *bindu* (Śiva), (b) *bīja* (Śakti), and (c) *nāda* (Śiva-Śakti).

From these tāntric spiritual developments, it can be safely asserted that the Trinity, Triangle and Uḍḍīyāna had originated in the upland Mahānadī valley and its early dwellers had attained great spiritual heights.

It seems that *kuṇḍalinī śakti* also was first experienced by the early upland dwellers because among the arts of pre-historic rock arts of Gurhāṇḍī in Kālāhāṇḍī district, line painting of Paśupati is found with a head, symbolized by a flower, which seems to mean the *sahasrāra cakra*,[17] (*Fig*. 1).

Another important finding is circular stone in two parts, 25 cm in diameter with a socket. It makes an overall shape of english numerical "8," thereby showing the union of male and female principals which developed *yoga* of sexual transformation. The author has collected such a stone set from the Mohangiri site (*Pls*. 16, 17). Baba Mishra and Pradeep Mohanty have also collected such a stone set from the Kharligarh site of Bolaṅgīr district (*Pls*. 18, 19). Both these sets are now preserved at Manikyapur Museum of Bhawanipatna.

14. Sadasiba Pradhan, *Rock Art in Orissa*, Aryan Books International, New Delhi, 2001, passim.
15. Dirk Janhoens, "Mantra and other constituents of Tāntric practice," *Hindu Tantrism, op. cit.*, Belgium, 1979, p. 98.
16. *Ibid*., 1979, p. 105.
17. Svāmī Satyānanda Sarasvatī, *Kuṇḍalinī Tantra*, Bihar School of Yoga, Munger, 1992, p. 200.

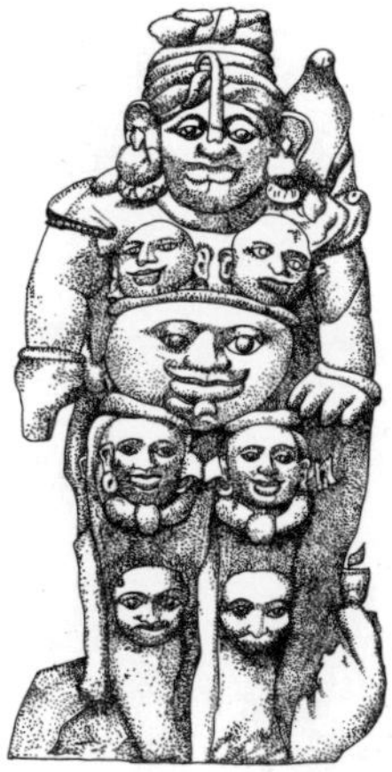

One half of such a stone socket has been found at the Pātālgaṅgā site, while there is information that such two stone sockets have been found within the ruins of the Śakti temple, on the left bank of the Udanti river, in Bargāon village of Nuāpāḍā district. Such an object has also been found from the layer III (early historic phase) at Veerapuram,[18] in Andhra Pradesh, where it is interpreted as a votive *liṅga*. But in fact, it is not a votive *liṅga*, rather a symbol of union of male and female principals, which developed the *haṭha yoga* practice of sexual transformation, as mentioned in the famous text, *Haṭha Yoga Pradīpikā*. Since the earliest spot of Uḍḍīyāna is found at the centre of the *yoni*, discovered from the Udanti river, it may be possible that the Uḍḍīyāna owes its name to the river "Udanti," a tributary of Tel, falling into the Mahānadī river on its right bank near Sonepur.

Later in the medieval period, it is known from the tradition embodied in the *Pāg-Sām-Jon-Zāñg*, that the tāntric Buddhism first developed in a place called Uḍḍīyāna, which is by far the most important among the four *pīṭha*s frequently mentioned both by Hindu and the Buddhist tantras.[19]

Scholars are not unanimous in identifying the Uḍḍīyāna-*pīṭha* (site), but the author claims that the entire Mahānadī river valley is Uḍḍīyāna-*pīṭha*, because, as mentioned earlier, the earliest finding of Uḍḍīyāna, has been discovered from the sand of Udanti river (*Pl.* 12). Further the earliest eight-handed Naṭarāja images with *ūrdhva-liṅga* (erected penis) belonging to the fifth and sixth centuries AD[20] have been found at Sirpur and Āsanapaṭ respectively, (*Pls.* 25, 26).

This study shows that a great spiritual tāntric-yogic concept developed in the Mahānadī valley which led to the evolution

18. T.V.G. Sastri, M.K. Bai & J.V.P. Rao, *Veerapuram*, Bhawani Printers, Hyderabad, 1984, passim.
19. N.K. Sahu, *Buddhism in Orissa*, Utkal University, Cuttack, 1958, p. 142.
20. *NIATAL*, 1994, pp. 159, 160, 164 and 165.

of the Jagannātha cult. A gigantic image of Tala with all the *haṭha* yogic features, found in Bilāspur district of Chhattisgarh province, has been identified as the composite tāntric-yogic figures of Mahākāla and Mahākālī by the author[21] (*Pl.* 27). This image has a *ūrdhva-liṅga* (penis erectus) and a tortoise like-head which symbolizes the *vajrolī mudrā*, i.e., the "thunderbolt attribute" in which muscles of the male sexual organ and the lower urinary tract contract to redirect sexual energy upwards. This is *haṭha yoga* and *tantra* practice.

The above discussed concept and practice of *tantra* had its origin in the Mahānadī valley and had attained refinement. It has greatly contributed the cultural and spiritual developments of the entire mankind.

II

Primal (Ādi) Yoni or Bhairavī Pīṭha (site) is located in Nuapada district

Nuāpāḍā District is situated on the extreme western border in the hinterland of Orissa. On the western border of this district, is the Sunabeda plateau, which runs north to south full of archaeological remains. The rest of the area is plain and hilly with the Chaura group of mountains. The rivers Jonk, Sundar and Udanti, and Tel, which are the tributaries of Mahānadī river flow on its right.

As mentioned before, Pātālgaṅgā in Nuāpāḍā district is the earliest Śakti *pīṭha* in Mahānadī valley or one of the earliest sites in the world (*Pl.* 9). As *tantra* gives prominence to the female energy of Śakti, the Śākta cult regards mother as the Supreme Being. Eight *yoni*s are discovered in Nuāpāḍā district so far. All these eight *yonis*, are the manifestation of Śakti in its Bhairavī form.

21. (i) J.P. Singh Deo, *Origin of Jagannāth Deity*, Gyan Publishing House, New Delhi, 1991, passim.
(ii) *ROII*, Delhi, 2000, pp. 127-34.

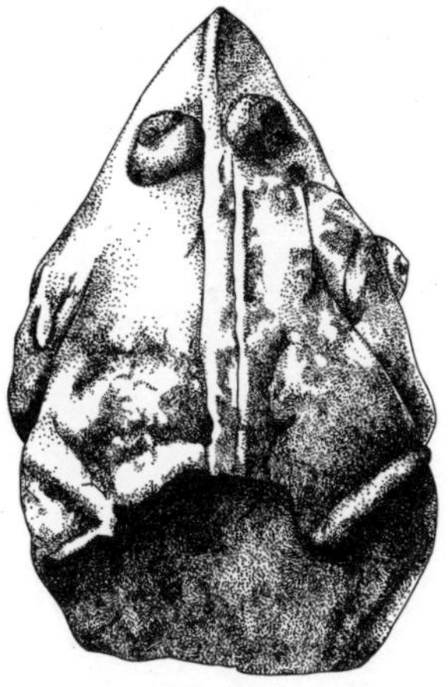

According to Don Mario Mazzoleni,[22] one of the objectives is to reveal the links which join mathematics to astronomy, astronomy to physics, physics to theology and so on.

> Another objective is to bring the scientific notion to the level and experience of the person learning it, and not vice versa. When teaching addition, you can reflect on the digit 1, which when added to itself grows to infinity, and this you can compare with the operation of God, who in his unity manifests Himself as many. The multiples of 9 always add up to 9. For example 27 or 72 always come to 9. From this observation, one can reflect on how the divine is unchanging, even though it loves to express itself through various forms. On the other hand the multiples of 8 are found to diminish; $8 \times 1 = 8$; $8 \times 2 = 16 = 7$; $8 \times 3 = 24 = 6$, etc. From this it can be deduced that 8 represents desire, which the more you multiply it, the less you get in the final value.

Eight is an important number, for God has 8 attributes. According to Svāmī Śivānanda[23] these are: *sarvajñatva* (omniscience, knowledge of the entire universe, their *jīva*s and their *karma*s), *sarveśvaratva* (supreme rulership of all, the power of dispensing fruits to all *jīvas*), *sarvāntaryamitva* (inner control of all names and forms and all *indriya*s and minds), *sarvakaraṇatva* (causality for the creation, preservation and destruction of all), *sarvaniyantritva* (doing everything without failure of *niyama*), *sarvakartṛtva* (the doing of all actions), *sarvaśaktimatva* (omnipotence), and *svatantratva* (absolute independence).

According to Jagadguru Svāmī Śrī Kṛpālujī Maharāja,[24]

---

22. Don Marie Mazzoleni, *A Catholic Priest Meets Sai Baba*, Sri Sathya Sai Book & Publications Trust, Prashanthi Nilayam, Andhra Pradesh, 1995, p. 205.
23. Svāmī Śivānanda, *Mind: Its Mysteries and Control*, The Divine Life Society, Shivanandanagar, 1974, p. 22.
24. Jagadguru Svāmī Śrī Kṛpālujī Mahārāja, *Philosophy of Divine Love (Prema-Rasasiddhānta)*, Sadhna Bhawan Trust, Mangarh, U.P., 2nd edn., 1996, p. 132.

> Becoming as motionless as a tree, sweating, horripilation, trembling, paleness, choked voice, tears and unconscious trance are the eight symptoms of divine ecstasy (*bhakti-rasāmṛta-sindhu*). Perceiving these eight symptoms of ecstasy, we can imagine the unfathomable Love that a saint possesses.

Śrī Svāmījī Mahārāja[25] of Datiā also states:

> The Lord's *prakṛti* or nature has eight chief aspects. The monosyllabic OM as the transcendental Brāhmaṇa has eight aspects very much like the Lord's. The *Mantrayoga Saṁhitā*, has defined them as Guruvij, Śaktivij, the Rāmavij, the Tejovij, the Kāmvij, the Yogavij, the Saktivij and Rakshavij. The eight monosyllabic symbols describing the eight chief *prakritis* or natures of the transcendental OM are *Aim, Hrim, Srim, Klim Krim, Trim, Strim* and *Hlim*.

The number 8 plays an important role in Hindu temple architecture also. Michael W. Meister[26] states that the square grid of the *vāstumaṇḍala* reflects the Vedic cosmology, which see the world as a square and in its construction could be related to the actual piling of bricks for the altar. Further, while studying the plan of temple architecture M.W. Meister[27] states:

> Underlying the plan for most temples in Central India in the seventh century is a *vāstupuruṣamaṇḍala* of 64 squares (8 × 8 = 64 squares), a ritual diagram prescribed for temples in the sixth century *Brihat Samhita,* as in later texts, but for which the origin goes back millennia to the construction of Vedic altars. This grid of eight by eight squares determined proportions and placement of parts for the square Nagara temple from the seventh to perhaps the eleventh century.

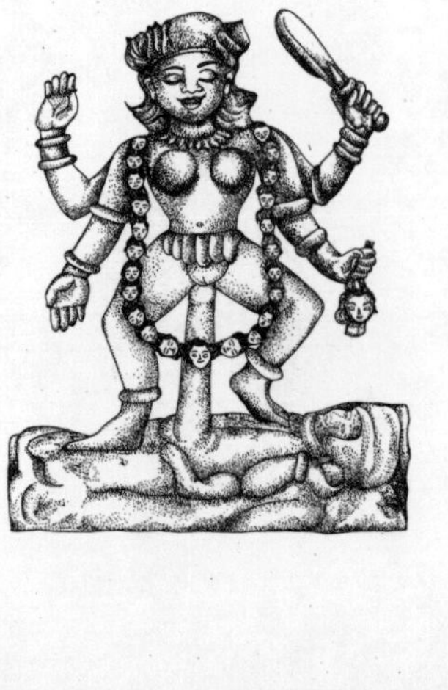

25. Śri Svāmījī Mahārāja, *Siddhānta Rahasya* (*Secrets of Spiritual Living*) Shri Pitambarapeeth Sanskrit Parishad, Datia, (M.P.), Chaitra Purnima, Samvat 2040, p. 42.
26. M.W. Meister, "Muṇḍeśvarī: Ambiguity and Certainty in the analysis of a Temple plan," *Kalādarśana* (*American Studies in the Art of India*), ed. J.G. Willams Oxford & I.B.H. Publishing Co., New Delhi, 1981, p. 83.
27. *Ibid.*, 1981, p. 79.

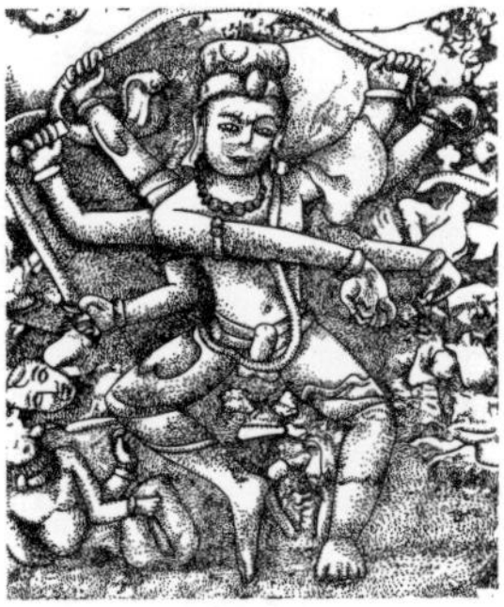

The origin of ten Wisdom Goddesses or *daśamahāvidyā* is from the *Śiva Purāṇa* (V.50).[28] They are Kālī, Tārā, Tripurasundarī, Bhuvaneśvarī, Bhairavī, Chinnamastā, Dhūmāvatī, Bagalāmukhī, Mātaṅgī and Kamalātmikā.

The *yantra* of the fifth Goddess Bhairavī of *daśamahāvidyā* is a triangle *yoni*. A triangle pointed downwards is the *yantra* of *yoni*. So, all the eight *yonis* discovered in Nuāpāḍā district symbolize the *yoni yantra*[29] and therefore are eight Bhairavīs.

According to David Frawley,[30]

> Bhairavī specifically means "terrifying" and is the powerful, awesome, or energetic form of the Goddess. She represents transforming heat or radiance Tejas, which is the primal power or divine energy. This we experience as a frightening thing because it burns away and destroys all the limitations and illusions of egocentric existence. . . . Bhairavī is the woman as warrior, who with her power of divine speech and spiritual fire eliminates all obstacles to the unfoldment of true awareness.

Pushpendra Kumar[31] describes Bhairavī or Tripura-Bhairavī thus:

> The fifth *mahāvidyā* Bhairavī is reddish like the morning sun. She is dressed in a silken cloth and wears a garland of heads on her neck. Her breast is anointed with *sindūra*. In her four hands she holds a rosary of beads, a book and the poses of granting boons and assurances. She has a crescent on her forehead. Her three eyes are as beautiful as the red lotuses, and there is a bejewelled crown over her head. A mild smile plays on her lips. As a Goddess she is Tripura-Bhairavī while as a *mahāvidyā* she is designated as Bhairavī only. This is a

28. *TYATWG*, 1996, p. 62.
29. *TYATWG*, p. 103, *bhairavī yantra*.
30. *TYATWG*, 1996, pp. 104-09.
31. Pushpendra Kumar, *Śakti Cult in Ancient India*, Bharatiya Publishing House, Vārāṇasī, 1974, p. 157.

benign manifestation of Śakti and is considered as the giver of knowledge.

According to tāntric literature *Śākta Pramoda*,[32]

> Bhairavī is the giver of knowledge. As the primal *yoni* or the Bhairavī site is found in Nuāpāḍā district of Orissa province. It can be claimed that *adi yoni* or the Bhairavī *Pīṭha* (site) is located in Nuāpāḍā district and knowledge was flashed or sparked from this area, which developed into imitative, repetitive, derigative, educative and intuitive knowledges (*Pl.* 12).

Because of this reason, the earliest archaeological remain of *kuṇḍalinī tantra*'s[33] *sahasrāra cakra*, is found in the rock art of Gurhāṇḍī in Kālāhāṇḍī district (*Fig.* 3).

According to Svāmī Satyānanda Sarasvatī,[34]

> *Sahasrāra* is not a *cakra* as is often thought. *Cakra*s are within the realm of the psyche. Consciousness manifests at different levels according to the *cakra* that is predominantly active. *Sahasrāra* acts through nothing and yet again, it acts through everything. *Sahasrāra* is beyond the beyond (*paratparam*) and yet it is right here. *Sahasrāra* is the culmination of the progressive ascension through the different *cakra*s. It is the crown of expanded awareness. The power of the *cakra*s does not reside in the *cakra*s themselves, but in *sahasrāra*.
>
> The literal meaning of the word *sahasrāra* is 'one thousand.' For this reason it is said to be a lotus with one thousand petals. However, while literally meaning one thousand, the word *sahasrāra* implies that in magnitude and significance it is vast — in fact, unlimited. Therefore, *sahasrāra* should more aptly be described as a lotus with an infinite number of petals, usually said to be red or multicoloured.

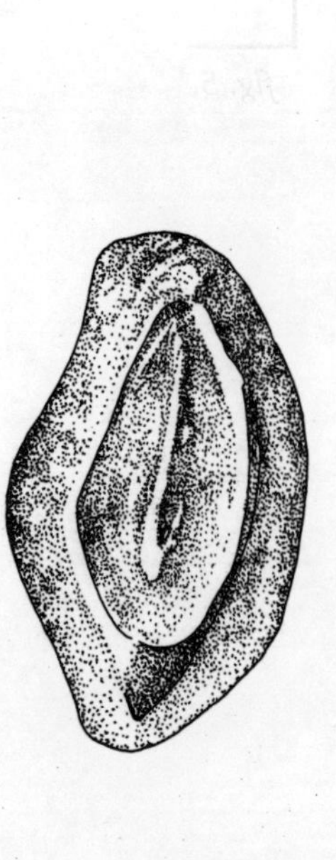

32. *Śākta Pramoda*, ed. Sri Venkatesvara Press, Bombay, 1951, p. 262.
33. *Śākta Pramoda*, Bombay, 1951, p. 262.
34. *Kuṇḍalinī Tantra*, Bihar School of Yoga, Munger, 1992, p. 201.

The pre-historic art of Yogīmaṭh donger (*Fig.* 2) shows the *yoga* concept of Creation and the Trinity conception of the early men. This is the potentiality and gift of the Nuāpāḍā district to the entire humanity. So, it can be claimed that Nuāpāḍā is the epicentre of Mahānadī river valley, from where spirituality and culture were flashed, focused and spread (*Fig.* 5).

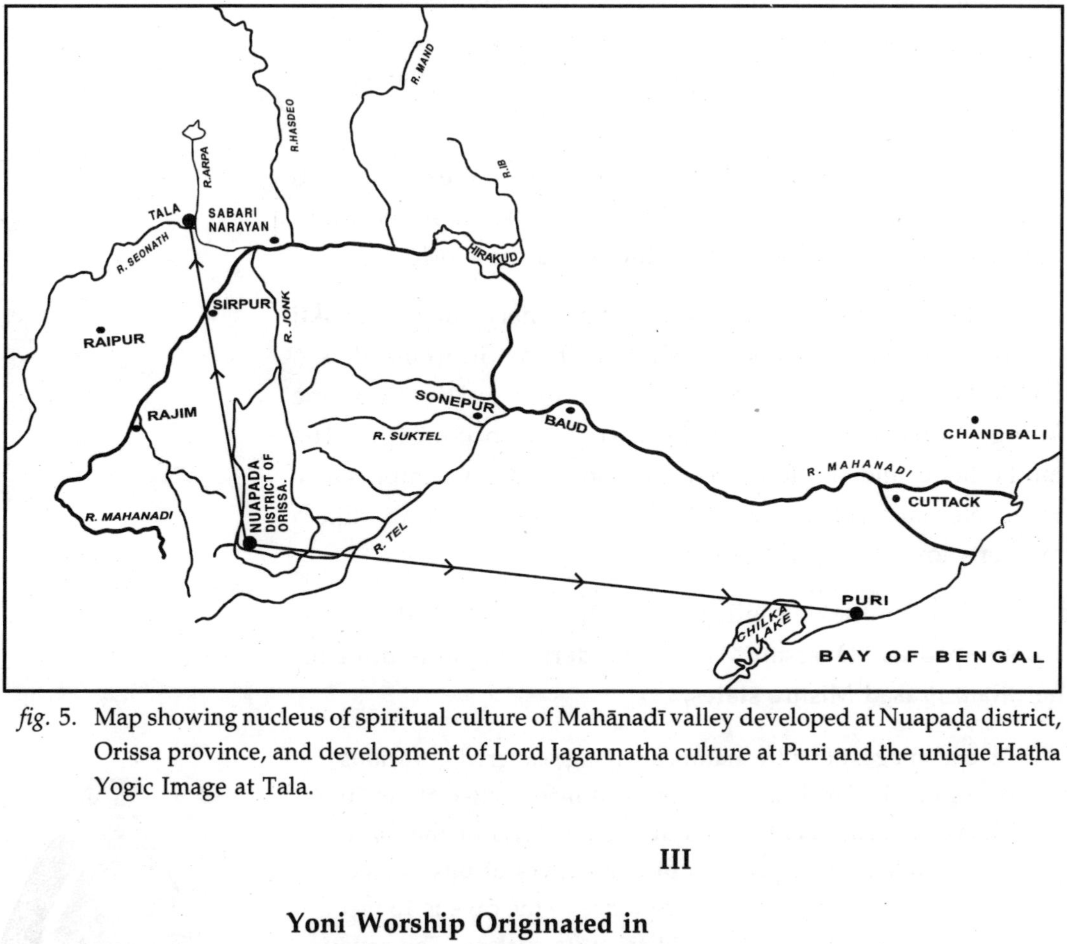

fig. 5. Map showing nucleus of spiritual culture of Mahānadī valley developed at Nuapaḍa district, Orissa province, and development of Lord Jagannatha culture at Puri and the unique Haṭha Yogic Image at Tala.

III

Yoni Worship Originated in Middle Right Mahānadī Valley

Early men of the middle Mahānadī river valley had developed a yogic vision which finds expression in the rock art, so widely found.

To know about the earliest *yoni* Śakti concept, attention

should be drawn to the period of geological formation. It is a fact that the course of human history in a region is in a considerable measure, shaped by its physical and geographical features, which are ultimately determined by the geological history it has passed through, in the dim vista of time.[35]

> *Yoni* is the female power in nature. The Supreme Being, wishing to begin creation, divided himself into two parts, Brahmā and Nature. From Brahmā originated all males while from Nature all females. The female is regarded as the real force in nature and most deserving of worship.

The *yoni* at Pātālgaṅgā (*Pl.* 9) is regarded as the earliest Śakti *pīṭha* of the Mahānadī river valley. There are many earthern vulvas or *yoni* sites elsewhere in India and the world.

Tantra gives prominence to the female energy or Śakti. Śakti (Kālī) of the Śakti cult is the Mother or the Supreme Being. Similarly, Śiva of the Śiva cult is the father or the Supreme Being. *Tantra*s attempt to blend these two concepts, the motherhood and the fatherhood of God and give importance to the eternal mother, for God's love for the creation is like a mother's love, deep and pure.

Yoni at Sindhekela village (*Pl.* 10) in Bolaṅgīr district is worshipped as "Dvārsanī," and a modern temple is built for her. Ram Prasad Mishra states,[36]

> Several images of tāntric nature are lying scattered in various places of Ghodar, Udaipur, Sihni and many other places in Titilagarh. A hillock located at the outskirts of the Sihni village called Ghusni Dungri by the natives of this village, contains a cave in its lap. The entrance to the cave is 13 feet in breadth and 8 feet in height from its surface. The cave seems to have been narrowed towards its inner side. The

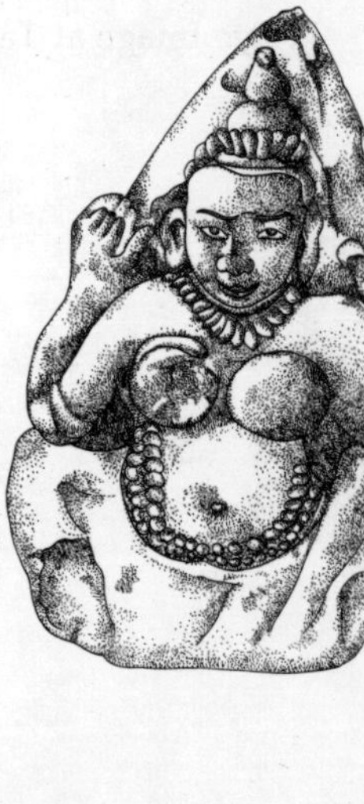

35. D.N. Wadia, "The Geological background of Indian History," *THACOTIP*, vol. I, *The Vedic Age*, 1965, p. 80.

36. R.P. Mishra, *Fragments of Indian Culture*, Punthi Pustak, Kolkata, 1995, p. 197.

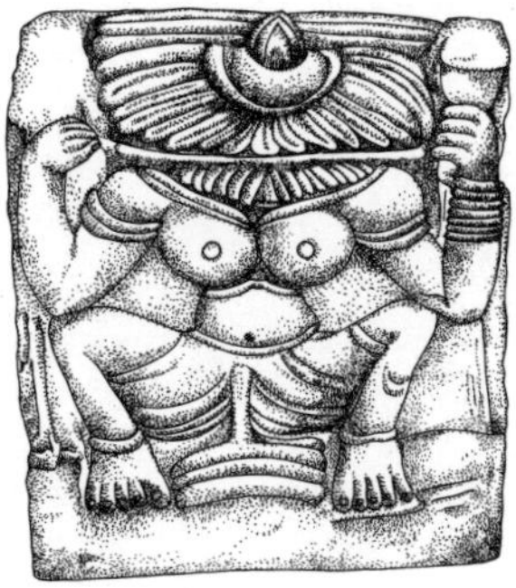

author during his travel to this place in 1983 had seen a broken image of Gaṇeśa measuring 1.6 feet in breadth and 1.4 feet in height and a carved figure of a *yoni* or female genitive organ, on a piece of stone measuring 1.3 feet in breadth and 3 inches in thickness and 1.6 feet in length. It is quite unfortunate for the culture of this region that the image of the Gaṇeśa and the carved figure of *yoni* have been missing from this place, what the author has observed during his visit to this place in 1987.

In this manner, most of the *yoni* traces are gradually getting lost, because of vagaries of nature and human vandalism. Sadāsiba Pradhān[37] reports of the findings of female genitals, or *yoni*s, in the form of rock art in Orissa. Host of triangles with or without a depression in the centre and resembling the female genitals are found in Vikramkhol,[38] Ulapgarh-Uṣākoṭi[39] and in Landimal (Uṣākoṭi-I), where they are profusely depicted in all the shelters, in all conceivable shapes and designs.[40] The representation of an anthropomorphic form, with a large vulva suspending at the bottom of the Rail Uṣākoṭi-XII engravings, deserves special mention, as it is depicted along with a male genital organ? It may be identified as the venus of the Uṣākoṭi group.[41] At Chormoda an apsidal/triangular pattern, composed of 17 cupules with a big cup-mark in the centre is an interesting specimen.[42] Engravings of seven triangles and other eroded specimens beyond recognition are found at Jhinkmoda.[43] Triangle engravings are found[44] at Jodabilmoda. At Imlimoda-

37. S. Pradhan, *Rock Art in Orissa*, Aryan Books International, New Delhi, 2001, passim.
38. *Ibid.*, pp. 28-29.
39. *Ibid.*, pp. 29-30.
40. *Ibid.*, p. 34.
41. *Ibid.*, p. 35.
42. *Ibid.*, p. 37.
43. *Ibid.*, passim. p. 39.
44. *Ibid.*

I at least 89 engravings are the usual female genital patterns in oval, apsidal and triangular shapes with or without a central line and a shallow depression at the lower edge or in the centre.[45] Imlimoda-II also has such triangles in all cenceivable forms. Traces of ocrhe are noticed in the grooves.[46] The female genitals predominate the triangular and serpentine engraving at Tongo[47] with honeycomb and traces of ochre as the marked decorative motifs. Though there is no discernible painting at Tongo, in one case a scooped out female genital pattern has been exquisitely painted in red and white.[48] Lekhamoda-III[49] and Rajbahal Uṣākoṭi are also replete with such triangular forms.[50]

Finally, Sadāsiba Pradhān[51] mentions that triangles resembling the female genitals are the main subject-matter of petroglyphs of Orissa.

The question arises why so many female genital depictions in the early geological formation, stone carvings and paintings are found in the central part of the Mahānadī river valley? As mentioned earlier, Bhairavī is the giver of knowledge and the *yoni* a *yantra* of Goddess Bhairavī in the tāntric literature, hence it can be construed that *yoga* was conceived and developed in the central Mahānadī river valley. The iconographical masterpieces representing the *haṭha* yogic features with sensual expressions are found in this area. Stones do not speak, only yogic masters show and interpret their expressions to the common man.

45. S. Pradhan, *Rock Art in Orissa*, Aryan Books International, New Delhi, 2001, passim. p. 40.
46. *Ibid.*
47. *Ibid.*
48. *Ibid.*, p. 42.
49. *Ibid.*, p. 44.
50. *Ibid.*
51. *Ibid.*, p. 46.

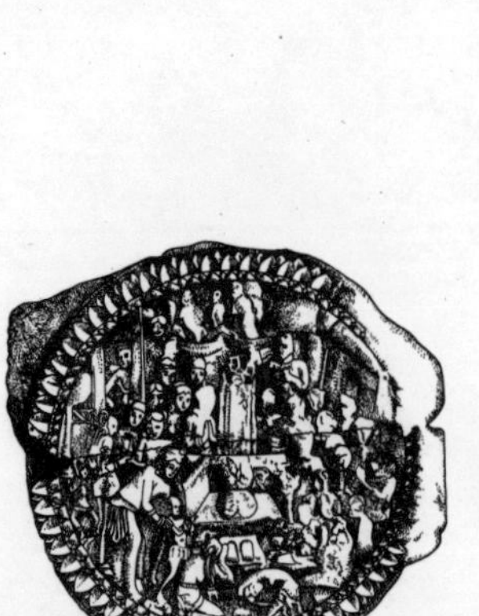

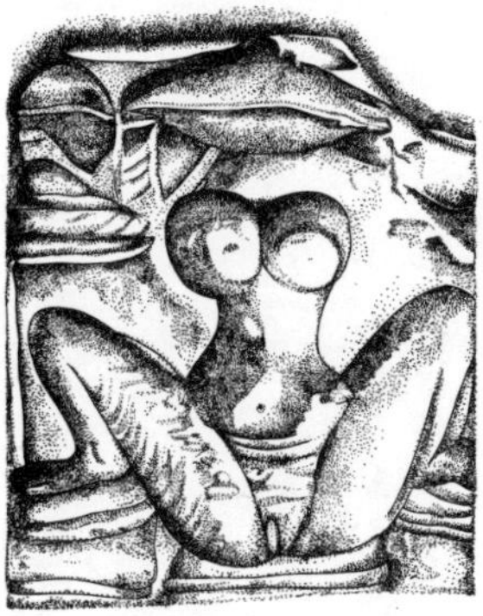

IV

Yoga of Sexual Transformation was Discovered in Mahānadī Valley

About purifying sexual energy, David Frawley[52] states,

> Our sexual energies in their ordinary expressions are not helpful for the practice of *yoga*, because they are directed outward and can be mixed with impurities or toxins of various sorts. First, our sexual energies must be purified and made subtle. According to the āyurveda seven tissues make up the body and are produced from the food that is digested and assimilated:
>
> 1. plasma, 2. blood, 3. muscle, 4. fat, 5. bone, 6. marrow and nerve tissue, 7. reproductive tissue.
>
> Each of these tissues is a transformation of the previous one, like milk becoming butter. Each become less in substance but greater in potency. For example, plasma is greater in quantity than the reproductive fluid, but the reproductive fluid contains much more concentrated energy.
>
> The reproductive fluid is the most potent ingredient in the body and the ultimate product of the digestive process. Though smaller in quantity than other bodily tissues, it has the greatest energy, it can produce new life and thus it also has the capacity to renew the life within the body itself. The energy of reproductive tissue is indispensable for achieving any internal transformation.
>
> While ordinarily we direct the sexual energy outward for procreative or pleasure purposes. *Yoga* practice directs this energy inward for revitalization and the development of higher consciousness. For this inner process to take place, the sexual energies must shift their location from their ordinary sites. It is not the outgoing sexual energies that are

52. *TYATWG*, Delhi, 1996, pp. 185-86.

united but their subtle counterparts. If sufficient amount of the reproductive fluid has not first been raised to the head and the energy of awareness has not been brought down to the base of the spine, we are not ready for the advanced practices of *yoga*.

The reproductive fluid must be distilled and in this process it rises to the brain and becomes *soma*. This requires the surrender of our desire for outer enjoyment, offering it into the fire of aspiration to discover the divine within. Our *soma* or desire for fulfilment must be redirected from its fixation on the outer world and the lower body centres to the Third Eye. Conversely *Agni*, the fire or power of perception and attention, must be directed from the head to the base of the spine, from its fixation on the outer world through the senses to its connection with the inner source of vitality. This requires calming the restless mind, withdrawing from sensory stimuli which keep our inquiring energy in the head, and discovering the deeper perception hidden at the root of the unconscious.

Many yogic practices are helpful in purifying sexual energy. Particularly when combined with the cultivation of devotion, *Āsana* (yogic postures) and *Prāṇāyāma* (breathing exercises) can be used to help redirect the reproductive fluid upward. *Mantra* and meditation and also music and chanting, help direct the mental fire inward and downward.

According to T.N. Mishra,[53]

Archaeological materials from the Indus valley civilization also point to the existence of a fertility cult in India from the proto-historic period. The discovery of numerous phalic stones and ring-stones, the figure of a male ithyphallic horned God (probably the prototype of Śiva) and the figure of a Mother Goddess are ample evidences to indicate the prevalence of the said cults. However, no representation of

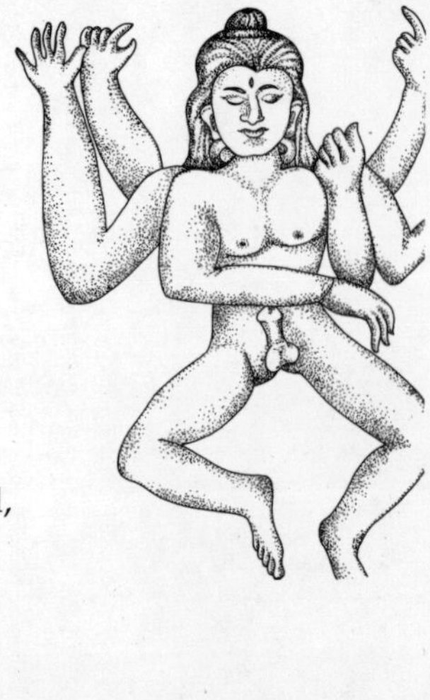

53. T.N. Mishra, *Impact of Tantra on Religion and Art*, D.K. Printworld, (P) Ltd., New Delhi, 1997, pp. 101-02.

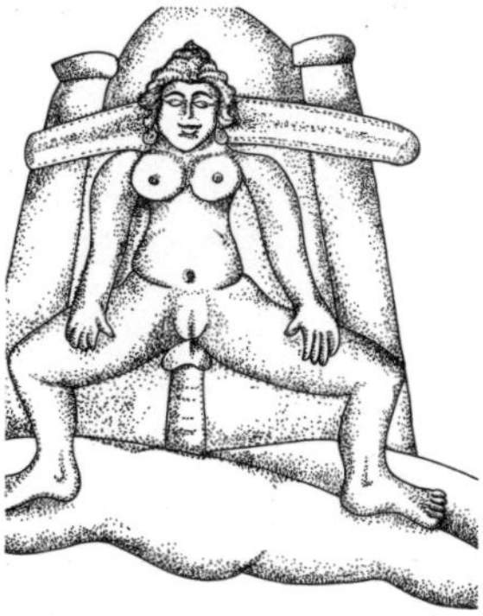

the sexual act has been reported in the art and ritual objects yielded by the Indus civilization. The earliest depiction of the sexual act among the objects excavated so far in india, is found on a pit of the chalcolithic period at Daimabad. Another early representation of sex has been noticed in the Kupgallu Cave in Mysore. Significant material for the possible connection of the depiction of erotic couples with fertility cult is available in the historical period. The secular subjects drawn from everyday life were introduced in the terracotta art and the stone monuments also. The religious theme gradually received an artistic treatment, with the result that it turned into an art motif. The process of secularization and sensualization of ritual or cultic objects is clearly noticeable in the ivory figure of Śrī found at Ter that has been assigned to the second century AD. Śrī was a Goddess of abundance, fertility, blissful prosperity, luck and beauty. Her fertility aspects are revealed in Śrī Sūkta, a Khil of the *Ṛgveda*.

These prove that the *yoga* of sexual transformation was discovered and was well known in peninsular India, even before the penetration of the Āryan culture.

Yogī Matsyendranāth who was born during the medieval period was a great exponent of *haṭha yoga*. According to Ram Prasad Mishra,[54]

> Younger Luipa or Matsyendranāth was the Nātha Siddha and was born in Cāndradvīpa, i.e., Chāndavāli — the Dhamra region of Baleswar (now Bhadark district area) in Orissa.

It was *yogī* Matsyendranāth who systemized the *yoga* of sexual tranformation by establishing "Nāthism," and the 64 *yoginī* cult.

According to the *Haṭha Yoga Pradīpikā*,[55] a *yoginī* is a lady who practices *vajrolī*, i.e., the *yoga* of sexual transformation. In

54. R.P. Mishra, *Sahajayāna — A Study of Tāntric Buddhism*, Punthi Pustak, Kolkata, 1991, p. 165.
55. *HYPBS*, Munger, 1993, p. 362.

Chapter 3, verse 99, it is mentioned, "If a woman practises *vajrolī* and saves her *rajas* and the man's *bindu* by thorough contraction, she is a *yoginī*." For this *yoga*, the *haṭha* yogic practices of *vajrolī-mudrā*, *sahajolī-mudrā* and *uḍḍīyāna-bandha* are required.

1. *Vajrolī-mudrā* — Thunderbolt attitude in which the muscles of the male sexual organ and lower urinary tract are contracted redirecting sexual energy upwards. A practice of *haṭa yoga* and *tantra*.
2. *Sahajolī-mudrā* — Practice of *vajrolī* by a woman, involving contraction of lower urinary muscles.
3. *Uḍḍiyāna-bandha* — Abdominal retraction lock; drawing in of the abdomen and stomach towards the backbone after exhaling.

With these three *haṭha* yogic practices the *yoga* of sexual transformation can be done. Śrī Svāmījī Mahārāj of Datiā[56] informs that in the practice of *haṭha yoga*, some of the gestures, postures and breathing exercises like the *bhastra-kumbhaka* (a breathing exercise in which one breathes like the iron-mongers bellows), *bhujaṅgāsana* (the serpent posture), *viparīta-karaṇa-mudrā* (reverse posture and gesture), *mahāmudrā* (the giant posture), etc., are very useful in *kuṇḍalinī* practice.

The *yoga* of sexual transformation helped in developing the "Kośali Style of Temple Architecture," based on the plan of two intersecting squares, meeting at 45° and thereby making a real view of eight-pointed star. It is considered to be *kāmakalā yantra*,

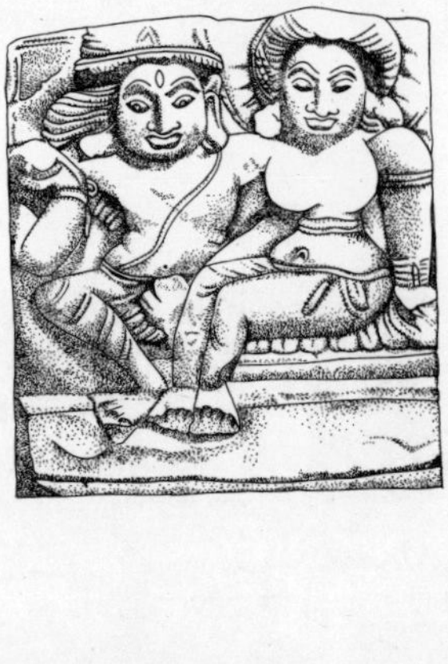

56. Śrī Svāmījī Mahārāja, *Siddhānta Rahasya* (*Secrets of Spiritual Living*), Shri Pitambarapeeth Sanskrit Parisad, Datia, M.P., Samvat 2040, pp. 50-51.

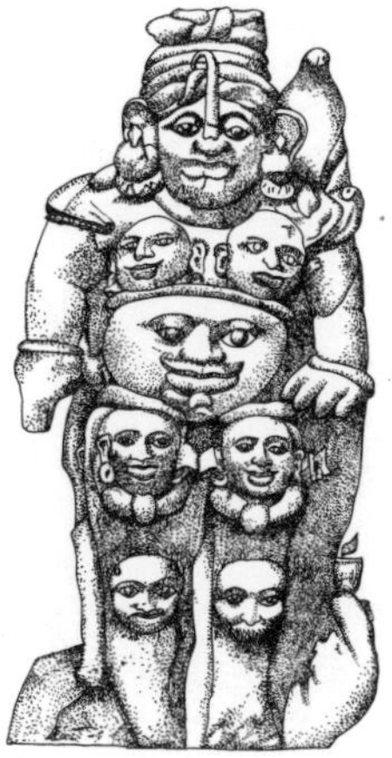

i.e., the desire fulfilling *yantra* (*Fig.* 6). The *yantra* plan of the Kośali *rekhā* temple influenced the development of the three tāntric temples standing in a triangular form or position at Bauḍ, which is the Bhairavī *yantra* itself. These three temples of Bauḍ, influenced the development of *pañcaratha* temples of coastal Orissa. This proves that the coastal temples of Orissa are based on the *kāmakalā yantra* and all the sculptural arts have a tāntric influence. Inside (*garbhagṛha*) of all such temples is a square. On the square an intersecting square has to be imagined which becomes the *kāmakalā yantra*. So, all Hindu temples are based on the *kāmakalā yantra*.

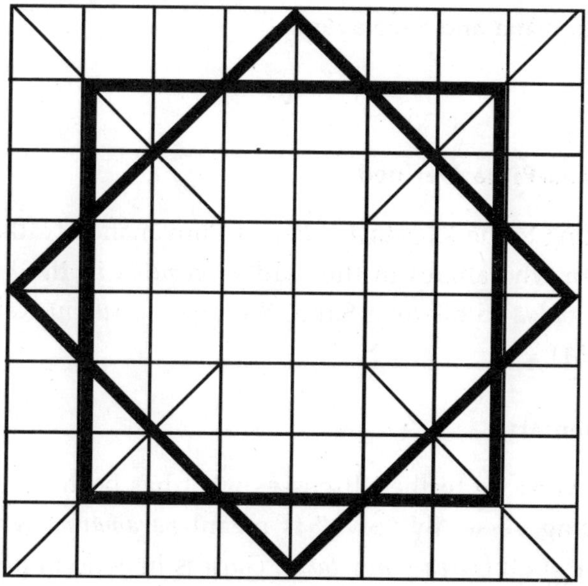

fig. 6. Plan of two squares, placed diagonally and intersecting each other at angles of 45 degrees. It is the *Kāmakalā yantra*, according to *Ānanda Laharī* and *Saundarya Laharī*, of Ādi Śaṅkarācārya.

Recently it has been discovered that the inner ground plan of the Rājarānī temple at Bhubaneswar is superimposed with *śrīyantra* or *śrīcakra*. *Śrī-yantra*[57] is a diagrammatic embodiment

57. Pronab Bandyopadhyay — *The Goddess of Tantra*, Punthi Pusktak, Kolkata, 1987, p. 48.

of the creative sexual activity of the universe. From this viewpoint the author[58] held that Orissa is the land of *kāmakalā*, i.e., erotic spiritual science, where the tāntric *yoga* of sexual transformation was re-discovered and is not "Kāmadeva's Pleasure Garden" as deemed by Thomas E. Donaldson.[59]

In the early medieval period the *yoga* of sexual transformation was popularized much and it was a period of religious eclecticism. Buddhism developed tāntric Buddhism and King Indrabhūti of Sambalaka in the Uḍḍīyāna-*pīṭha*, i.e., Mahānadī river valley, during the eighth century AD, became the first propounder of Vajrayāna, which later developed into Kālacakrayāna and Sahajayāna.

V

Uḍḍīyāna-Pīṭha Defined

According to the *Kāmakalā-Vilāsa* of Puṇyānanda Nātha,[60] Śiva, the *guru* who abides in the Uḍḍīyāna-*pīṭha* in the *kṛta-yuga*, impart *vidyā* to his own Śakti, the *vimarśa-rūpiṇī* Kāmeśvarī. (verse 51).

Commentary

In this verse he further discusses what has been stated in the preceding verse. By "Śiva" is meant *paramātmā* who is the Creator of all (*sarva-pravartaka*). *Guru* is he who imparts *jñāna* (*jñānopadeṣta*). So it has been said that "the *guru* is the means (of success)" (*gurur upāyaḥ*); (*Kulārṇava-Tantra*, XVII.7).

The word *gu* signifies darkness and the word *ru* signifies

58. J.P. Singh Deo, *Tāntric Art of Orissa*, Kalpaz Publications, Delhi, 2001, p. 209.
59. T.E. Donaldson, *Kāmadeva's Pleasure Garden: Orissa*, B.R. Publishing Corporation, Delhi, 1987, passim.
60. Sir John Woodroffe (Translated with Commentary), *Kāma-Kalā-Vilāsa*, Ganesh & Co. Pvt. Ltd., Madras, 1971, pp. 234-35.

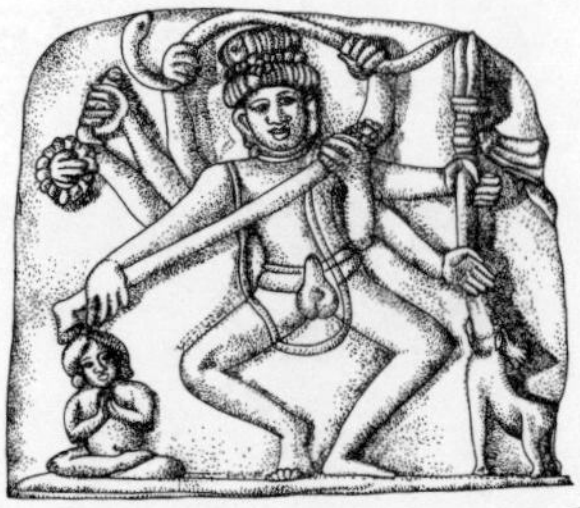

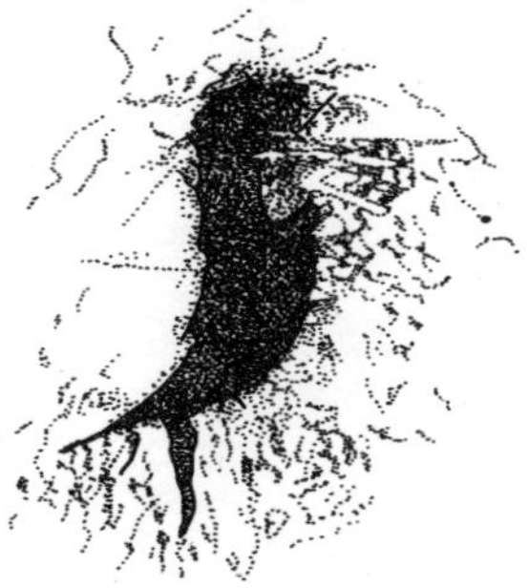

that which dispels it. *Guru* is thus so-called because he dispels darkness.

Who abides in the Uḍḍīyāna-*pīṭha* (*āsinaḥ śrīpīṭha*), by this is meant that the abode of Śiva is the Uḍḍīyāna-*pīṭha* in the inner most triangle.

By the *kṛta-yuga* (*kṛta-yuga-kāle*) we are to understand that it was in the beginning of *kṛta* or *satya* age that Śiva imparted the *vidyā* or knowledge which is fully established in all the Upaniṣads and by which a man can realize his oneness with the *ātmā* (*ātmaikya-pradāyinī*).

Did impart (*dadau*). Fully instructed (*upadideśa*). Her, his own Śakti (*tasyai svaśaktyai*). The emphasis on Her is to draw the reader's attention to the fact that it is She who gives boundless happiness to all creatures (*sarva-bhūtānāṁ niravadhi kūnarda-dāyinī*). His own Śakti (*svaśakti*). By this we are to understand that it is She who enables the Lord to manifest His own being (*svasvarūpa-sattā saṁpradātrī*). So it has been said:

> Even the supreme if disunited from Śakti is unable to do anything. O Parameśvarī! He is capable (of action) if He is united with Śakti.
>
> *Vimarśa-rūpiṇī*. She is so-called because she is the supreme Śakti which is (literally is the resting place of) the supreme manifesting bliss, (*anuttarānanda-viśrānti-sthāna-bhūta-śākti-para-rūpiṇī*). So it has been said, (*saṁketa-paddhati*). "The letter *a* is the first of all and is *prakāśa* and the supreme Śiva and the letter *ha* is the last which is *kalā* and is called *vimarśa*."
>
> *Kāmeśvarī*. She is so called because she at all times and in every way grants all objects of desire (*sarvābhiṣṭa-pradāyinī*) and is one with one's own *ātmā* (*svātma-bhūtā*).

Teun Gourdriaan[61] states that in the Śrīvidyā theory, Uḍḍīyāna

61. Teun Goudriaan, "Tantrism in History," *Hindu Tantrism*, Handbuch Der Orientalistik-II. Ast., IV, Band, 2 ABSCHN, Leiden/Koln, E.J. Brill, Belgium, 1979, p. 38 and p. 64.

is located within the central triangle of the *śrī cakra* (*Kāmakalā-Vilāsa*, 51); an indication of the ever increasing tendency towards interiorization and symbolization of outside realities.

While giving description of the shape of the *śrī-yantra*, Grace E. Cairns[62] states,

> The central feature of the *śrī cakra* is the series of symbolic interlocking triangles in the centre. These are surrounded by two circles of lotus petals bordered by three circular lines. Outside there is a square with four gateways. One at each of the cardinal points. The interlocking triangles are composed of five inverted triangles, the Śakti triangles, and four upright triangles, the Śiva triangles. The centre triangle formed by interlocking Śakti triangles, called the *kāmakalā* triangle, is the core of the diagram where the entire universe symbolized by the *śrī cakra* emanates. In its centre is the *mahābindu*, the *sarvānandamaya cakra* of this *yantra*. . . . *Sarvānandamaya*, the first and innermost *cakra*. This is the place of the *mahābindu*, seat of Mahāśakti herself where she is in blissful union with Śiva. The aspirant merges himself into the Divine Union, but must go beyond to the *nirguṇa Brahman* within the void that is beyond the *mahābindu*, to realize his identity with the two-in-one, the one that transcends the space-time world.

The centre triangle of *śrī-yantra* has in its centre the *mahābindu*, which is the *yantra* of Bhairavī, the fifth Goddess of *daśamahāvidyā*.[63]

It can be thus claimed that *mahābindu* is found at the centre of Bhairavī *yantra* and *śrī-yantra*, which is the Uḍḍīyāna-*pīṭha*, according to the tāntric-yogic view (*Pl.* 12).

With the development of tāntric *haṭha yoga*, the science of *yoga*, which purifies the physical body by means of *ṣaṭkarma*, *āsana*, *prāṇāyāma*, *mudrā*, *bandha*, concentration as a prelude to *rāja yoga* and *samādhi*, the *yoga* of sexual transformation evolved.

---

62. G.E. Cairns, *Man as Microcosm in Tāntric Hinduism*, Manohar, New Delhi, 1992, p. 58.
63. *TYATWG*, 1996, p. 103.

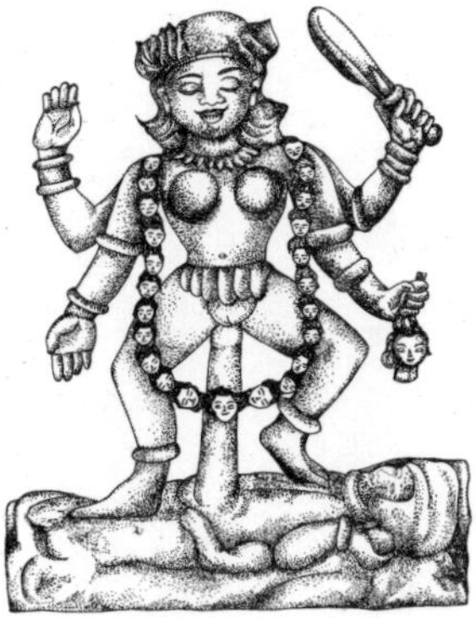

Interaction between man and woman, *tantra* wise, has three purposes — pleasure, procreation and *samādhi*.[64]

When sex energy is utilized for *samādhi*, self-realization, realization of God or from sex to super consciousness, *haṭha yoga kriyā* (a dynamic yogic practice) has to be performed which includes the *vajrolī-mudrā, sahajolī-mudrā, khecarī-mudrā* and *uḍḍīyāna-bandha.*

Of the above four *haṭha* yogic *mudrās* three has already been explained and the *khecarī-mudrā* require explanation. According to *Haṭha Yoga Pradīpikā:*[65]

The *khecarī-mudrā* is an attitude of dwelling in the supreme consciousness.

(a) *Khecarī-mudrā* is turning the tongue backwards into the cavity of the cranium and turning the eyes inwards towards the centre of the two eyebrows (*Haṭha Yoga Pradīpikā*, verses 32-36).

(b) The tongue should be exercised and milked and the underneath part cut away in small degrees. Indeed *khecarī* is perfected when the tongue touches the centre of the two eyebrows.

(c) With a clean thin blade, gently cut away the membrane under the tongue. Cut in by a fine hair's breadth each time.

(d) Then rub in a mixture of powdered rock salt and turmeric. After seven days again cut a hair's breadth.

(e) One should continue doing this regularly for six months, then the membrane at the root of the tongue will be completely severed.

For those who cannot practice *khecarī-mudrā*, it doesn't matter.

64. J.P. Singh Deo, *Tāntric Art of Orissa*, Kalpaz Publications, Delhi, 2001, p. 31.

65. *HYPBS*, Munger, 1993, pp. 564, 558, 278-79 and 563.

Vajrolī-mudrā or *sahajolī-mudrā* and *uḍḍīyāna-bandha* have to be perfected, so that the *yoga* of sexual tranformation can be easily done.

By constant practice of the *vajrolī-mudrā*, a male individual can suck one's penis inside the body, like tortoise withdraws its head, neck and legs inside its shell. The same *sahajolī-mudrā* can be done by a female, but female sexual organs are inside the body and they can't be seen. For those who practice the *vajrolī-mudrā* and *sahajolī-mudrā*, the final *uḍḍīyāna-bandha*, i.e., sucking of the sexual ejaculation and organism upwards, into *iḍā*, *piṅgalā* and *suṣmunā nāḍī*s before it is discharged (i.e., male semen and female ovum), are to be done.

The *ūrdhva-liṅga* (erected penis) of Lord Śiva (*Fig*. 7) symbolizes the upflow of semen to different *cakra*s of *kuṇḍalinī* for different *samādhis*. *Samādhi* means culmination of meditation, state of oneness of mind with the object of concentration, supernatural consciousness, by the eight stages of *aṣṭāṅga yoga*.

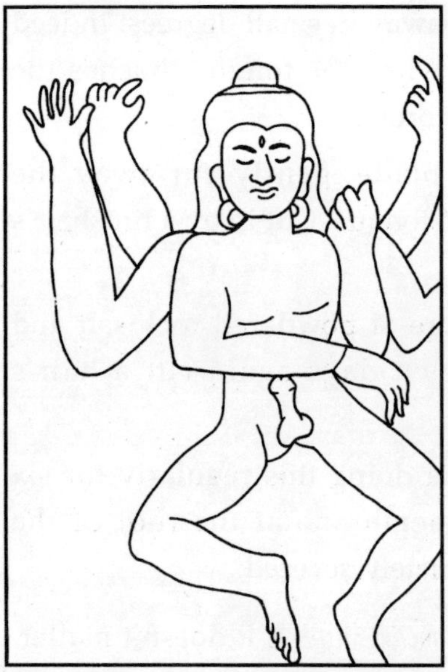

fig. 7. Monolithic four-handed Naṭarāja Image with *Ūrdhva-liṅga*. Find spot: Tandel Donger (Hill) in Dungripali village, Nuāpāḍā district. Mediaeval period.

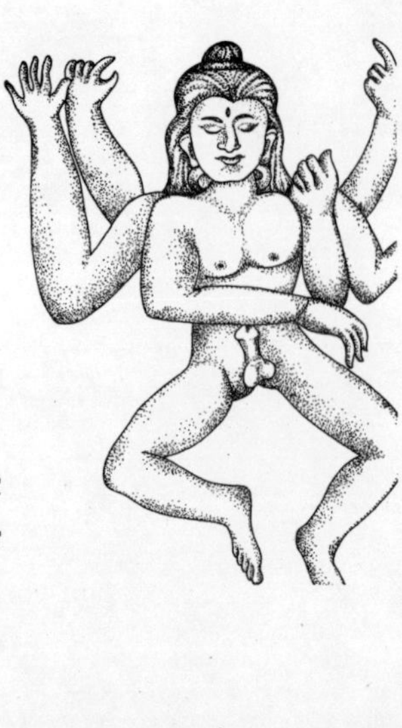

A unique image of Lord Śiva with all the tāntric *haṭha* yogic features carved throughout the body is found at Tala, in Bilāspur

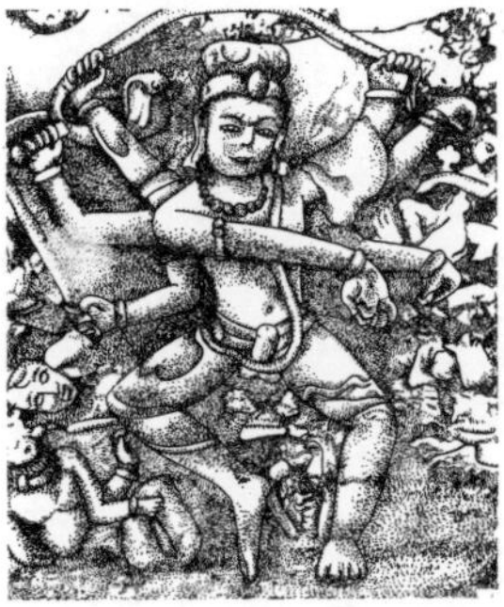

district of Chhattisgarh province (*Pl.* 27). It is nine feet in height and five tons in weight. It has been identified as "Composite tāntric yogic figure of Mahākāla and Mahākālī," by the author.[66] The significance is that the *ūrdhva-liṅga* (erected penis) edge of this huge image has tortoise like head and neck, which symbolizes *vajrolī-mudrā* and *uḍḍīyāna-bandha*. All these discoveries definitely prove that the whole Mahānadī river valley is the great Uḍḍīyāna-*pīṭha* (site), so greatly adored both by the tāntric Hindus and Buddhists. Therefore N.K. Sahu[67] states that it is known from the tradition embodied in the *Pāg-Sām-Jon-Zāñg* that tāntric Buddhism first developed in a place called Uḍḍīyāna, which is by far the most important among the four *pīṭhas* (Uḍḍīyāna, Pūrṇagiri, Kāmākhyā and Sirihaṭṭa) frequently mentioned both by the Hindus and the Buddhist *tantras*.

Overall findings, observations and study of the author[68] show that no definite period of composition of the tāntric yogic works are known, however the systematic form of tāntric *yoga* and *haṭha yoga* began to emerge in India sometime in the sixth century AD. It was the period of religious eclecticism. For survival probably Buddhism developed tāntric Buddhism. The study claims that the whole Mahānadī river valley is Uḍḍīyāna-*pīṭha* (site).

An interesting discovery has been made by scholars[69] about the most beautiful Rājaranī temple at Bhubaneswar. The mystery about the most beautiful and magnificent edifice has been enhanced by the fact that at present it contains no deity in the

66. J.P. Singh Deo, "Composite Tāntric Yogic Figure of Mahākāla and Mahākālī," *ROII*, Delhi, 2000, pp. 127-34.

67. N.K. Sahu, *Buddhism in Orissa*, Utkal University, 1958, p. 142.

68. J.P. Singh Deo, *op. cit.*, Delhi, 2001, pp. 201-02.

69. B. Baumer and R.P. Das (ed. & tr.), *Silparatnakośa* (*A Glossary of Orissan Temple Architecture*), Indira Gandhi National Centre for the Arts, New Delhi and Motilal Banarsidass, Delhi, 1994, pp. 146-53.

cella. Some scholars accept it, as a Vaiṣṇava temple, while others claim it, to have been a Śaiva temple. K.C. Panigrahi[70] has given much successful explanations and has proved Rājarānī temple, to have been Indreśvara temple, as mentioned in *Ekāmra Purāṇa*, *Svarṇādri-mahodaya* and *Kapila-Saṁhitā*, a Śaiva shrine.

The most interesting fact in proving the Rājarānī temple to have been a Śaiva shrine is that, in the latest study of *Śilparatnakośa*, of Sthāpaka Nirañjana Mahāpatra, it has been proved that the outer ground plan of Rājarānī temple is Mañjuśrī ground plan, while the inner chamber (*garbhagṛha*) or the inner ground plan has the *śrīcakra* superimposed on it. As studies show, Lord Śiva loves to abide in the Uḍḍīyāna-*pīṭha*, which is located as *bindu alias* centre point, within the innermost triangle of *śrīcakra*. So, it is an additional proof to claim that in origin, Rājarānī temple is a Śiva temple, with Uḍḍīyāna-*pīṭha* located at the inner centre of the *garbhagṛha* or the inner sanctum.

Theologically, the central *mahābindu*s are found at the centre of the *yantra*s of all the Goddesses of *daśamahāvidyā*, who are (1) Kālī, (2) Tārā, (3) Tripurasundarī, (4) Bhuvaneśvarī, (5) Bhairavī, (6) Chinnamastā, (7) Dhūmāvatī, (8) Bagalāmukhī, (9) Mātaṅgī, and (10) Kāmakalātmikā.[71] All these *mahābindu*s can be claimed as Uḍḍīyāna-*pīṭha*s where Lord Śiva abides and which are located in the *yantra*s of *daśamahāvidyā*.

Śāradātilaka (I.78), also records that from the *saguṇa* Śiva rise *śakti*, *nāda* and *bindu*. This *bindu* is threefold: (a) *bindu* (Śiva), (b) *Bīja* (Śakti), and (c) *nāda* (Śiva-Śakti).[72]

---

70. K.C. Panigrahi, *Archaeological Remains at Bhubaneswar*, Orient Longmans, New Delhi, 1961, pp. 94-98.

71. *TYATWG*, 1996, pp. 63, 75, 85, 95, 103, 111, 121, 129, 137 & 145.

72. Dirk Jan Hoens, "Mantra and other constituents of Tāntric Practice," *Hindu Tantrism*, Handuch Der Orientalistik-II, ABT, IV, Band, 2 ABSCHN, Leiden/Koln, E.J. Brill, Belgium, 1979, p. 105.

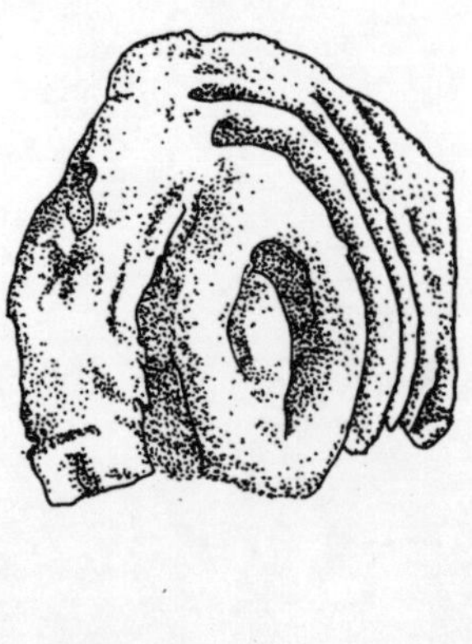

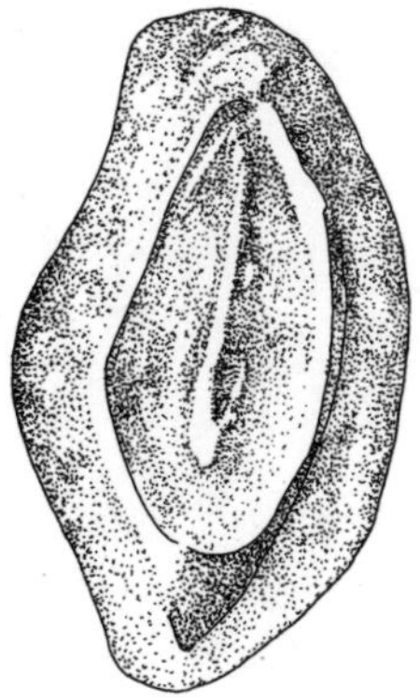

VI

Uḍḍīyāna-Pīṭha (site) Identified

J.A. Schoterman[73] states that the relation of the *yoni* with the present *kali-yuga* has been worked out more thoroughly in the *Samayācaratantra* (*Fig.* IIB), where we find the four *yuga*s, the four *pīṭha*s and four parts of the body of Śakti interrelated:

1. Pūrṇagiri : *Kṛta-yuga* : The complete body of Śakti.
2. Uḍḍīyāna : *Tretā-yuga*: The head of Śakti.
3. Jālandhara: *Dvāpara-yuga*: The breasts of Śakti.
4. Kāmapīṭha: *Kali-yuga*: The *yoni* of Śakti.

The correct reading of Oḍḍiyāna in the *Samayācaratantra* should be Uḍḍiyāna because Oḍḍiyāna, has no tāntric or yogic meaning, while Uḍḍīyāna is a *bandha* (abdominal retraction lock), a *haṭha yoga sādhanā*, as mentioned in the *Haṭha Yoga Pradīpikā* (Chapter 3, verses 55, 56, 57, 58 and 59).

H.N. Cakravarty[74] states, The *Yoginī-Hṛdaya*, gives an account of four *pīṭha*s designated by Kāmarūpa, Pūrṇagiri, Jālandhara and Oḍḍīyāna, representing four elements with their respective shapes and colours (*Yoginī-Hṛdaya* I. 42 cd 43).

> Square and circular associated with six dots, the shape of a half-moon, triangular — these are the shapes in their respective order, that is, of the earth, water, fire and air. The colours of them are yellow, smoky, white, red and without any colour. The *pīṭha*s viz., Kāmarūpa and so on emerge from the principal *bhū*, earth, Pūrṇagiri consists of the principal water, Jālandhara of fire, Oḍḍīyāna of air. These *pīṭha*s are

---

73. J.A. Schoterman, *The Yoni Tantra*, Manohar Publications, New Delhi, 1980, pp. 22-23.

74. H.N. Cakravarty, "The Pentadic Universe in the Śaivāgamas," *Prakṛti — The Integral Vision*, vol. 3 (The Āgamic Tradition and the Arts), Kapila Vatsyayan (General editor), Indira Gandhi National Centre for the Arts, New Delhi, D.K. Printworld, (P), Ltd., New Delhi, 1995, pp. 34-35.

physically located in different parts of India on one hand, while on the other they are meditated upon as located in Mūlādhāra and so on.

H.N. Cakravarty has also done the same mistake. Most probably, the scribers of tāntric texts have done the mistake of writing Uḍḍīyāna as Oḍḍīyāna, or it is a reading mistake. These texts have been re-written many a times, before they have come to us. So, there is every chance of mistakes cropping up.

The question arises why the Uḍḍīyāna-*pīṭha* is most important? Without answering this basic question scholars are only trying to identify the Uḍḍīyāna-*pīṭha*. Uḍḍīyāna-*pīṭha* is associated with a *haṭha yoga bandha* which is a binding, a bondage, a posture in which organs and muscles are contracted and controlled, creating a psycho-muscular energy lock, which redirects the flow of energy or *prāṇa* in the body and locks it into a specific area. So, the Uḍḍīyāna-*pīṭha* is that place where the *Uḍḍīyāna-bandha* of *haṭha yoga* developed.

M. Sylvan Levi,[75] L.A. Waddel,[76] P.C. Bagchi,[77] F.W. Thomas[78] and S.C. Das[79] suggest the location of the Uḍḍīyāna-*pīṭha* in Swat of Kabul, while Hara Prasad Sastri,[80] K.K. Kara,[81] N.K. Sahu,[82] Chandra Cakravarty[83] and others like H.C. Das,[84] R.P. Mishra[85] and few others identify Oḍḍīyāna or Uḍḍīyāna with Orissa.

75. *Journal Asiatique*, 1951, pp. 105-07.
76. L.A. Waddel, *Tibetan Buddhism*, p. 26.
77. P.C. Bagchi, *Indian Historical Quarterly*, vol. VI, pp. 576-78.
78. F.W. Thomas, *Journal of Royal Asiatic Society*, 1906, pp. 461-578.
79. B. Bhattacharya, *An Introduction to Buddhist Esoterism*, pp. 44-45. (View of Sri S.C. Das quoted).
80. *Ibid.*, p. 44.
81. K.K. Kara, *Ascharja Charya Chaya*, Odisha Sahitya Akademi, Bhubaneswar, 1969, pp. 1-14.
82. N.K. Sahu, *op. cit.*, chapter IX, 1958, pp. 141-55.
83. C. Cakravarty, *Sex Life in Ancient India*, Firma K.L.M., Kolkata, 1963, pp. 93-95.

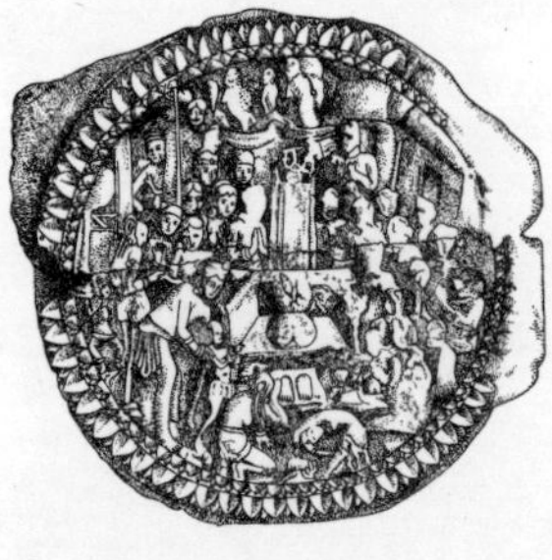

→

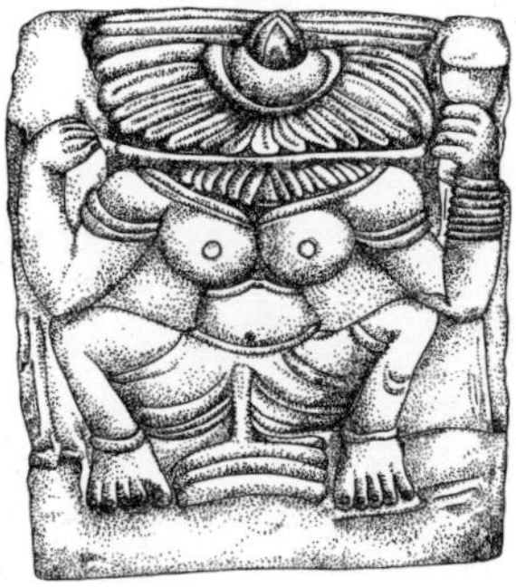

With the development of human thought process and dawn of civilization, growth took place in various fields. Many types of *yoga*s, a state of union between two opposite poles, viz., Śiva and Śakti, body and mind, individual and universal awareness, were developed. *Yoga* is a process of uniting opposing forces in the body and mind in order to realize the spiritual essence of being and existence. Many types of *yoga*s like *jñāna-yoga*, *rāja-yoga*, *bhakti-yoga*, *karma-yoga*, *haṭha-yoga*, *kuṇḍalīṇi-yoga*, *tantra-yoga*, *japa-yoga* and *laya-yoga* developed in India.

Tantra-yoga is a certain mystic process of generating spiritual energy forces and vibrations within, with the help of *mantra*, *yantra* and *devatā* theory, as also of relating these to the forces without, through the symbology of specific sounds, formulas, diagrams and rituals intended to liberate human beings from confinement to the lower nature and raise them to the regions of the higher nature.

Interaction between man and woman, *tantra*-wise, has three purposes: pleasure, procreation and *samādhi*. *Tantra*-wise sexual intercourse with a female partner is a mechanism for enhancing ecstatic enjoyment, and it does not conceive sex, as a quick scurry to orgasm or ejaculation. Control of seminal fluid is thought to restrain all passions and lead to achievement of desirelessness. *Mithuna* is sexual union for pleasure but *maithuna* is not for pleasure but a union for *samādhi*, i.e., *yoga* of sexual transformation. According to *Haṭha Yoga Pradīpikā*:

> He who controls the *bindu* and keeps his own *rajas* separated through *vajroli* is known as a *yogī*. His *rajas* can never be

---

84. H.C. Das, *Cultural Development in Orissa*, Punthi Pustak, Kolkata, 1985, p. 150.

85. (i) R.P. Mishra, *Sahajayāna — A Study of Tāntric Buddhism*, Punthi Pustak, Kolkata, 1991, p. 41.

    (ii) R.P. Mishra, "Samvalaka Tantra — Rajarsi Indrabhuti and His Influence on Culture of Western Orissa," *Souvenir, Loka Mahoshaba — 2001*, ed. Nilamadhab Panigrahi, Sambalpur, 2001, pp. 125-33.

> destroyed and in his body the *mada* merges in the *bindu*. If in *vajroli* the *bindu* and *rajas* can be kept separately in one's own body, then by the practice of *yoga*, all kinds of *siddhis* can be obtained. This is applicable to female also.[86] That woman who is able to keep her *rajas* above by means of retention of the orgasm, is the real *yoginī*. This practice of *vajroli* gives *siddhis* to the body — it becomes handsome, smooth, bright and attractive. This is the divine practice of *yoga* that gives liberation through enjoyment.

This signifies to a tāntric *haṭha yogī* that the vital energy or *ojas* should not be wasted in sensual enjoyment, because *ojas* is the unfoldment of the refined consciousness. So, in *tantra* there is sexual transformation to different *samādhis*.

For the practice of *yoga* of sexual transformtion *uḍḍīyāna-bandha* or abdominal retraction lock of *haṭha-yoga* is required. According to the *Haṭha Yoga Pradīpikā:*[87]

> *Uḍḍīyāna-bandha* is so-called by the *yogīs* because through its practise the *prāṇa* (concentrated at one point) rises through *suṣumnā*. — Verse 55, Chapter 3

> The *bandha* described is called the rising or flying *bandha*, because through its practise, the great bird (Śakti) flies upward with ease. — Verse 56, Chapter 3

Uḍḍīyāna-bandha changes the course of the downward moving *apāna vāyu* and unites it with *prāṇa vāyu* and *samāna vāyu* in the naval centre. When the two opposite energies of *apāna* and *prāṇa* meet in the naval region, there is an explosion of potential force, which travels upward through *suṣumnā nāḍī*. Powered by *udāna vāyu*, it is taken up into the higher centres. Of course, this is a major event in the course of one's *sādhanā* and it does not take

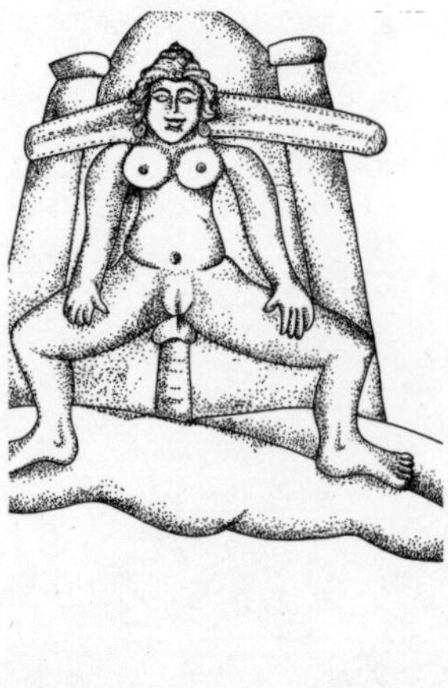

86. Svāmī Muktānanda Sarasvatī, *Nawa Yoginī Tantra*, Bihar School of Yoga, Munger, 1983, pp. 64-65.
87. *HYPBS*, Munger, 1993, pp. 299-303.

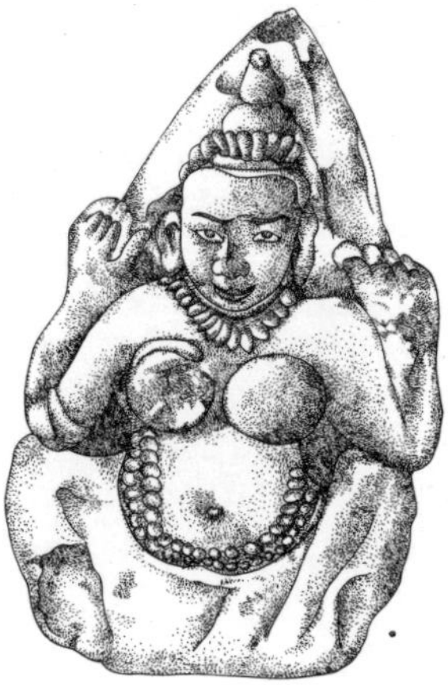

place with one or two rounds of practice. It requires a patient and ardent performance in combination with other techniques.

> Pulling the abdomen back in and making the navel rise is *Uḍḍīyāna-bandha*. It is the lion which conquers the elephant, death. — Verse 57, Chapter 3

It is advised by *haṭha-yogīs* that *jālandhara-bandha* must always be performed after the practice of *uḍḍīyāna-bandha*. *Jālandhara-bandha* controls the blood pressure.

A unique image, which the author has identified as "Composite tāntric yogic figure of Mahākāla and Mahākālī," is found at Tala site of Bilāspur district. It has the depiction of all the *haṭha*-yogic conceptions, on his body,[88] (*Pl.* 27).

When one practices the esoteric *haṭha-yoga* of *uḍḍīyāna-bandha*, one should maintain *kūrmasthiti*, as advised by *tantra rāja tantra*.[89] He who does *japa* (i.e., esoteric yogic practices like *uḍḍīyāna-bandha*, etc.) without knowing *kūrmasthiti*, not only fails to get the fruit thereof but also suffers destruction (Verse 88). Therefore, should *kūrma* be known first. *Kūrma* is of four kinds, the first being *para kūrma*. This, which is steady (*sthira*) and extends to 50 *koṭis* (500,000,000) of *yojanas* (between 8 and 9 miles), supports Pṛthvī. The others are *deśagata*, *grāmaga* and *gṛhaga*. Just as the Supreme Tortoise supports the whole universe, the others support particular countries, village and dwellings.

Four *kūrmas* or tortoises are chiselled in the north-west direction on the stone basement of the ruined Bhairava temple at Mohangiri site of Kālāhāṇḍī district.

Further, the two earliest Naṭarāja image with *ūrdhva-liṅga* (erected penis); one dated to the fifth century AD, found at Śrīpur

88. J.P. Singh Deo, "Composite Tāntric Yogic Figure of Mahākāla and Mahākālī," *ROII*, Delhi, 2000, pp. 127-34.

89. Sir J. Woodroffe, *Tantraraja Tantra*, Ganesh & Co. Madras, 1971, p. 33.

(*Pl.* 25) and the another dated sixth century AD, found at Āsanapaṭ site of Keoñjhar district (*Pl.* 26); prove that *uḍḍīyāna-bandha haṭha yoga* practice was invented or founded in the Mahānadī river valley.[90] All these narrations prove that the Uḍḍīyāna-*pīṭha* was and is the Mahānadī river valley which comprised South Kośala, parts of Utkala and parts of Kaliṅga states during ancient and medieval periods of Indian history.

Once the Mahānadī valley is accepted as the Uḍḍīyāna-*pīṭha* (site), the question arises why this name has been forgotten? A major part of the Mahānadī valley comprises the modern Orissa. As such the proper name would have been "Uḍḍisa," and its language not Oriyā but "Uḍḍiā." While the name "Uḍḍiā" has a tāntric *haṭha*-yogic concept, "Oriyā" has no yogic meaning. Uḍḍiba is to fly, i.e., to fly sexual energies up by the tāntric *haṭha*-yogic practices. How all this happened has been explained by N.K. Sahu:[91]

> The word "Uḍisa" of Afif is quite likely the developed variant of the word "Ursfin" of Ibn Khurdadhbih (ninth century AD) and "Urshin" of the Hudad-al-Alam (tenth century AD), the Chinese form of which is Wu-cha (Wu-ta) of Yuan Chwang (seventh century AD), the original being Oḍra or Oḍradeśa in medieval epigraphs and ancient literature. On the other hand, the word "Oḍra-Viṣaya," of the Soro Copper Plate inscription (seventh century AD) and subsequent medieval epigraphs, expressed as "Urda-bishau" in Alberuni's account (AD 1025), and as "Oḍḍa-viṣaya," in Tirumadai inscription (AD 1025) of Rājendra Cola, takes the form of "Oḍivisā," or "Uḍivisā," in the traditional records consulted by Lama Tāranāth and the author of *Pāg-Sām-Jon-Zāñg,* falling back on "Uḍḍisa" in the tāntric literature of late medieval time. The *Tantrasāra* in its two *Pīṭhatattvanyāsas* refers to God Jagannātha as "Uḍḍiśa-nātha," while the *Jñānārṇava*,[92] declares "Uḍḍisa," as one of the Śākta-*pīṭha*.

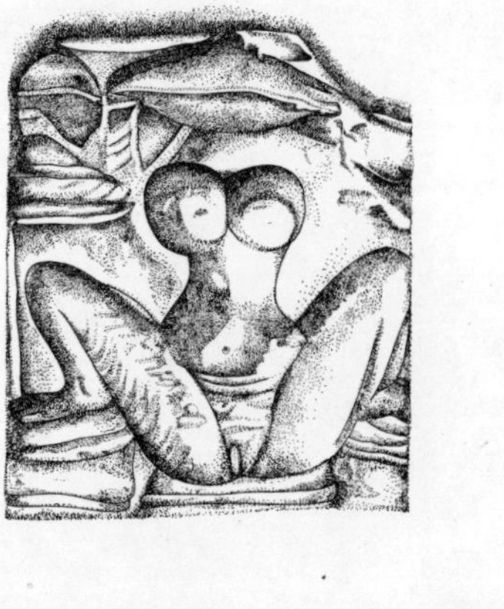

90. *NIATAL*, 2nd edn., 1994, pp. 159-60 and 164-65.

91. N.K. Sahu, *Utkal University History of Orissa*, vol. I, Utkal University, 1964, pp. 153-54.

→

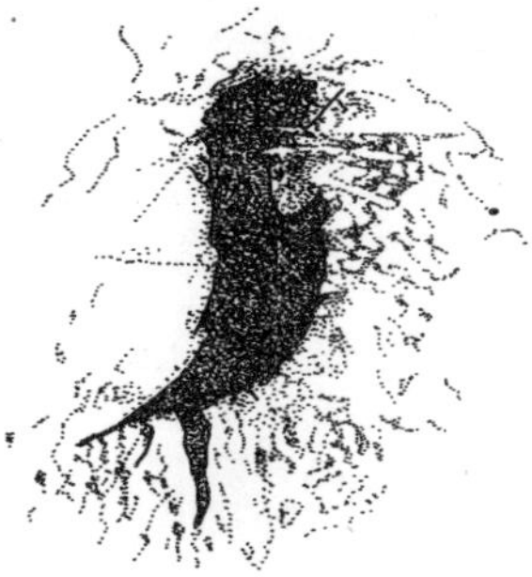

> It is thus evident that the word "Uḍḍisa," or "Uḍisa" had already developed by the fifteenth century AD, and the poet Saralādāsa naturally makes "Uḍisā," or "Oḍisā" synonymous with Oḍrarāṣṭra. The "Oḍrarāṣṭra — Oḍisā," of Saralādāsa is also represented as Oḍisā-rājya, in the proclamations of Gajapati Kapileśvaradeva (AD 1435-1467) during whose reign the poet flourished. From this time onwards the word "Oḍisa," denoting to the entire land of the Oriyā people, came in common use.

In this manner the impact of *uḍḍīyāna-bandha*, Uḍḍīyāna-*pīṭha* (site) and the *yoga* of sexual transformation were forgotten.

VII

Study of Lāṭa-mudrā, Vajrolī-mudrā, Sahajolī-mudrā and Uḍḍīyāna-bandha

Yoga is the means for awakening or realization. *Yoga* is usually defined as union. It is the union between limited self (*jīva*) and the cosmic self (*ātman*). As separation develops because of *māyā*, there should be an aim or goal of union. *Māyā* is no illusion or false notion, it is a power, according to the *Śvetāśvatara Upaniṣad*. From this Upaniṣad, which belong to the *Kṛṣṇa Yajurveda* (vide R.S. Nathan, *Our Heritage*, Book 1, Central Chinmaya Mission Trust, Mumbai, 1986, p. 120, Appendix), *māyā* is a power of god through which this world is created. Since the material objects and the mind have the same source, both help each other. God on the other hand is a divine entity, hence the mind is not naturally attracted to him.[93] In fact, separation does not exist. The aim of *yoga* is to unite a human being with cosmic consciousness, i.e., the limited self-consciousness with greater self-consciousness. So *yoga* is the path to perfection. The meaning of *yoga* can also be denoted by the words unity and

---

→ 92. D.C. Sircar, "The Śākta Pīṭhas," *Journal of Royal Asiatic Society, Bengal*, vol. XIV, pp. 20-21.

93. Sri Kripaluji Jagadguru Maharaj, *Philosophy of Divine Love*, Sadhna Bhawan Trust, Mangarh, U.P., 2nd edn., 1996, p. 59.

oneness, because the practice of *yoga* aims at rooting out the ego. Once the ego is transcended, one realizes one's inner, real nature. This definition of *yoga* is a spiritual one. *Yoga* therefore brings harmony between thoughts, words and deeds.[94]

There are nine kinds of *yoga*. They are *jñāna-yoga, rāja-yoga, bhakti-yoga, karma-yoga, haṭha-yoga, kuṇḍalinī-yoga, tantra-yoga, japa-yoga* and *laya-yoga*.[95] *Haṭha-yoga, kuṇḍalinī-yoga* and *tantra-yoga* are intermingled or inter-connected.

For *haṭha yoga*[96] *āsanas, ṣaṭ karmas, prāṇāyāmas, mudrās, bandha* and *samādhis* are described. *Tāntrika yoga* had early origin, because *kuṇḍalinī*, is a gift of *tantra* to human beings.[97] The earliest trace of *yoga* can be traced in the pre-historic paintings of palaeolithic and neolithic ages at Guḍahāṇḍī and Yogīmaṭh rock-shelters in western Orissa.

In the rock-shelter art of Yogīmaṭh donger in Nuāpāḍā (*Fig.* 2), discovered by the author, on 21 December 1970,[98] the paintings of bulls, triangles, rings, *ḍamarus* and triple-lines (trinity) are interesting. This painting of the neolithic period speaks of the prevalence of phallism and the first trinity concept of cosmic life, by an early *yogī*.

The opinion of Svāmī Satyananda Sarasvati[99] may be quoted here thus:

> There are also minor references to *haṭha yoga* in the ancient Upaniṣads and Purāṇas. The Upaniṣads date back earlier than the Buddhist period, which was around the sixth century

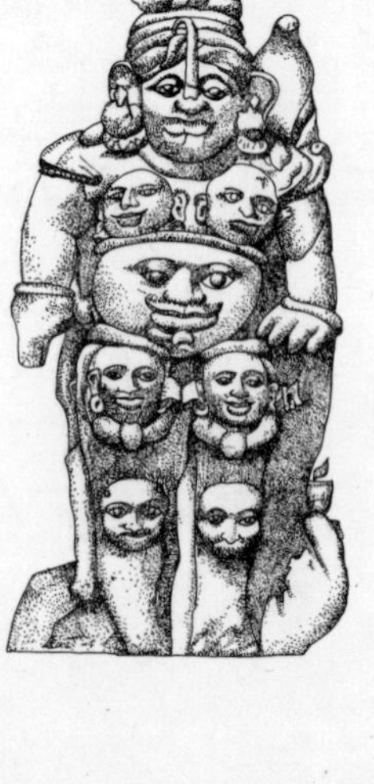

94. J.P. Singh Deo, *Tāntric Art of Orissa*, Kalpaz Publications, Delhi, 2001, p. 197.
95. *Ibid.*, p. 29.
96. *HYPBS*, Munger, 1993, passim.
97. Svāmī Satyānanda Sarasvatī, *Kuṇḍalinī Tantra*, Bihar School of Yoga, Munger, 1992, passim.
98. J.P. Singh Deo, *Cultural Profile of South Kośala*, Gyan Publishing House, New Delhi, 1987, p. 20.
99. *HYPBS*, Munger, 1993, p. 1.

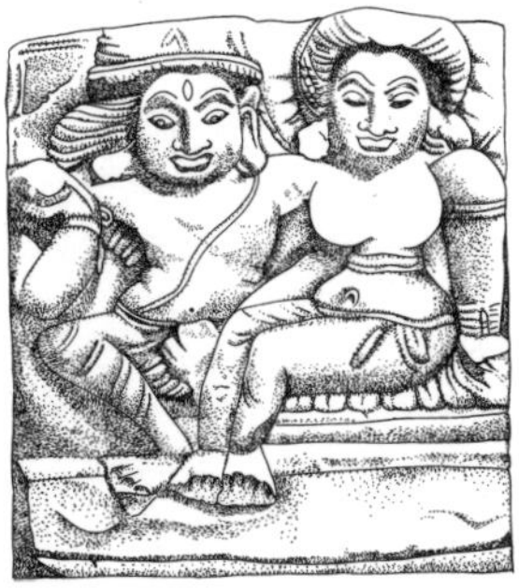

BC. The reference made in the Upaniṣads indicate that the science of *haṭha yoga* was known much before this period. There is another very important text known as *Śrīmad Bhāgavatam*, the story of Kṛṣṇa. In this voluminous book, there are references to *haṭha yoga* in several chapters.

Evidence of *haṭha yoga* have also been found in the Pre-Colombian culture of the Americans. Even now at St. Augustine, a southern province of Colombia in South America, there are large stone figures and carvings depicting *haṭha yoga* practices. However, the systematic form of *haṭha yoga* began to emerge in India sometime in the sixth century AD.

By the sixth century AD a lot of spiritual evolution had already taken place in India, over many centuries. Two great men were born in India in the sixth century BC one is internationally known as Buddha and the other was Mahāvīra, the founder of the Jain sect, a tradition in the Indian culture. They performed severe austerities and both of them preached non-violence, *ahiṁsā*. . . .

After about 500 years or so, the popularity and influene of Buddhism declined and so did these tāntric sects and other practices. Then in the fourth, fifth and sixth centuries AD, after the period of Buddhist decadence in India, some great *yogī*s took this science and set out to purify the tāntric system. Matsyendranāth, Gorakhanāth and a few other *yogī*s in the tradition found that this important science was being ignored by the serious minded people and was being wrongly taught by others. So they separated the *haṭha yoga* and the *rāja yoga* practices of *tantra* from the rest and they left out the rituals of *tantra* altogether, and they did not even mention it.

The beauty lies in the fact that the revitalization of *yoga* took place in the Mahānadī river valley, as *yogī* Matseyendranāth was born at Candradvīpa identified with Candravali-Dhamra region of Bhadrak district in Orissa.[100] *Yogī* Matseyendranāth

100. R.P. Mishra, *Sahajayāna — A Study of Tāntric Buddhism*, Punthi Pustak, Kolkata, 1991, p. 165.

established Nāthism and systematized 64 *yoginī tantra* in his famous book, *Kaulayānanirṇaya.*[101] The great disciple of *yogī* Matseyendranāth was *yogī* Gorakhanāth, whose disciple Swātmarāma produced a complete work on *haṭha yoga*, named *Haṭha Yoga Pradīpikā*. *Āsanas* like *svastikāsana* (auspicious pose), *gomukhāsana* (cow's face pose), *vīrasana* (hero's pose), *kūrmāsana* (tortoise pose), *kukkuṭāsana* (cockeral pose), *uttānakūrmāsana* (stretching tortoise pose), *dhanurāsana* (bow pose), *matsyendrāsana* (spiritual twist pose), and many *āsanas* are taught in *haṭha yoga* for different benefits.

The *yoga* of sexual transformation or from sex to superconsciousness is also a part of *haṭha yoga*, which had early origin, as known from the discovery of stone sockets from Mohangiri site in Kālāhāṇḍī district, Kharligarh in Bolaṅgīr district,[102] and Bargāon and Pātālgaṅgā of Nuāpāḍā district.

Before dealing with the *mudrās* and *bandha*, related to *haṭha yoga* it is worth quoting a passage from *Mahānirvāṇa Tantram*,[103] thus :

> The river Ganges, the Mahānadī, the residence of the spiritual guide and the celebrated shrines, these are the *tirthas* or the holy places of pilgrimage in the *kali yuga*.

To practise the *yoga* of sexual transformation *lāṭa-mudrā*, *vajrolī-mudrā*, *sahajolī-mudrā* and *uḍḍīyāna-bandha* are required to be perfected by the either sex. So, it is worth knowing about them.

Lāṭa-Mudrā

In the entire Mahānadī valley, lot of images of Umā-Maheśvara, Lakṣmī-Nārāyaṇa and Gaṇeśa with his Śakti, are found. In the

101. H.C. Das, *Tāntricism: A Study of the Yoginī cult*, Sterling Publishers, New Delhi 1981, p. 3.
102. J.P. Singh Deo, "Study on Identification of Uḍḍīyāna-*pīṭha* (site)," *Souvenir-2002*, Loka Mahoshaba, Sambalpur, 2002, pp. 133-35.
103. Manmatha Nath Dutt, *A Prose Translation of Mahānirvāṇa Tantram*, Chowkhamba Sanskrit Series Office, Vārāṇasī, 1979, p. 135.

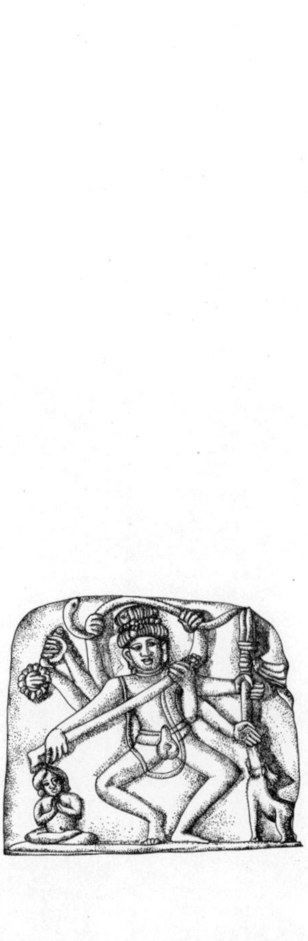

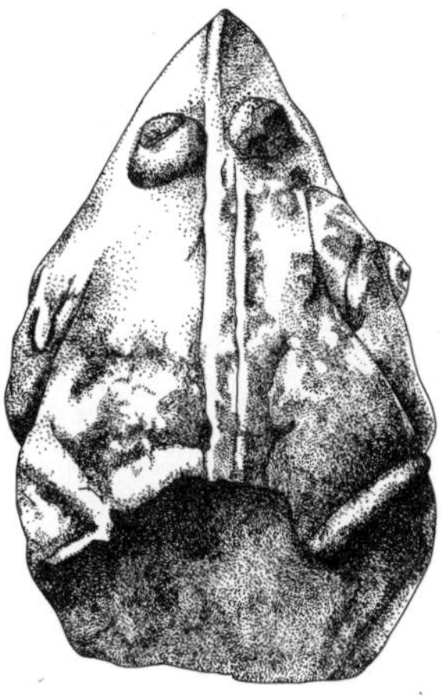

haṭha yogic concept they are performing the *lāṭa sādhanā*. The earliest Umā-Maheśvara image with *ūrdhva-liṅga* (erected penis) has been found at Belkhaṇḍī site which is now preserved at Manikyapur Museum, Bhawanipatna. One earliest Lakṣmī-Nārāyaṇa image, dated eighth-ninth centuries AD,[104] is also found at the same site and this too has been preserved at the Museum of Bhawanipatna.

With the development of Vaiṣṇava *tantra*, Lakṣmī-Nārāyaṇa images, like those of Umā-Maheśvara, were made during the Gaṅga period in Orissa, the traces of which can be seen in the Lakṣmī-Nārāyaṇa images at Liṅgarāja of Bhubaneswar, Lakṣmīnagar, Caurasī, the Maṭh of Thakurpatna in Prācī valley, Pratāpanagarī, Konduli, Cuttack town and Belkhaṇḍī.

Lāṭa-mudrā is also called *Śiva lāṭa-mudrā* by a Śaiva (*Pl.* 28). Robert E. Svoboda[105] and his tāntric master (*guru*) Vimalānanda described it thus:

> When a man and a woman come together for *Śiva lāṭa-mudrā*, the woman must sit on the man's left thigh and hold his penis with her right hand. He must cup her left breast with his left hand. Like a creeper she drapes herself around him, clinging tightly like a delicate vine, and he permits himself to be clung to, offering her support.
>
> There are three types of *Śiva lāṭa-mudrā* — mudane, spiritual and one which is beyond both the mundane and the spiritual. The mundane gives maximum sexual excitement, the spiritual is for *sādhanā* and "beyond" is too advanced to be

---

104. (i) J.P. Singh Deo, "Uma-Mahesvara Image of Belkhandi is the earliest Uma-Mahesvara Image with Ūrdhva-liṅga (Penis-erectus) in Orissa," *Souvenir — Kālāhāṇḍī Utsav 1999*, District Council of Culture, Bhawanipatna, 1999, pp. 23-26.

(ii) J.P. Singh Deo, "Earliest Laxmi-Narayan Sculpture of Orissa is in Kālāhāṇḍī district," *Souvenir — 2002 — Kālāhāṇḍī Utsav*, Bhawanipatna, passim.

105. E. Robert Svoboda, *Aghora* (*At the left hand of God*), Rupa & Co. New Delhi, 1993, pp. 271-72.

dealt here with. In all types the female counts *japa* with her left hand, the male with his right. The *mantras* are specific for each type. He forgets who he is, and she forgets who she is. He thinks, "I am Lord Śiva in the form of Bhairava (the fearful Lord) and this is my Śakti, my Bhairavī." She thinks, "This is my Lord Śiva, and I am his grand consort, his Bhairavī (the fearful Goddess)."

If the couple is doing it for mundane purposes they must concentrate on exciting each other. Without realizing it, she will begin to breathe through her left nostril and will direct that Śakti to him. His right nostril will be working and that Śakti of his will be directed to her. Hypersecretion of all glands will result and at the moment of greatest excitation, the cessation of breathing occurs for a moment. Then the male mounts and discharges his semen convulsively. Because of hypersecretion he will now eject three teaspoonsful of semen as opposed to his normal one teaspoonful. Because the vagina and cervix have become utterly loose and dilated, the sperm will go directly into the mouth of the cervix. The result is a child, if this is done at the right time of the month. This is the *brahmacarya* appropriate to the ordinary householder because by such sex, satiation occurs for a month or more and *ojas* is not wasted by frequent orgasms.

The spiritual *Śiva lāṭa-mudrā* is quite different. The Śiva must control his Śakti very carefully to ensure that she does not become sexually excited. The couple should be able to sit together for at least three hours, without the least excitation, no twitching or oozing. The girl must understand that she will not get an ordinary orgasm this way. If she waits patiently she will eventually get a super orgasm which will make her forget sex forever. If this *mudrā* is done properly she will go into *bhava samādhi*. Her emotions will crescendo until her mind becomes totally one-pointed, directed towards Śiva, and she will partly forget her worldly existence for a while. Even *mahābhava-samādhi*, which I call emotional highlights, is possible — total immersion in Śiva but with retained awareness of the Bliss. Wonderful!

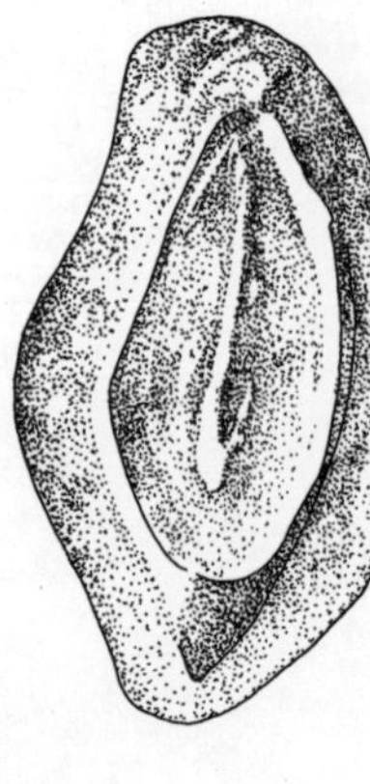

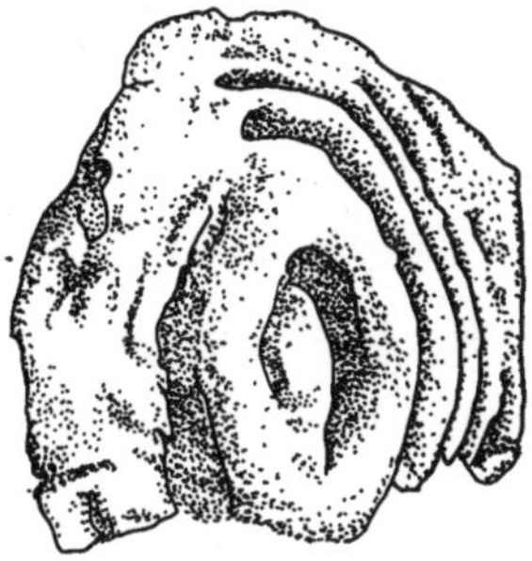

Be reminded that *tantra*-wise, sex has three purposes — pleasure, procreation and *samādhi*. *Haṭha* yogic practices of *vajrolī-mudrā*, *sahajolī-mudrā* and *uḍḍīyāna-bandha* of *haṭha yoga* are required when sex is utilized for *samādhi*. To be observed in a particular type of consciousness is called *samādhi*. *Samādhi* takes place with the rise of *kuṇḍalinī śakti* in the human body.

These *mudrā*s and *bandha* should be learnt from a proficient *guru* or master, else they would prove dangerous healthwise.

As the early images of Lord Śiva practising *uḍḍīyāna-bandha* are found in the Mahānadī valley, and also the one found at Tala in Chhatisgarh which is marked with yogic depictions and *ūrdhvamedhas*, the whole Mahānadī valley should be identified as Uḍḍīyāna-*pīṭha* (site). This identification supersedes educative knowledge and is given with intuitive knowledge of the author.

Now, with the growth of media, human beings are no more followers of dogmatic faiths or religions. People want practical experiences which intuitive yogic knowledge can give. With these practical yogic and spiritual tāntric knowledge, temple architecture in Kośali and Kaliṅga styles,[106] developed in the whole Mahānadī valley. Hence, the maximum number of manuscripts of *Śilpa Śāstra*, are found in Orissa.[107]

The present is a period of spiritual, yogic and cultural revival. The situation, through which all the religions are passing, has been well described by Ram Swarup:[108]

> A fateful thing has been happening. The east is waking up from its slumber. The wisdom of Hinduism, Buddhism,

---

106. J.P. Singh Deo, *Tāntric Art of Orissa,* Kalpaz Publications, Delhi, 2001, pp. 147-96.

107. R.P. Das, "The Study of Śilpa Śāstra," *Reference Orissa*, ed. A.N. Tiwari, Enterprising Publishers, Bhubaneswar, 1999, pp. 174-81.

108. Ram Swarup, "Introduction to the Reprint," *Mohammad and The Rise of Islam*, D.S. Margoliouth, Voice of India, New Delhi, reprint 1985, p. XX.

Taoism and Confucianism is becoming available to the world. Already, it is having a transforming effect on the minds of the people, particularly in countries where there is freedom to seek and express. Dogmas are under a cloud, claims on behalf of the last prophethood and only sonship, hitherto enforced through great intellectual conditioning, brow-beating and the big stick, are becoming unacceptable. Religions of proxy are in retreat. More and more men now seek authentic experience. Borrowed creed will not do. Men and women are ceasing to be obedient believers and are becoming seekers. They no longer want to be anybody's sheep, now that they know that they can be their own shepherds. An external authority, even when it is called God in certain scriptures threatening and promising alternately, is increasingly making less and less impression, people now realise that Godhead is their own true, secret status and they seek it in the depth of their own being. All this is in keeping with the wisdom of the east.

VIII

Study on benefits of Uḍḍīyāna-bandha and its Acquaintance with Mahānadī Valley

Uḍḍīyāna-bandha is a *haṭha yoga* practice. It means "Abdominal retraction lock, drawing in of the abdomen and stomach towards the backbone after exhaling." By utilizing the *haṭha* yogic *uḍḍīyāna-bandha,* one can perform the *yoga* of sexual transformation. According to *tantra,* sex has three purposes and they are: (1) pleasure, (2) procreation, and (3) *samādhi.* When sex is utilized for *samādhi* or super consciousness, *uḍḍīyāna-bandha* is required. In *kali-yuga* (age) everything is exciting, therefore *uḍḍīyāna-bandha* and its benefits should be properly understood by all.

Uḍḍīyāna-bandha is described in verses 55, 56, 57, 58, 59 and 60 of *Haṭha Yoga Pradīpikā.*[109] Thus:

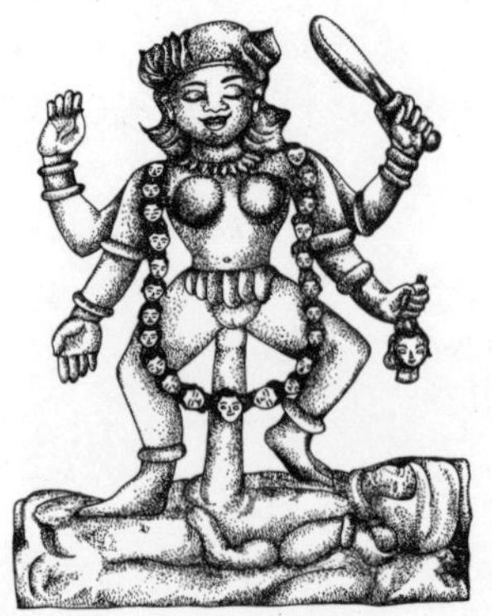

109. *HYPBS,* Muger, 1993, pp. 299-303.

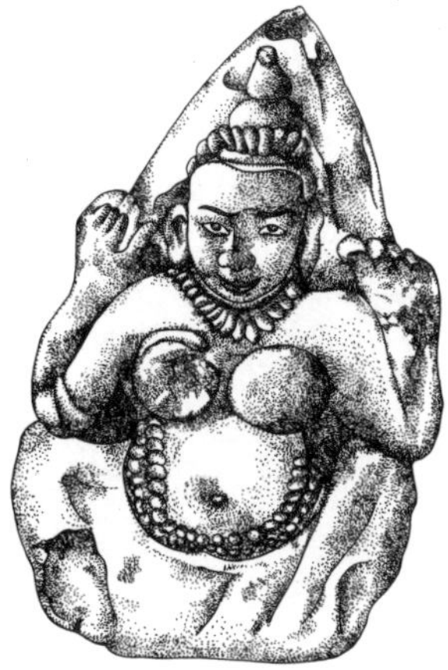

1. *Uḍḍīyāna-bandha* is so-called by the *yogīs* because through its practise the *prāṇa* (is concentrated at one point and) rises through *suṣumnā*. (verse 55)
2. The *bandha* described is called the rising or flying *bandha*, because through its practice, the great bird (Śakti) flies upward with ease. (verse 56)
3. Pulling the abdomen back in and making the navel rise is *uḍḍīyāna-bandha*. It is the lion which conquers the elephant, death. (verse 57)
4. *Uḍḍīyāna-bandha* is easy when practised in accordance to the instructions of the *guru*. Even an old person can become young when it is done regularly (verse 58).
5. The region above and below the navel should be drawn backwards with effort. There is no doubt that after six months of practice, death is conquered (verse 59).
6. Of all the *bandhas*, *uḍḍīyāna* is the best. Once it is mastered, *mukti* or liberation occurs spontaneously. (verse 60)

As said earlier, *uḍḍīyāna-bandha* is the abdominal retraction lock, a practice of *haṭha yoga*. *Uḍḍīyāna* means "to rise or fly." In the practice of *uḍḍīyāna-bandha*, the abdominal nerves (organs) are pulled up and thereby creating a natural upward flow of energy. Hence, it is often translated as the stomach lift. *uḍḍīyāna-bandha* changes the course of the downward moving *apāna vāyu* and *samāna vāyu*, in the navel centre. When the two opposite energies of *apāna* and *prāṇa* meet in the navel region, there is an explosion of potential force, which travels upward through *suṣumnā nāḍī*. Powered by *udāna vāyu*, it is taken up to the higher centres. Of course, this is a major event in the course of one's *sādhanā* and it does not take place with one or two rounds of practice. It requires patient and ardent performance in combination with other techniques.

Uḍḍīyāna-bandha involves the sucking in and pulling up of the abdomen and stomach. It can be done while sitting, standing or lying flat on the back. Initially, it should be practised while standing. It must always be done empty stomach and the bowels should preferably be evacuated first.

The most important lesson is that "*jālandhara* must always be done with *uḍḍīyāna*." When *haṭha yoga* is practised, it gives *viparīta* movement to the functioning of the whole human body. Therefore, blood pressure develops. *Jālandhara bandha*, popularly known as throat lock, controls blood pressure in the physical body. In the *Haṭha Yoga Pradīpikā*,[110] *jālandhara bandha* is described thus:

> Contracting the throat by bringing the chin to the chest is the *bandha* called *jālandhara*. It destroys old age and death. (verse 70)
>
> That is *jālandhara bandha* which catches the flow of nectar in the throat. It destroys all throat ailments. (verse 71)
>
> Having done *jālandhara bandha* by contracting the throat, the nectar does not fall into the gastric fire and the *prāṇa* is not agitated. (verse 72)

With this much of information about the *uḍḍīyāna* and *jālandhara bandhas*, it should be made clear that if *bandhas* are to be practised perfectly, they must be learned from a *guru* or qualified teacher. In *yoga* texts, full details are always omitted and if *yoga* is practised according to the instructions given in books, one will never be able to perform it, according to one's need and capacity. A proficient *guru* and regular practice[111] are the two basic requirements for the achievement of perfection in *yoga*.

According to *haṭha yoga*, the human body is an instrument and as *vāyu* is already dealt with, it is proper to have knowledge

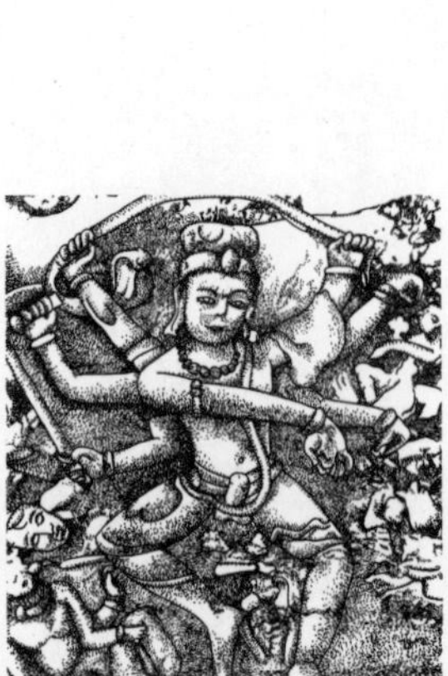

110. *HYPBS*, Muger, 1993, p. 315.
111. *HYPBS*, Muger, 1993, p. 302.

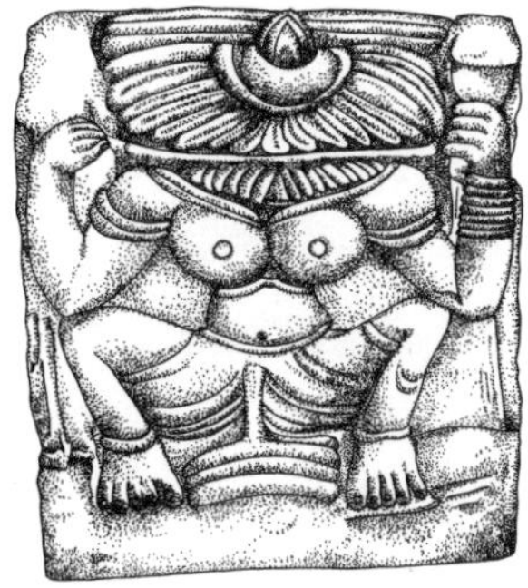

of the *mahābhūtas* (i.e., *ākāśa, agni, vāyu, vyāna* and *samāna*). Mukund Lath states,[112]

> The body, being made up of the five *mahābhūtas*, imbibes properties from them, too. These again are a mixed bag. *Ākāśa* imparts to it sound, the power of hearing (*śrotra*), hollowness (*susiratā*) and interestingly, a distinct identity in space (*vaiviktya*). But it also imparts a conscious property: subtlety of understanding. *Agni* is responsible for the eyes, form and colour, the quality of "ripeness" or "maturity," the state of being "cooked" (*pāka*); it is not clear whether the *pāka* spoken of here is a quality of organic entities or also of entities, such as *manas* and *buddhi*. *Agni* also causes bile as well as the property of making manifest (*prakāśatā*) — a property which is patently a property of consciousness — as well as head sharpness and energy. It is also the source of other inner qualities: bravery, anger and intelligence. *Vāyu* or wind is responsible for the awareness of touch and the *karmendriya* of touch. Besides, it is also responsible for the various movements of the body. Ten modifications of *vāyu* (*vāyuvikr̥tayāla*) reside within the human frame and are responsible for various bodily movements and functions. These are the well known *prāṇa, apāna, samāna, udāna* and *vyāna*, which are the five major *vāyus*. There are five others which are more minor roles. The ten *vāyus* help in carrying out various functions with and within the body, functions both voluntary and involuntary. *Apāna*, for example expels urine and excreta. *Vyāna* is stationed at the eyes, the ears, the nose as well as the ankles and the waist. Its role is not quite clear from Śārṅgadeva's account. Perhaps it helps other *vāyus* in carrying out functions such as smelling, bearing, batting of the eyes (for which one of the five minor *vāyus* is said to be responsible); The functions like those of the *indriyas* have in some sense both the aspects of being intentional and unintentional. But its functions in the ankles and the waist,

112. Mukund Lath, "The Body as an instrument (A Theoretical choice made by Śārṅgadeva)," *Prakr̥ti — The Integral Vision*, vol. 3 (*The Agamic Tradition and the Arts*), Kapila Vatsyayan, (General editor), D.K. Printworld (P) Ltd., New Delhi, 1995, pp. 105-06.

> whatever they are, are in no way within our control. *Samāna* performs functions which are purely organic and involuntary. Moving all over the body through *nāḍīs* or arteries numbering 72,000, it distributes all over the body the juices resulting from food and drink.
>
> The chief of the *vāyus* is *prāṇa*. From its station below the navel, it moves to the navel, the nose and the heart. It is responsible for breathing in and out, coughing and emitting sound.

Shri Svāmījī Mahārāja of Datiā[113] states,

> This gross physical body is made up of five elements. The seven components of this body are the juices, blood, flesh, fats, bones, marrows and semen. The three elements — air, fire and water called *vat, pitta* and cough in *Āyurveda* (Indian Medical System), blent in proper proportions keep the body fit and in proper shape. There dwell five vital breaths in the body, namely *prāṇa, apāna, samāna, uḍāna* and *vyāna*. There exist also five countributory or collateral breaths known as *Nāga, Karma, Devdatta, Krikala* and *Dhananjaya*. The five senses of cognition are the eyes, the nose, the ears, the skin and the tongue. The five senses of action are speech, hands, feel, rectum and genitals. These senses are directed by the mind conjointly with the self or *ātman*. The physical body of man is 90 fingers in height.

The body as an instrument had its origin in Vedic culture.[114] A man is dissected as a five-layered being: (1) food sheath, (2) vital air sheath, (3) mental sheath, (4) intellectual sheath, and (5) bliss sheath. It should not be forgotten that though no social sanction was received, people continued to practise *tantra*, with the rituals and continued to attach to it a philosophical content.

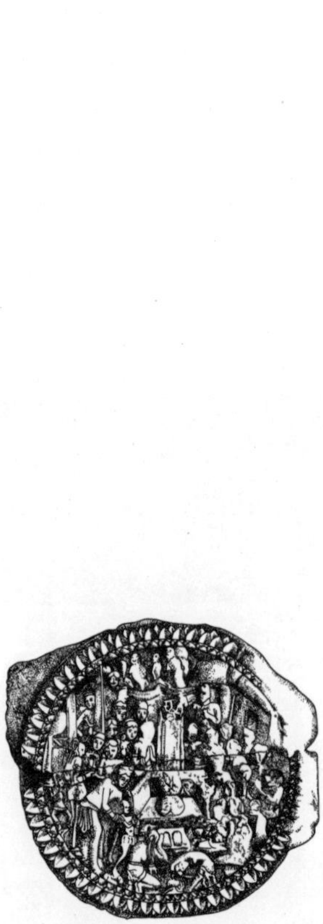

113. Shri Svamījī Mahārāja, *Siddhānta Rahasya* (*Secrets of Spiritual Living*), Shri Pitambarapeeth Sanskrit Parishad, Datia (M.P.), Chaitra Purnima, Samvat 2040, pp. 52-53.

114. Svāmī Chinmayananda, *Vedānta The Science of Life*, part I, Central Chinmaya Mission Trust, Bombay, 1983, pp. 131-61.

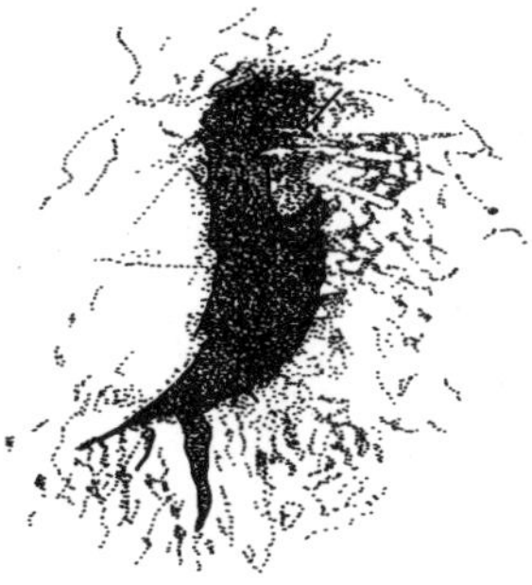

Tantra was and is a parallel cultural current along with the philosophical one in the Indian culture.[115] R.K. Upadhyaya[116] states that the *ipsissima verba* of the allegorical utterances of the *tantra śāstra* may be quoted for its confirmation, "The Vedas, the *śāstra*s and the Purāṇas are like a public woman, but the doctrine revealed by Śambhu, i.e., the *Tantra* remains veiled like a chaste housewife." The obvious import of it is that under no circumstances the secret doctrines of *tantra*s should be disclosed to the laities.

The origin of *tantra* is lost in mystery, but it is a branch of knowledge which offers a systematic and scientific method by which great spiritual powers can be achieved in human life for realization of the self that leads one to salvation.[117] *Kuṇḍalinī* is a gift of *tantra* to mankind or human beings.[118] For the rise of *kuṇḍalinī* and to receive intuitive knowledge or *samādhis, yoga* is the path.

As mentioned earlier *haṭha yoga* was popularized by *yogī* Matsyendranāth in post-Gupta period, and he was born in Candradvīpa, which has been identified as Candradvīpa or Candravali-Dharma region of Orissa, i.e., the Candbali-Dhamra region of the old Kanika estate, now located on the seacoast of Bhadrak district. It seems therefore that Nāthism as a School of Śaivism originated in Orissa and as its neighbourhood, Delhi, was the primal seat of this School, the Nāthas treated Kurukṣetra as the seat of their primal Lord of Ādinātha Śiva.[119]

---

115. *BSOIHAC*, vol. I, (*Beginning of Life, Culture and History*) Thane, 1997, p. 462.
116. R.K. Upadhyaya, *The Concept of God in Śaiva Tantra*, Jnananidhi Prakashan, Muzaffarpur, 1984, p. 22.
117. J.P. Singh Deo, *Tāntric Art of Orissa*, Kalpaz Publications, Delhi, 2001, p. 21.
118. Svāmī Satyananda Saraswati, *Kuṇḍalinī Tantra*, Bihar School of Yoga, Munger, 1992, passim.
119. J.P. Singh Deo, *op. cit.*, 2001, p. 89.

H.K. Mahatab[120] confirms that evidence of the Nātha *dharma* in Orissa can be traced to the last quarter of the eighth century AD. A statue of Matsyendranāth in the form of Padmapāṇi Avalokiteśvara in the forests of Rājnagar under the Deravisi Block of Kendrapārā sub-division (now district) is still worshipped by Nāthas of the surrounding villages. The inscription on both sides of the statue is in Kuṭilalipī or proto-Uḍralipī. The present Oriyā script was not evolved by then and the period of that script is accepted to be in between the sixth and eleventh centuries. The prototype of the same statue is seen at Kendrapārā bus stand with the same inscription and another at Trilocanpur village under Mahājājpur gram panchayat near Bahagram is also worshipped by Nāthas of the surrounding villages.

These three statues of Matsyendranāth clearly shows that Matsyendranāth was associated with that area and his birth place as identified by Ram Prasad Mishra,[121] was in the Candavali-Dhamra region of Bālāsore (now Bhadrak district). Since Matsyendranāth was associated with the whole Mahānadī valley as a great yogi there is one "Matsyendranāth Ghāṭ," along the Mahānadī river, near Sonepur town. One Matsyendranāth temple exists at Amarkaṇṭaka.[122] The most important disciple of *yogī* Matsyendranāth was Gorakhanāth, who rose to greater spiritual heights, than his *guru*. *Yogī* Gorakhanāth's disciple was *yogī* Swātmārāma, who wrote the famous *haṭha* yogic script, *Haṭha Yoga Pradīpikā.*

It is a paradox that the earliest sculptural arts of India, depicting the practice of *uḍḍīyāna-bandha,* with *ūrdhva-liṅga* (penis erected) are found on the eight-handed Naṭarāja images

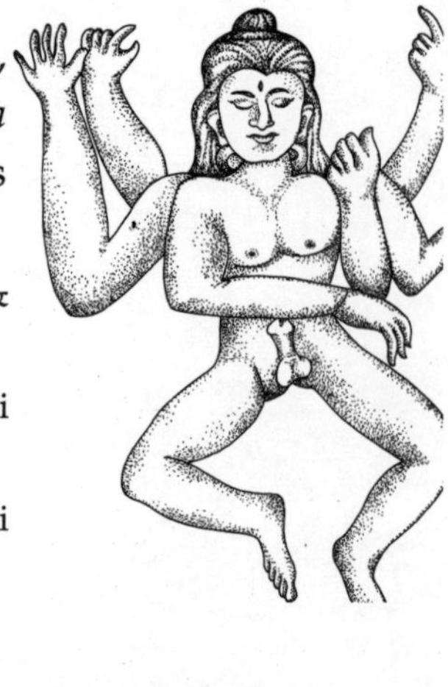

120. H.K. Mahatab, "Culture of Orissa," *OHRJ*, vol. XXX, Nos. 2, 3 & 4, 1984, p. 10.

121. R.P. Mishra, *Ṣahajayana — A Study of Tāntric Buddhism*, Punthi Pustak, Kolkata, 1991, p. 165.

122. Minoti Cakravarty — *Religious Life in the Kalachuri Empire,* Punthi Pustak, Kolkata, 1999, vide: Illustration No. 42.

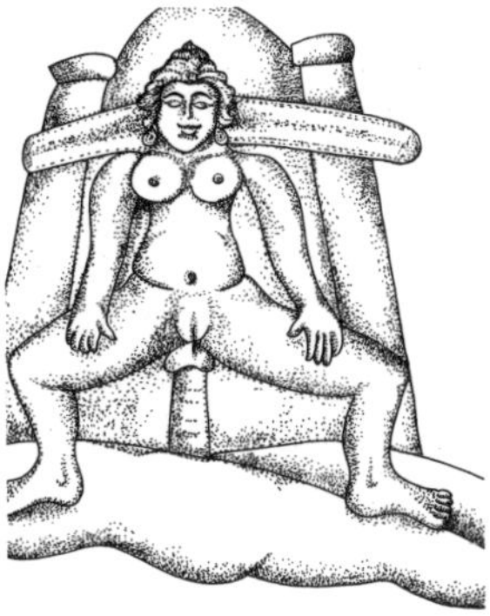

at Sirpur (ancient Śrīpur), dated to fifth century AD (*Pl.* 25) and Āsanapaṭ (*Pl.* 26), dated to sixth century AD in the far extended Mahānadī valley.[123] In the same yogic legacy of "the *yoga* of sexual transformation," a masterpiece image, depicting all *haṭha* yogic features, is found at Tala in Bilāspur district of Chhattisgarh province. The author[124] has identified it as "composite tāntric-yogic figure of Mahākālī and Mahākāla." It is nine feet in height and five tonnes in weight. This image of Śiva from Tala proves that the *haṭha yoga* had its beginning and quittance in the Mahānadī valley (*Pl.* 27).

Rock arts and temple sculptures are dumb without the power of speech. They can't speak rather they are the yogic expressions with features of their own meaning. A human being has to develop a yogic vision, through knowledge and wisdom, to understand them. The sensuous quality of tāntric art, which developed in the Mahānadī valley, to its logical culmination, completely shattered aesthetic barriers and exposed the ultimate realization that life is art. There is an ecstasy of joy in all plastic possibilities, which mankind could make. The female and male figures united together in a creative force to awaken their inner spirit are symbols of transcendent union. The tāntric arts of the Mahānadī valley are dynamic and sublime representations, which emphasize that human beings have the quality to plunge, dive or strike to the inner moods through *yoga* for self-realization.

IX

Uḍḍīyāna-pīṭha Represent Air Element

The human body is full of matter. Svāmī Chinmayananda[125] states,

---

123. *NIATAL*, New Delhi, 1994, pp. 159-60 and pp. 164-65.

124. J.P. Singh Deo, "Composite Tāntric Yogic Figure of Mahākāla and Mahākālī," *ROII*, Delhi, 2000, pp. 127-34.

125. Svāmī Chinmayananda, *Vedānta The Science of Life*, Part I, →

Matter, as we now know it, is perceivable and so is gross. For everything gross, there must be a previous subtle state of existence. Therefore, the gross matter is made up of its subtler components called in Vedānta as *tanmātras*. These *tanmātras* are each constituted of the three *gunas*. These *tanmātras* or subtle elements are five in number corresponding to the perceivable five gross elements of space, air, fire, water and earth which together constitute the perceived gross world.

Abhinavagupta[126] quoted *Kālottara*, and mention:

The earth, the water, the fire, the air and the void — these indeed, are the five principles by which the entire universe is pervaded.

The five constitute the physical objects is known to all but it is not known to all that they are the manifestation of consciousness. The Supreme Consciousness manifests itself or rather extends in five different ways. These ways are five outlets through which Śiva, the Supreme Consciousness, expresses himself though basically remaining as being Consciousness, Bliss, Knowledge and Activity. These are known to the Śaivas as the five faces of Śiva, the Lord.

H.N. Chakravarty[127] further states,

The *Yoginī Hṛdaya* gives an account of four *pīṭhas* designed

→ (*Understanding Human Nature*), Central Chinmaya Mission Trust, Bombay, 2nd edn, 1983, p. 115.

126. "Kalottara," as quoted in "Tantraloka of Abhinavagupta, XI.19." Vide H.N. Cakravarty, "The Pentadic Universe in the Śaivagamas," *Prakṛti, The Integral Vision*, vol. 3, Kapila Vatsyayan, (General editor), Indira Gandhi National Centre for the Arts, New Delhi and D.K. Printworld (P) Ltd., New Delhi, 1995, pp. 28-29.

127. Vide H.N. Cakravarty, "The Pentadic Universe in the Śaivagamas," *Prakṛti, The Integral Vision*, vol. 3, Kapila Vatsyayan, (General editor), Indira Gandhi National Centre for the Arts, New Delhi and D.K. Printworld (P) Ltd., New Delhi, 1995, pp. 34-35.

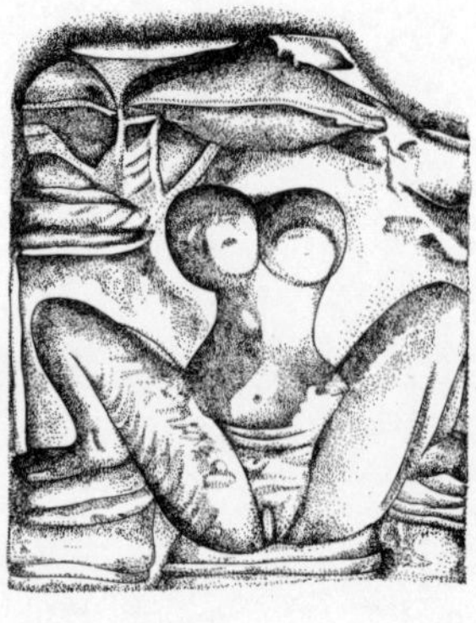

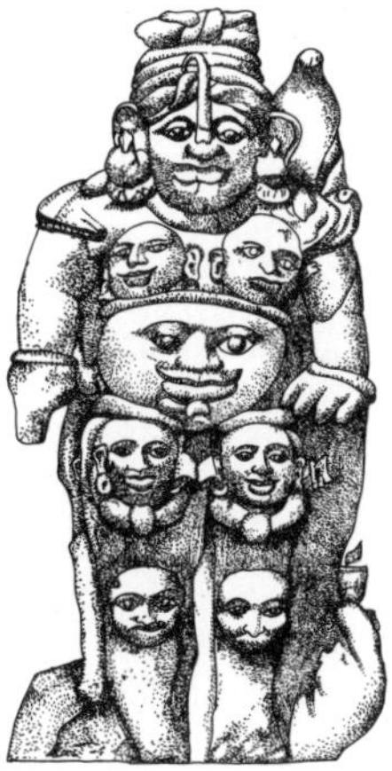

by Kāmarūpa, Pūrṇagiri, Jālandhara and Oḍḍīyāna representing four elements with their respective shapes and colours thus:

caturasraṁ tathā binduṣaṭkāyuktam ca vr̥ttakam,
ardhacandram trikoṇam ca rūpāṇyeṣāṁ kramenatu,
pīto dhūm rasthatha śveto rakto'rūpam ca kīrtitam.

— *Yoginī Hr̥daya, I.42cd-43*

Square and circular associated with six dots, the shape of a half moon, triangular — these are the shapes in their respective order, that is, of the earth, water, fire and air. The colours of them are yellow, smoky, white, red and without any colour. The *pīṭhas*, viz., Kāmarūpa and so on emerge from the principle *bhū*, earth, Pūrṇagiri consists of the principle water, Jālandhara of fire, Oḍḍīyāna of air. These *pīṭhas* are physically located in different parts of India on one hand, while on the other they are meditated upon as located in *mūlādhāra* and so on.

Further, *uḍḍīyāna-bandha*, which is *haṭha* yogic practice is concerned with the *yoga* of sexual transformation, i.e., pulling up the semen of male or ovum of female, before they are ejaculated and discharged. This *yoga* is possible with the use of *vāyu* or air in the human body. Therefore, it seems that the *Yoginī Hr̥daya*, is very correct when it mentions that the Uḍḍīyāna-*pīṭha* represents the air element.

Uḍḍīyāna-bandha is abdominal retraction lock, a practice of *haṭha yoga*. *Uḍḍīyāna* means "to rise or fly." In the practice of *uḍḍīyāna-bandha*, the abdominal nerves including the organs are pulled up thereby creating a natural upward flow of energy. It is hence often translated as the stomach lift. *Uḍḍīyāna-bandha* changes the course of the downward moving *apāna vāyu* and unites it with *prāṇa vāyu* and *samāna vāyu*, in the naval centre. When the two opposite energies of *apāna* and *prāṇa* meet in the naval region, there is an explosion of potential force, which travels upward through *suṣumnā nāḍī*. Powered by *udāna vāyu*, it is taken up to the higher centres. Of course, this is a major event in the course of one's *sādhanā* and it does not occur in one or two rounds of practice. It requires a patient and ardent performance in combination with other techniques.

According to yogic texts,[128] there are ten *vāyus* in human body, which are responsible for various bodily movements and functions. These are the well known *prāṇa, apāna, samāna, udāna* and *vyāna,* which are the five major *vāyus*. There are five others which are mere roles. These ten *vāyus* help in carrying out various functions with and within the human body, which functions both voluntarily and involuntarily.

X

Kūrmaśiti is a gift of Kālāhāṇḍī district to Mankind

Ṛgveda (5.60.5) declares, "Here, there is none greater, none smaller. All have gathered together here for advancing common welfare of all." The studies of Vedas show that the Vedas constitute the root of all religious, social, cultural, political and economic thoughts of mankind. The existential blissful consciousness is the source of all creation. The energy of the Lord or by whatever name one recognizes it, is Truth, Beauty and Goodness. The Vedas are His breath, man His expression. The tenets of the Vedic Sanātana *dharma* with its scientific yogic rationalism can help human beings in the flowering of their genius to its fullest potential. The fundamental truths of life is revealed to us by the Vedas, which can make our lives healthy, wealthy and wise.

The greatest fact of the Vedic culture or Sanātana *dharma* is that it has the capacity to absorb every truth into its fold because it is based on truth.

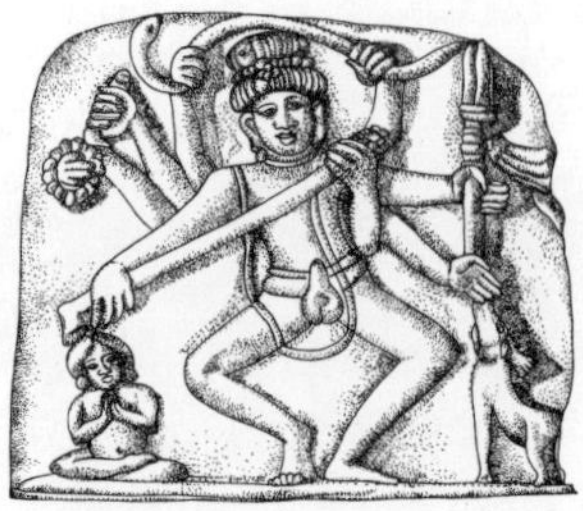

128. Mukund Lath, "The Body as an Instrument, (A Theoretical choice made by Śārṅgadeva," *Prakṛti, The Intergral Vision*, vol. 3 (*The Āgamic Tradition and the Arts*), ed. Kapila Vatsyayan, D.K. Printworld (P) Ltd., New Delhi, 1995, pp. 105-06.

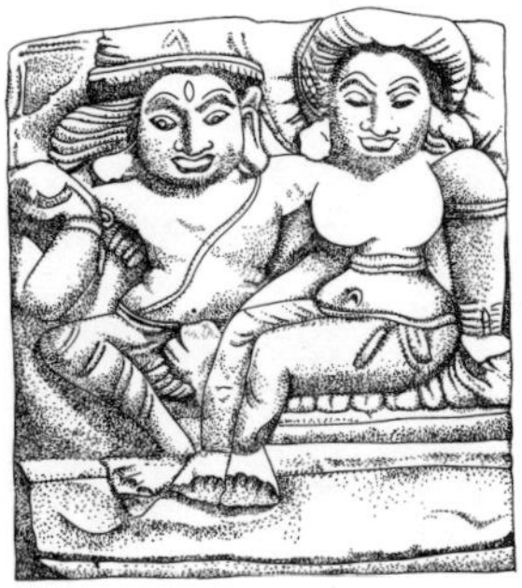

In the philosophy of *tantra*,[129] human being is divine and only the divine can worship the divine or realise the divine. Thus *tantra* represents the essence of Vedic mysticism in a nutshell. According to *tantra*, a human body is an epitome to the cosmic body.

Chāndogya Upaniṣad says, as a human being thinks that one becomes. According to the *Viśveśvara Tantra*, "What is here is there, what is not here is nowhere." The different types of consciousness has to be realized through *yoga*, within the human self, which is called theosophy in the english language.

The knowledge which is acquired from teachers and from books is imitative, repetitive, derivative and educative. Another knowledge which is above these types of knowledge is intuitive. Only intuitive knowledge reaches the reality or truth.[130] Intuitive knowledge can be acquired only through *yoga*. There are different types of *yogas*, as *karma-yoga*, *jñāna-yoga*, *haṭha-yoga*, *rāja-yoga*, *mantra-yoga*, *laya-yoga*, esoteric *yoga* or the *yoga* of sexual transformation, etc.[131]

According to one of the *haṭha* yogic text, *Tantrarāja Tantra*,[132] it is mentioned,

> He who does Japa without knowing *Kūrmasthiti* not only fails to get the fruit thereof but he meets with destruction (V.88). Therefore should *kūrma* be first known. *Kūrma* is of four kinds, the first being the *para kūrma*. This which is steady (*sthira*) and extends to 50 *koṭis* (500,000,000) of *yojanas*

129. Svāmī Satyananda Saraswati, *A Systematic Course in the Ancient Tāntric Techniques of Yoga and Kriya*, Bihar School of Yoga, Munger, 1989, passim.

130. J.P. Singh Deo, *Origin of Jagannāth Deity*, Gyan Publishing House, New Delhi, 1991, p. VII (Preface).

131. Paramahamsa Niranjanananda, *Yoga Darshan* (*Vision of the Yoga Upaniṣad*), Sri Panchdashnam Paramahamsa, Alakhbara, Deogarh, Bihar, 1993, passim.

132. Sir John Woodroffe (ed.), *Tantraraja Tantra* (*A Short Analysis*), Ganesh & Co., Private Ltd., Madras, 1971, p. 33.

> (between eighth and ninth miles) supports *pṛthvī*. The others are *deśagata, grāmaga* and *gṛhaga* which just as the Supreme Tortoise supports the whole universe, the others support particular countries, villages and dwellings.

This statement of *tantra* shows that higher *sādhanā*s should be kept secret. Only through the secret *sādhanā*s, which is called esoteric rites, one can achieve higher consciousness.

Archaeological concepts of *yoga* are found in the hilly, forest and isolated areas of India. It is strange that Mohangiri site of Kālāhāṇḍī district in Orissa is a site of such archaeological tāntric-yogic importance.

Kedarnath Mahapatra[133] brought Mohangiri site into limelight and states,

> The broken Śiva temple at Mohangiri in the extreme north-east corner of this state bordering the Gañjam district and standing not very far from the famous Khingghat is a noteworthy monument of this area. It belongs to the Paraśurāmeśwar type of temples in Bhubaneswar and is similar to the twin temples at Gandharadi of Bauḍ State on the bank of the Mahānadī. The place Mohangiri seems to have strategic importance in those days of yore, as it was situated on the highway passing from Kaliṅga (Gañjam side) to Kośala (Kālāhāṇḍī Patna side) and this temple was erected to serve the purpose of a guide as well as a place of worship for the travellers passing through this way.

At the site of the dilapidated temple of Mohangiri, two small inscriptions are found. One is of "Sphita Candra," who belonged to Mudgalakula and the other of "Vydha Bhairava," who was probably the presiding deity. Details about the Mudgala dynasty, which ruled the north-east portion of Orissa, as known from Soro copper-plates, dated to the sixth century AD and how they shifted

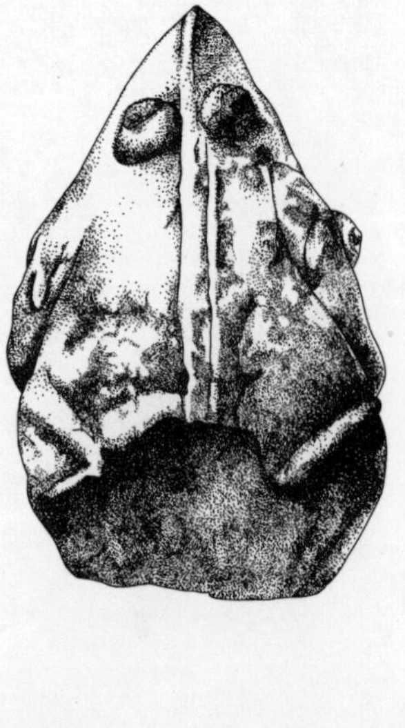

133. K.N. Mahapatra, "History of the Kālāhāṇḍī State before the Rise of the Gaṅga power," *The Journal of the Kalinga Historical Research Society*, vol. I, no. 4, March 1947, p. 268.

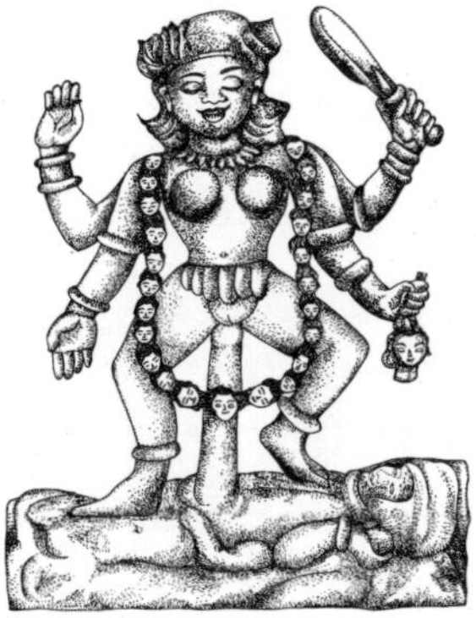

to the west into the hilly and forest tract of Kālāhāṇḍī region in medieval period are not yet known.[134] On palaeolithic consideration, the two small inscriptions of Mohangiri site dated to the tenth century AD.

While collecting antiquities in 1992, to start a multipurpose museum at Bhawanipatna, the author had visited the Mohangiri site. It was apparent from the ruins of the Śiva or the Bhairava temple at Mohangiri that it faced east and stood on a stone platform. At the north-west portion of the platform or stone basement, four tortoises were chiselled. The name "Vydha Bhairava," found in the inscriptions proves that the site was important because the tāntric-yogic and esoteric *sādhanās* were practised here which are inner, secret, mysterious *sādhanās*. The most esotoric *sādhanā* is the *yoga* of sexual transformation, or the *haṭha yoga* practice of the union of male and female principals. The remnant of four chiselled tortoises, found on the platform of the Śiva or Bhairava temple, now named Dhabaleswar Śiva temple, at Mohangiri reminds the author about the secret doctrinaire of *Kūrmaśiti*, as mentioned in the *Tantrarāja Tantra*, a *haṭha yoga* manual, meant for daily *sādhanās* of the Nātha *haṭha yogīs*. The existence of four tortoises in different sizes chiselled in one line at Mohangiri site, is Kālāhāṇḍī's gift to the esotoric *haṭha yoga* of the Nātha *dharma*.

According to the *Haṭha Yoga Pradīpikā*, Chapter I, verses 5-9,[135] the *mahāsiddhas* (great masters), having conquered time (death) by the practice of *haṭha yoga*, roamed about the universe. The *Mahānirvāṇa Tantra*[136] also states that the river Ganges, the Mahānadī, the residence of the spiritual guide, and the celebrated shrines, these are the *tīrthas* or the holy places of pilgrimage in the *kali-yuga*.

---

134. J.P. Singh Deo, *Cultural Profile of South Kośala*, Gyan Publishing House, New Delhi, 1987, p. 165.

135. *HYPBS*, Munger, 1993, p. 29.

136. Manmatha Nath Dutt, *Mahānirvāṇa Tantram*, Chowkhamba Sanskrit Series Office, Vārāṇasī, 1979, p. 135.

Yogī Matsyendranāth is the founder father of Nāthism and in recent years Ram Prasad Mishra[137] has established that younger Luipa or Matsyendranāth was the Nātha *siddha* and was born in Candradvīpa, the Cāndavāli-Dhamra region of Bālāsore (now Bhadrak) in Orissa. To emphasize his view, the author points out that there are lot of ruins connected with Matsyendrnāth in the Mahānadī valley. The Matsyendranāth *ghāṭ* on Mahānadī river in Sonepur site and the existence of Matsyendranāth temple at Amarkaṅṭak.[138] may be cited as examples. H.K. Mahatab[139] says,

> Evidences of the Nātha *Dharma* in Orissa can be traced since the last quarter of the eighth century. A statue of Matsyendranāth in the form of Padmapāṇi Avalokiteśvar in the forests of Rajnagar under Deravisi block of Kendrapara sub-division (now district) is still worshipped by the Nāthas of the surrounding villages. The inscription on both sides of the statue is in Kutila-lipi or proto-Udra-lipi. The present Oriya script was not evolved by then and the period of that script is accepted to be inbetween sixth and eleventh centuries AD. The prototype of the same statue is seen at the Kendrapārā bus stand with the same inscription and another at Trilocanpur village under Mahājājpur Gram Panchayat near Bahugram is also worshipped by the Nāthas of the surrounding villages. This proves that towards the last quarter of the ninth century AD. Matsyendranāth and Gorakhanāth were worshipped in Orissa, as the incarnations of Viṣṇu and Śiva respectively. The most ancient specimens of Oriya prose and poetry are ascribed to be the work of Gorakhanāth and other Nātha-Siddhas.

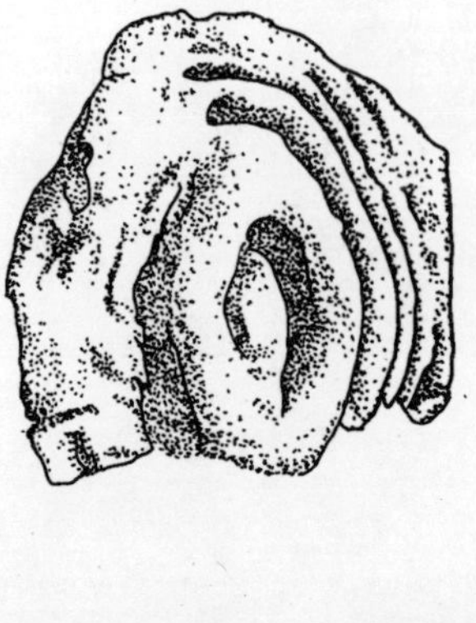

137. R.P. Mishra, *Sahajayāna — A Study of Tāntric Buddhism*, Punthi Pustak, Kolkata, 1991, p. 165.

138. Minoti Cakravarty, *Religious Life in the Kalachuri Empire*, Punthi Pustak, Kolkata, 1999, vide: Plate No. 42.

139. H.K. Mahatab, "Culture of Orissa," *OHRJ*, vol. XXX, nos. 2, 3 and 4, 1984, p. 10.

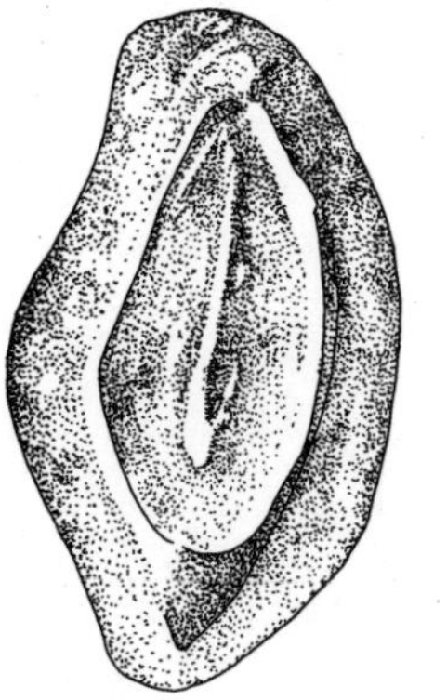

The theory of *Piṇḍa-Brahmāṇḍa* (cosmos in microcosm) of Gorakhanāth serves as the backbone of Orissan Vaiṣṇava philosophy of Pancasakha literature as in the case of Nirguna Santh Kavyas of Hindi, Punjabi and Gujarati literature of the ancient and medieval periods.

The discussion shows that when Nāthism and *haṭha yoga* spread all-over India during the early medieval and middle medieval periods, the forests and hill tracts of Kālāhāṇḍī were not isolated. Many *siddha haṭha yogī*s lived in this region and the four chiselled tortoises on the north-west portion of the pavement or stone plinth of the Śiva/Bhairava temple at Mohangiri, is an archaeological art discovery, proving the prevalence of the *Kūrmaśiti* practice in those days. In modern days, a temple has been built on the ruin and is named as "Dhabaleśvar temple of Mohangiri."

XI

Yoginī Tantra and Yoni Tantra Originated in Central Right Mahānadī River Valley

Usually the tāntric texts are not found in good Sanskrit language, because most of the later works were written by *sādhaka*s and *yoga* participants and not by the Sanskrit scholars.

J.A. Schoterman[140] a critical editor of the *Yoni Tantra*, states that six of its manuscripts are written in Bengālī script which he has edited. He holds that the most important in determining the origin of the text in *paṭala* IV:

kocākhyāne ca deśe ca yonigartasmipataḥ ॥ 2 ॥
gaṅgāyāḥ paścime bhāge mādhavī nāma viśrutā ।

gatva tatra maheśāni yonidarśanamānasaḥ ॥ 3 ॥
ahaṁ cātra niśam devī yonipūjanatatparaḥ ।

140. J.A. Schoterman, *The Yoni Tantra*, Manohar, New Delhi, 1980, pp. 3-4 and p. 9.

bhikṣācāraprasaṅgena gacchāmi ca divāniśam ॥ 4 ॥
mādhaviyonisadṛśīnāsti yonir mahitale ।
tatkucaa kaṭhinau durge yonistasyāḥ supinata ॥ 5 ॥

We are thus informed that in a country called Koca, near Yonigarta, on the *paścima* side of the river Ganges, a certain Mādhavī is known to exist whose *yoni* is unequalled on earth; it is an object of constant veneration for Mahādeva, who is the narrator in this fourth patala of the *Yoni Tantra*. The country called Koca is unmistakably modern Cooch Bihar, north of Bangla Desh. . . . Thus summarizing this section on the origin of the *Yoni Tantra,* he concludes that its origin is in the region of Cooch Bihar near Yonigarta/Kāmarūpa centring around the cult of Mādhavī.

J.A. Schoterman[141] states that the story of Revatī/Mādhavī in the *Yoginī Tantra* can be regarded as an illustration of a common phenomenon, e.g., the embedding of a foreign/local deity into an established religious system: (SC: the worship of Kāmākhya). . . . Throughout the story she is referred to with non-descript denominations: Yoginī, Satī, Brāhmikā and Sādhvī. Only once she is called Revatī (XIII, 2b), which is again a non-committal name. Revatī is best known as the wife of Balarāma, and as a *yoginī* she is mentioned among the 64 *yoginī*s (*Agni Purāṇa*, LII, CXVIL, 21, and *Caturvargacintāmaṇi*, p. 102).[142] Only at the end of the story it seems her real name Mādhavī is mentioned, when *īśvara* urges *devī* to accept Mādhavī and her son Venusiṁha (vide supra). It is very plausible that the story told in connection with the *yoginī* Revatī/Mādhavī in the *Yoginī Tantra* refers to the Mādhavī of the *Yoni Tantra*.

In the Oriyā language lexicon,[143] the word Mādhavī, means,

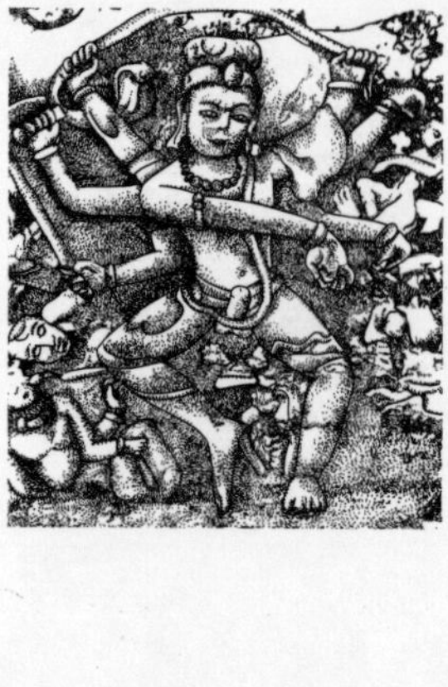

141. J.A. Schoterman, *The Yoni Tantra,* Manohar, New Delhi, 1980, pp. 7-8.

142. Pandit Kanhaiyālala Misram who translated the *Yoginī Tantra,* into Hindi, takes *Yoginī* as her name.

143. Gopal Chandra Praharaj, *Pūrṇachandra Orḍiā Bhāṣakoṣā,* vol. V (Consonants, Pha — Ma), Cuttack, 1936, pp. 6459-60.

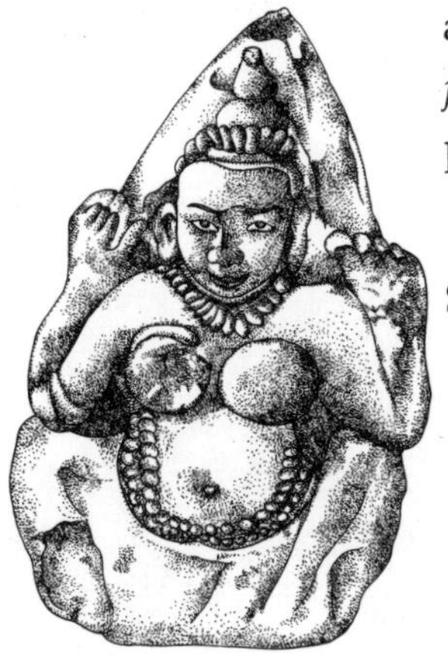

a flowering creeper; the spring creeper; *hiptage madablata, jasminum arborescens;* clustered hiptage; (*kīrtikar*), the holy basil plant, Lakṣmī, the name given to females.

While dealing with the evaluation of the *Yoni Tantra,* J.A. Schoterman[144] remarks,

> The *Yoni Tantra* had its origin in the region of Cooch Bihar and can be placed in a Vaiṣṇava environment around the worship of the Goddess Mādhavī. This Mādhavī may be regarded as the Vaiṣṇava counterpart of the Śaiva Kāmākhya in Kāmarūpa. The *Yoni Tantra* seeks to surpass its Vaiṣṇava limitations by allaying itself with the Kulācāra, thus trying to find a more general acknowledgement beyond the boundaries of "Sectarianism." In this context one should place the conspicuous absence of any direct reference to Kāmākhya or Kāmarūpa. Furthermore, the superficiality of the *Yoni Tantra* should be mentioned with regard to the Śakti, the *śaśaka* and the ritual itself, comparing the *Yoni Tantra* with other texts dealing with the same subject. . . . If provides, us with information on that side of tāntric *sādhanā* which is only hinted at in the texts, but which has remained virtually unknown.

Two manuscripts of *Yoni Tantra,* written in Oriyā are also found in Orissa. J.A. Schoterman[145] informs,

> To our knowledge there exist only two other manuscripts of the *Yoni Tantra,* which were, however, inaccessible to us. They are included in the "Descriptive Catalogue of Sanskrit Manuscripts of Orissa, vol. V)," compiled by Śrī Mahesh Prasad Dash, Curator of the Orissa State Museum (Bhubaneswar, 1965). As far as the text of the two MSS is reproduced in the catalogue, they show some variant readings not accounted for in the MSS we have used. The first MS No. T.35(b) is written on palm-leaf in Oriyan Script: it is complete in eight chapters, and was probably written in

144. J.A. Schoterman, *op. cit.,* Manohar, New Delhi, 1980, pp. 32-33.
145. *Ibid.,* 1980, pp. 38-39.

> the eighteenth century AD according to the catalogue. The second MS No. T/9 (c), is also written on palm-leaf in Oriyan script. It is, however, incomplete: the last *paṭala* is omitted. According to Śrī Mahesh Prasad Dash, it was written in the eighteenth century. The most significant fact with regard to this second MS is its title. In the catalogue this MS is called *Yoginī Tantra*, a name given by the text itself (*iti yoginī tantre prathamaḥ paṭalaḥ*, etc.). From the lines quoted in the catalogue, however, it becomes evident that the text is actually the *Yoni Tantra*, and not the *Yoginī Tantra*.

With this information it can be surmised that the composition of the *Yoni Tantra* was done in late medieval and early modern period, within last five hundred years. *Yoni Tantra* seems to be a development of *Yoginī Tantra* text, because according to a earlier tāntric-yogic text, the *Haṭha Yoga Pradīpikā:*,[146]

> If a woman practises *vajroli* and saves her *rajas* and the man's *bindu* by thorough contraction, she is a *yoginī*.
>
> — verse 99, chapter 3

While dealing about the ritual of the *yoni pūjā*, J.A. Schoterman[147] states,

> As we have seen, the main purpose of performing the *yoni pūjā* in that *Yoni Tantra* is the production of the *yoni tattva*. The *Yoni Tantra* nor the *Bṛhadyoni Tantra* explain how the *sādhaka* is supposed to extract this *yoni tattva* from the *yoni* of his Śakti. Probably this is accomplished by means of the *vajroli-mudrā* (cf. (i) *Śiva Saṁhitā*, IV, 52 ff, (ii) *Haṭha Yoga Pradīpikā*, III, 82-89, and (iii) D.N. Lorenzen, *The Kāpālikas and Kālāmukhas*, New Delhi, 1972, p. 96).

This discussion shows that both the tāntric texts, *Yoginī Tantra*, and *Yoni Tantra*, are concerned practically with the *yoga* of sexual transformation particularly with the *vajrolī haṭha yoga-mudrā*. *Vajrolī-mudrā*, as earlier discussed, is a "thunderbolt attitude"

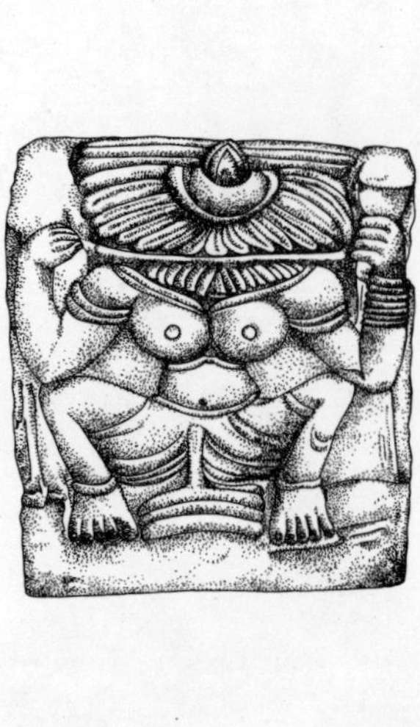

146. *HYPBS*, Munger, 2nd edn., 1993, p. 362.
147. J.A. Schoterman, *op. cit.*, 1980, pp. 28-29.

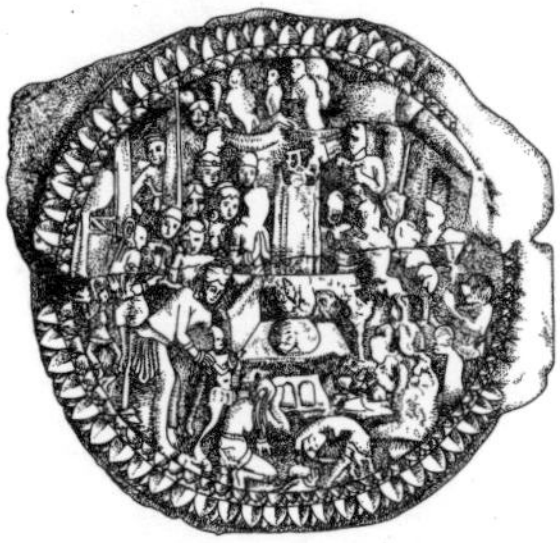

in which the muscles of male sexual organ and lower urinary tract are contracted, redirecting sexual energy upwards.

Sahajolī-mudrā is the *haṭha yoga* practice of *vajrolī* by a woman, involving contraction of the lower urinary muscles.

Central Mahānadī valley consists of Sonepur, Bolaṅgīr, Nuāpāḍā and Kālāhāṇḍī districts in Orissa province. The author's field survey has reveiled finds of eight *yonis* in Nuāpāḍā district. One of them consists of *yoni* triangle *yantra* with a *bindu* (dot) at the centre, which is the *bhairavī yantra*. The earliest *yoni* among these findings is the naturally formed *yoni*, under a bamboo thicket and worshipped as "Dwārsani," near Pātālgaṅgā site. These finds prove that the *yoga* of sexual tranformation was discovered in this region because here we find the earliest concepts of *yoga* like the Paśupati line drawing with *sahasra-padma* head of a human figure in the rock art of Gurhāṇḍī in Kālāhāṇḍī district, and the yogic conception of trinity and creation in the rock art of Yogīmaṭh Donger in Nuāpāḍā district, which has been discovered by the author on 21st December, 1970.[148]

Stone sockets in two parts in semi-circular shapes are found at the Mohangiri site of Kālāhāṇḍī district (*Pl.* 16). They represent the union of male and female principals and their shape owes its origin to the Rock Art of Yogīmaṭh Donger (*Pl.* 1). Such a set of sockets has been discovered at Kharligarh site of Bolaṅgīr (*Pls.* 18 & 19) district and both these sets are preserved at Manikyapur Museum of Bhawanipatna. Two such sets are found within the dilapidated Śakti temple, on the left bank of the Udanti river, within Bargāon village area. One half of such a socket is found at Pātālgaṅgā site in Nuāpāḍā district. One such sockets set is discovered from layer III (early histroic phase) from Veerapuram in Guṅṭūr district of Andhra Pradesh, where it is interpreted as a votive *liṅga*.[149]

148. J.P. Singh Deo, *Cultural Profile of South Kośala*, Gyan Publishing House, New Delhi, 1987, p. 20.

149. T.V.G. Sastri, M.K. Bai & J.V.P. Rao, *Veerapuram*, Bhavani Printers,

→

These stone sockets are the earliest findings of the union of male and female principals. According to T.N. Mishra,[150] however, no representation of the sexual act has been reported in the art and ritual objects yielded by the Indus civilization. This proves that *yoga* of sexual transformation first developed in peninsular India and most emphatically in Nuāpāḍā region of the central right Mahānadī valley.

It has been already dealt that a *yoginī* is a lady, who practices the *yoga* of sexual transformation. Because of the popularity of this *yoga*, H.C. Das[151] states,

> Matsyendranāth in view of popularity of this cult gained over the period, systematised and expounded it in this cult gained over the period, systematized and expounded it in his famous work *Kaulayānanirṇaya*, which has become the authoritative text of the cult.

According to R.P. Mishra,[152] the concepts of *yoginī*s in India began to grow in the lap of Śāktism from the sixth century AD onwards. . . . *Ādipīṭha* of 64 *yoginī*s is with the Someśvara-*liṅga*, as decribed in the *Yoginī Tantra*, which is probably a work of the eleventh century AD.[153] As Someśvara Temple[154] is found at Rānīpur-Jharial site of Bolaṅgīr district, it may be accepted that the first 64 *yoginī* temple was built at Rānīpur-Jharial site and from here this cult spread to different parts of India and abroad.

The *summum bonum* of the spiritual yogic concept of both

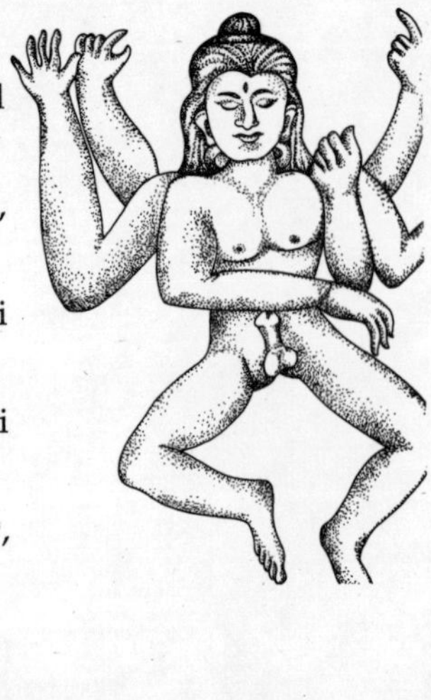

→ Hyderabad, 1984, passim.

150. T.N. Mishra, *Impact of Tantra on Religion and Art*, D.K. Printworld (P) Ltd., New Delhi, 1997, p. 101.

151. H.C. Das, *Tāntricism: A Study of Yoginī Cult*, Sterling Publishers, New Delhi, 1981, p. 3.

152. R.P. Mishra, *Fragments of Indian culture* (*Ranipur-Jharial*), Punthi Pustak, Kolkata, 1995, p. 203.

153. R.P. Mishra, *Fragments of Indian culture* (*Ranipur-Jharial*), Punthi Pustak, Kolkata, 1995, pp. 207-08.

154. Dipakranjan Das, *Temples of Orissa: The Study of a Sub-style*, Agamkala Prakashan, Delhi, 1982, pp. 26-29.

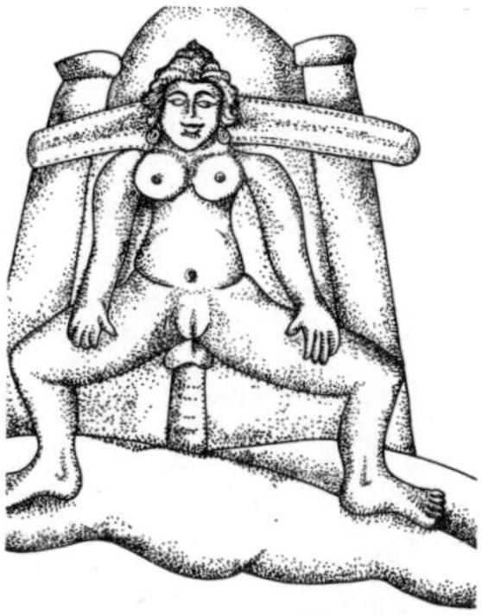

the *Yoginī Tantra* and the *Yoni Tantra,* is the *yoga* of sexual transformation or from sex to super-consciousness. So, it seems that both these *tantra*s originated and developed in the central right Mahānadī river valley and gradually shifted to Bengal, Cooch Bihar, Kāmākhyā, coastal Orissa and other parts.

The country of Koca, on the *paścima* (west) of Gaṅgā river, as mentioned in *Yoni Tantra* should have been Kośala country, i.e., South Kośala. It seems to be a spelling mistake or vague negligence of the unqualified writer of *Yoni Tantra,* which was composed under the Vaiṣṇava influence in the late medieval period. According to J.A. Schoterman,[155] the establishment of Vaiṣṇava Tāntric literature can be attributed to the late medieval period (thirteenth century AD and onwards), especially the post-Caitanya centuries.

So, it can be surmised that the central right Mahānadī river valley had contributed much to the origin of esoteric yogic *sādhanā*s, which spread to other parts and its glorious spiritual achievements are now forgotten, lost and bereft of recognition. Present period is the time of revival of Indian culture, i.e., Vedic culture, therefore such archaeological discoveries reflect the true or real importance of the soil where such serene spiritual *yoga*s were founded and developed.

With this background the author[156] is of the opinion that no definite periods of composition of the tāntric-yogic works are known, however the tāntric-*yoga* and *haṭha yoga* began to emerge in a systematic form in India, i.e., Bhārata, sometime within fifth-sixth centuries AD. It was the period of religious eclecticism.

---

155. J.A. Schoterman, *op. cit.,* 1980, p. 17.

156. (i) J.P. Singh Deo, *Tāntric Art of Orissa,* Kalpaz Publications, Delhi, 2001, pp. 201-03.

 (ii) N.K. Sahu, *Buddhism in Orissa,* Utkal University, Cuttack, 1958, passim.

 (iii) S.K. Moharana, *Tāntric Buddhism,* Aryan Books International, New Delhi, 2001, passim.

Probably for its survival, the Buddhism developed tāntric Buddhism.

Tāntric Buddhism was developed in the central left bank of the Mahānadī river, comprising Sambalpur area. King Indrabhūti of Sambalaka in Uḍḍīyāna was the founder of tāntric Buddhism, Vajrayāna and Kālacakrayāna, which was developed by Pito. Lakṣmīkara was the sister of king Indrabhūti, who married Prince Sevola, the son of king Jalendra of Laṅkāpurī, identified with modern Sonepur, situated on the central right bank of Mahānadī river, near its confluence with the tributary Tel river. Lakṣmīkara popularized Sahajayāna. As a whole, all branches of tāntric Buddhism deals with the *yoga* of sexual transformation and *haṭha yoga*.

This discussion proves that the central portion of both the right and left middle valley of the Mahānadī river had contributed to the development of tāntric *haṭha yoga* and the *yoga* of sexual transformation for the entire humanity, specially of the *kali-yuga* (*kali* age).

XII

Study of Śyāmākālī and Dakṣinākālī

Kālī is the primal manifestation of Śakti, the divine mother, destroyer of time, space and object, i.e., ignorance. Time is the great womb and hence has a feminine quality.[157] *Tantra* gives importance to the motherhood of *Brahman* (Godhood), because mother's love for children is more than the father's.

N.N. Bhattacharyya[158] states,

> In principle Kālī is one, and there can be nothing apart from her. But, according to the capability and desire of the worshipper, she may be conceived of in innumerable forms.

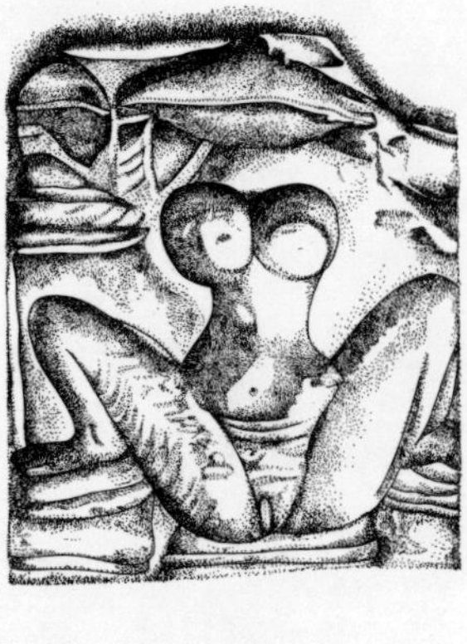

157. *TYATWG*, Delhi, 1996, p. 66.

158. N.N. Bhattacharyya, *History of the Tāntric Religion*, Manohar Publication, New Delhi, 1987, p. 349.

According to the *Toḍalatantra*, her well-known forms are eight — Dakṣiṇā, Siddhā, Guhyā, Śrī, Bhadrā, Cāmuṇḍā, Śmaśāna and Mahā. The *Mahākāla Saṁhitā* gives nine names, Dakṣiṇā, Bhadrā, Śmaśāna, Kalā, Guhyā, Kāmakalā, Dhanā, Siddhi and Caṇḍikā. The *Jayadrathayāmala* mentions Kālīkā, Dambara, Rākṣasī, Indivara, Dhanadā, Ramaṇī, Īśāna, Jīvā, Vīryā, Prājñā and Saptāṇa. The *Śaktisaṅgama* mentions Haṁsā and Vaśikaraṇā.

Of all these forms, Dakṣiṇākālī or Śyāmā is the most important. In her *dhyāna*, quoted in the *Tantrasāra*, she is described as having terrible appearance — a fierce face, four hands, untied hair, and a garland of severed heads, around the neck. In her lower and upper left hands, she holds a freshly severed head and a sword, and in the lower and upper right hands she exhibits *abhaya* and *varada* poses. Naked, dark as dense cloud in complexion, her body is streamed with blood which oozes from the garland of several heads that she wears. Two corpses serve as her ear-rings. Terrible in face and teeth, she has well developed breasts, her girdle is made of hands cut off from the bodies of corpses. Her face is smiling, but it is stained with blood falling from both corners of her mouth. She screams terribly. She lives at the cremation ground. She has three eyes resembling the orb of the rising sun. Her united hair hang to the right. She stands on the chest of Śiva lying as a corpse. She is engaged in *viparīta-rati* (inverted sexual intercourse also called *puruṣāyita*) with Mahākāla (Śiva),[159] (*Pl.* 29)

Śmaśāṇa Kālī or Śivā resembles Daksiṇākālī. She is also engaged in *viparīta-rati,* with Mahākāla (*Fig.* 8). According to the description of her in the *Tantrasāra*, her sacred thread is a snake, and physical features being more or less the same as those of Dakṣiṇākālī. She, however, is surrounded by jackals and *yoginī*s and is intoxicated as result of drinking wine. Siddhakālī is also a form of Dakṣiṇākālī.

159. *The Niruttara Tantra,* Paṭala-II, gives a slightly different version of this Dhyāna.

The *Tantrasāra* of Kṛṣṇananda Āgamavāgīśa is the most comprehensive and popular of the numerous digests known in India.[160] In the eighteenth century AD a famous *tāntrika yogī* and scholar by the name of Kṛṣṇananda Āgamavāgīśa came from Navadvīpa to Halisahar. He was a famous devotee of Kālī and had written the *Tantrasāra*.[161]

The iconography of Dakṣiṇa Kālī and Śyāmākālī are the same in *viparīta-rati* (*Pl.* 29). In the *haṭha yoga* practice of *vajrolī, sahajolī* and *uḍḍīyāna-bandha, viparīta-rati* takes place in the final stage and then only the *yoga* of sexual transformation takes place. Though *viparīta-rati* is not mentioned directly, it is taught in practice by tāntric *gurus* or masters.

While dealing with the forms of Kālī, Sarbeswar Satpathy,[162] describes,

> Of all these forms Dakṣiṇākāli or Śyāmākālī, as quoted in the *Tantrasāra,* has been described as having a terrible appearance, a fierce face, four hands, untied hair and a garland of severed heads around the neck. In her lower and upper left hands she holds a freshly cut severed head and a sword and in the lower and upper hands she exhibits *abhaya* and *varada* poses. Naked, dark as dense cloud in complexion, her body is streamed with blood which oozes from the garland of severed heads that she wears. Two corpses serve as her ear- rings. Terrible in face and teeth, she has well-developed breasts, her girdle is made of hands cut-off from the bodies of corpses. Her face is smiling, but it is stained with blood falling from both corners of her mouth. She screams terribly. She lives in the cremation ground. She has three eyes resembling the orb of the rising sun. Her untied hair hung to the right, she stands on the chest of Śiva lying as a corpse. She is engaged in *viparīta-rati* (inverted sexual

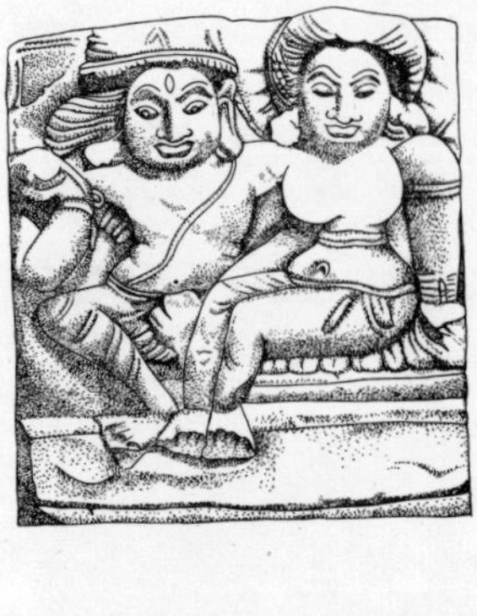

160. Editions in Bengali script by Rasikmohan Chatterji, Kolkata, 1880, Vangavasi Press, Kolkata, 1929.
161. U. Elizabeth Harding, *Kālī* (*The Black Goddess of Daksineswar*), Motilal Banarsidass, Delhi, 1998, pp. 215-17.
162. S. Satpathy, *Śakti Iconography in Tāntric Mahāvidyās*, Punthi Pustak, Kolkata, 1991, pp. 120-21.

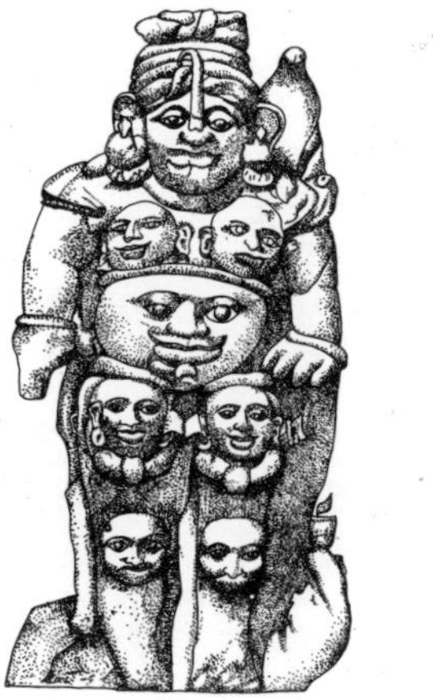

intercourse) called *puruṣāyita* with Mahākāla. This inverted sexual intercourse gives the clue that the *Mahāvidyā-upāsanā* symbolized the principle of involution, i.e., withdrawal of prapance to its source by means of yogic process.

Of all the forms of Kālī, Dakṣiṇa Kālī is very popular and is also known as adyākālī. Dakṣiṇa Kālī is worshipped at Purī, Pratāpapura and Kandadora village in Gañjam district; and Paikpāḍā in Raigarh district as *pārśva-devatā* in a niche of the Kedāreśvara Mahādeva temple at Ichhāpur in Kālāhāṇḍī district and also in the Tārā-Tāriṇī temple of Bhawanipatna, as a deity on the Baneswar temple campus at Bonai and many other places.

According to Chandra Shekhar Rath,*

> Even *tantra* has a prominent place in the system of rituals followed in the Jagannātha temple. The exponents of *tantra* consider Puri as a major *tantra kṣetra* where Vimala is Bhairavī and Jagannātha is Bhairava in the *tantra* School. By another interpretation Jagannātha who is gender-free is conceived as Dakṣiṇā Kālīkā.

According to H.C. Das,[163]

> The oldest shrine of Kālī in Orissa is located in the Puri town near the old palace of the Raja. She is locally known as Śyāmākālī and is worshipped according to the tāntric rites. She is four-armed standing in *pratyālīḍha* posture on the bosom of Śiva and engaged in cohabitation in a reverse manner. In her left hands she holds a sword and a severed human head, while the right hands are in *abhaya* and *varada* poses. She is three-eyed and is surrounded by howling jackals

* C.S. Rath, "Lord Jagannātha, A Legend and a Symbol — An Interpretation," in *Studies in the Cult of Jagannātha*, ed. K.C. Mishra, Institute of Orissan Culture, Bhubaneswar, 1991, pp. 7-15.

163. (i) H.C. Das, *Iconography of Śākta Divinities*, vol. I, Pratibha Prakashan, Delhi, 1997, pp. 20-21 & p. 26.

(ii) H.C. Das, *Daśamahāvidyās* (Oriya), S.B. Publications, Cuttack, 1983, p. 89.

> and vultures. This is a life size image exhibiting exquisite workmanship. The image on stylistic grounds can be attributed to the fifteenth century AD. A local tradition relates that the Gajapati Kapilendra Deva installed the Goddess after his successful expedition to the south. She conforms to the *dhyāna* of Dakṣiṇākālī.

According to the archaeological field survey conducted by the author, the oldest Śyāmākālī of present Orissa seems to be a monolithic Śyāmākālī found on the Tandel donger (mountain), near Dungaripali village of Nuāpāḍā district (*Fig.* 8). It seems to be a workmanship of the early medieval period. Śyāmākālī is worshipped at Kuśaṅga in Bolaṅgīr district. The iconography of Śyāmākālī is described in the *Śyāma Rahasya Tantra*.[164]

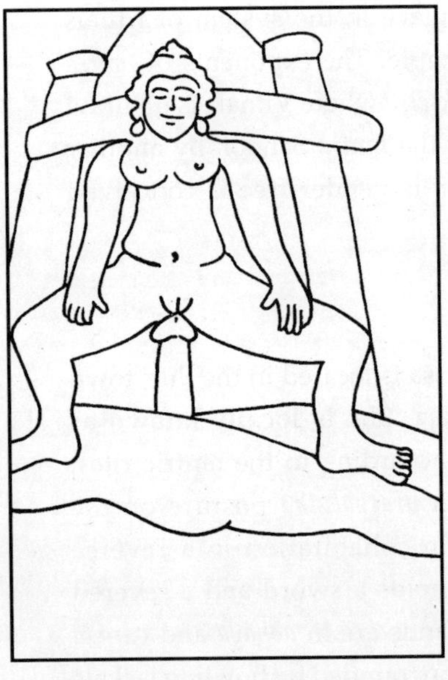

fig. 8. Monolithic figure of Śyāma Kālī in *viparīta-rati* (opposite sexual pose). Find spot: Tandel Donger (Hill) in village Dungripali, Nuāpāḍā district. Mediaeval period.

Further, Śiva and Śakti in sexual union or *viparīta-rati*, are found at:[165]

1. Ambikā Devī temple of Debakuṇḍa, in Mayūrbhañj

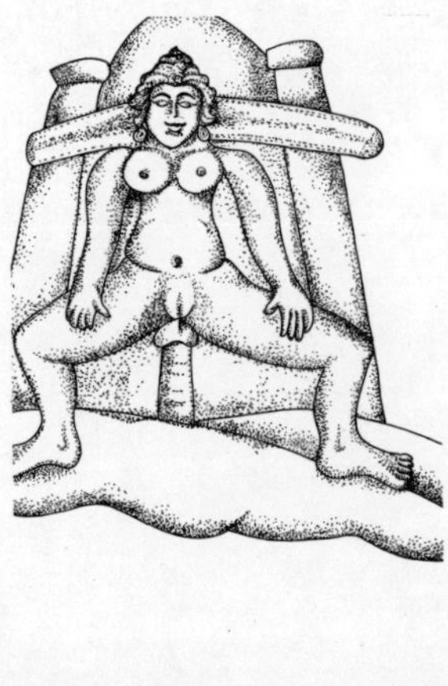

164. Pandit Harisadakarji Sastri (ed.), *Śyāma Rahasya Tantra* (Sanskrit), Sanskrit Pustakalaya, Haridwar, 1911, passim.

165. J.P. Singh Deo, "Tāntric Sculptures in Nuāpāḍā District, Orissa," *OHRJ*, vol. XLII, nos. 1 to 4, pp. 101-02.

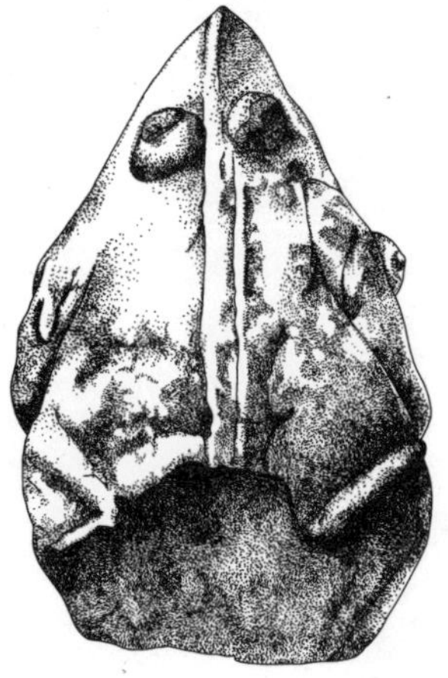

district, discovered by late Kumar Prafulla Chandra Bhañja Deo, a tāntric scholar.

2. Kālī temple at Pitala in Gañjam district.
3. Budharāja deity (Śiva and Śakti in union) at Aṭgāon, Bolaṅgīr district.
4. Sambaleśvarī Devī temple of Sonepur.

The poses of Śiva and Śakti in *viparīta-rati* or cohabitation in reverse manner, found in Orissa, denotes the *yoga* of sexual transformation, i.e., from sex to super-consciousness or divine *maithuna*, as prescribed in *haṭha yoga* and taught by *haṭha yogī* masters in an esoteric manner (*Pl*. 29 and *Fig*. 8).

XIII

Śūnya or Void in Yogic-Tāntric Śaivism of Mahānadī River Valley

Prabhat Mukherjee[166] has stated that the concept of Brahmā or Absolute Monism of the Upaniṣads was beyond comprehension. According to the Yājñyavalka, *ātman* is unknowable and transcendental. All that can be said of it, is *neti, neti*, i.e., no, no.

> Śūnyavāda or the theory of void is a contribution of the Nāgārjunīya philosophy. Void, according to Nāgārjuna, is not nothingness, but that which is devoid of all attributes by which we try to describe it. Thus it is neither existent or non-existent. Acyutānanda in his *Śūnya Saṁhitā* refers to Nāgānti Vidyā or Nāgārjunīya knowledge.
>
> In Orissa, in the eighth century, an esoteric system known as Vajrayāna, was superimposed on Mahāyāna which radically altered its characteristics. *Bodhī Citta* or perfect wisdom is attained by the knowledge of things as pure void. The concept

166. P. Mukherjee, "The theory of void according to Śūnya Saṁhitā," *Bharati-Utkal University Journal Humanities*, vol. IV, July, 1971, p. 1.

of *Śūnya* was identified with *Vajra* which is imperishable as void.

The Muslim conquest of Northern India gave a death blow to Buddhism. The Buddhist theory of void influenced Śaivism and Vaiṣṇavism, before Buddhism was totally lost in Hinduism.

The view of Prabhat Mukherjee that Śūnyavāda or the theory of void is a contribution of the Nāgārjuniya philosophy, can't be accepted.

Nāgārjuna[167] is assigned the period *circa* second century AD while Patañjali[168] is assigned the period second century BC. In the *Yoga Sūtras*, Patañjali has dealt with *śūnya*, i.e., void.

Paramahamsa Svāmī Satyananda Sarasvati[169] states,

In the *Yoga Sūtras* of Patañjali you will not come across the word *kuṇḍalini*, as this text does not directly deal with *kuṇḍalinī yoga*. However, not every saint, *ṛṣi* or teacher has referred to *kuṇḍalinī* by this name. *Kuṇḍalinī* is the subject-matter of *tantra*. When Patañjali wrote the *Yoga Sūtras* 2,600 years ago, it was during the period of Buddha and about four centuries before the great era of philosophers. At that time, *tantra* had a very bad reputation in India, because the gifts of *kuṇḍalinī*, the *siddhis*, were being misused for petty purposes and people were being exploited. Therefore, *tantra* and tantric terminology had to be suppressed, and in order to keep the knowledge alive, an entirely different language had to be adopted. . . . In *tantra*, the *sahasrāra* is the highest point of awareness, and in Patañjali's *Rāja Yoga*, the highest point of awareness is *nirvikalpa samādhi*. Now, if you compare the descriptions of the *sahasrāra* and *nirvikalpa samādhi*, you will find that they are the same. And if you compare the

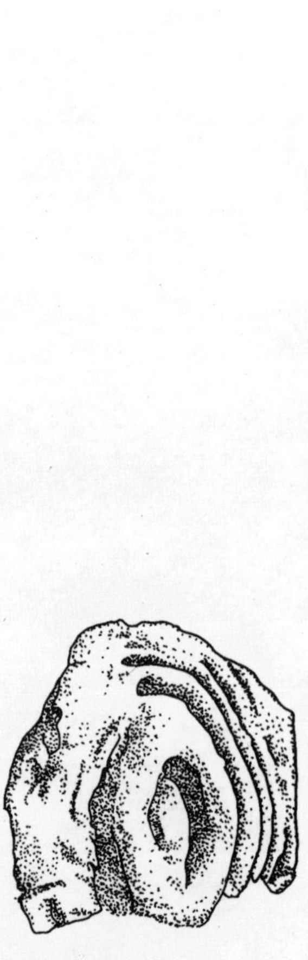

167. *THACOTIP*, vol. II, *The Age of Imperial Unity*, 1968, p. 210.

168. *Ibid.*, 1968, p. 107.

169. Svāmī Satyananda Saraswati, *Kuṇḍalinī Tantra*, Bihar School of Yoga, Munger, pp. 203-05.

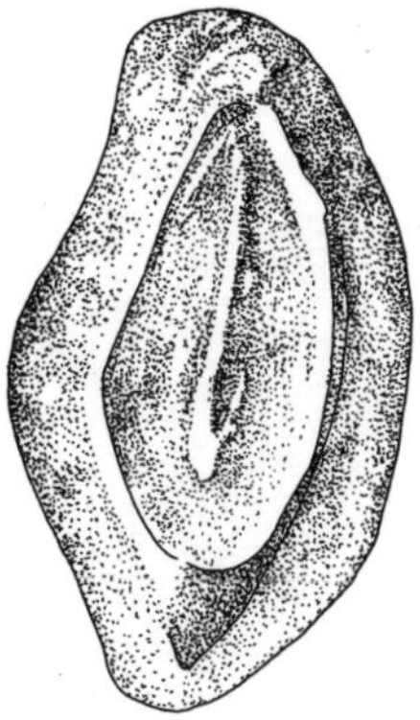

> experience of *samādhi* described in the *Rāja Yoga* with the descriptions of *kuṇḍalinī* awakening, you will find that they are also the same. It should also be noted that both systems talk of the same types of practices.

Kuṇḍalinī and *śūnya* or void are mentioned in the *Śiva Saṁhitā*[170] (chapter V, verse 127) thus,

> Owing to this (*vidyā*) man wanders in the circle of the universe; the *yogī*s, therefore, do not desire to keep up this circulation; all the *nāḍī*s are bound by eight knots: only this *kuṇḍalinī* can pierce these knots and pass out of the *brahmarandhra*, and show the way to salvation.

Śiva Saṁhitā[171] (chapter V, verse 161) mentions,

> The great void, whose beginning is void, whose middle is void, whose end is void, has the brilliancy of tens of millions of suns, and the coolness of tens of millions of moons. By contemplating continually on this, one obtains success.

During the second century AD, Nāgārjuna popularized the theory of Śūnyavāda or void. The existence of a line of the Sātavāhana kings holding sway over South Kośala (modern Chhattisgarh and the adjoining region) is suggested by a tradition recorded among others, by the Chinese pilgrim Hiuen Tsang. According to this tradition, when Nāgārjuna (*circa* second century AD) lived in a monastery built by Aśoka to the south of the capital city of Dakṣiṇa Kośala, the king of the land was So-to-po-ha, i.e., Sātavāhana.[172] This shows that Nāgārjuna had popularized the theory of *śūnya* or void, in the Dakṣiṇa Kośala area, which comprised the whole upper Mahānadī river valley and central India.

---

170. Srisa Chandra Vasu, *The Śiva Saṁhitā*, Munshiram Manoharlal Publishers Pvt. Ltd., New Delhi, 1990, p. 74.

171. Srisa Chandra Vasu, *The Śiva Saṁhitā*, Munshiram Manoharlal Publishers Pvt. Ltd., New Delhi, 1990, p. 79.

172. D.C. Sircar, "The Sātavāhanas and the Chedis," *THACOTIB*. vol. II, *The Age of Imperial Unity*, Bombay, 1968, p. 210.

About the fifth or sixth century AD *tantra* as a special religious or philosophical concept gradually came into use and *kuṇḍalinī tantra* became popular. According to Svāmī Śivānanda,[173]

> The spinal cord was called *suṣumnā nāḍī* by the *yogīs* of yore. . . . Within this *suṣumṇā* there is a *nāḍī* by name *vajra* which is lustrous as *sūrya* (sun) with rājasic qualities. Again, within this *vajra nāḍī* there is another *nāḍī*, called *citrā*. It is of *sāttvic* nature and of pale colour. The qualities of *agni*, *sūrya* and *candra* (fire, sun and moon) are the three aspects of *śabda-Brahman*. Here within this *citrā*, there is a very fine minute canal (which is known as *analis centralis*). This canal is known as *brahma nadī* through which *kuṇḍalinī*, when awakened, passes from the *mūlādhāra* to the *sahasrāra cakra*. In this centre exist all the six *cakras* (lotuses: viz., *mūlādhāra, svādhiṣṭhāna, maṇipūra, anāhata, viśuddhi* and *ājñā*).

Further Svāmī Śivānanda[174] states,

> When *kuṇḍalinī* is awakened it passes on from the *mūlādhāra* to the *sahasrāra* through all the *cakras*. At every centre to which a *yogī* directs the *kuṇḍalinī*, he experiences a special form of *ānanda* (bliss) and gains special *siddhis* (psychic powers) and knowledge. He enjoys the supreme bliss when *kuṇḍalinī* is taken to the *sahasrāra cakra*.
>
> The following are some other *cakras*: Ādhāra (another name of *mūlādhāra cakra*), Amrita, Ananda, Lalita, Balwana, Brahmadvara, Chandra, Dipaka, Karnamula, Gulhaha, Kuladipa, Kundali, Galabaddha, Kaladaada, Kaladhwara, Karangaka, Kalabhedra, Lalana, Mahotsaha, Manas, Talana, Mahapadma, Niradhara, Naukula, Prana, Soma, Triveni, Urdhvarandhra, Vajra, etc. Some of these names refer only to the six important *cakras* only. There are also many minor

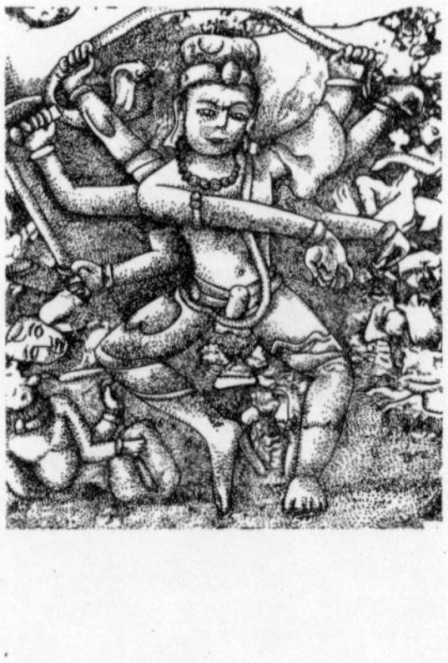

---

173. Svāmī Sivananda, *Kuṇḍalinī Yoga*, The Divine Life Society, Sivanandanagar, 1971, pp. 36-37.

174. Svāmī Sivananda, *Kuṇḍalinī Yoga*, The Divine Life Society, Sivanandanagar, 1971, pp. 46-47.

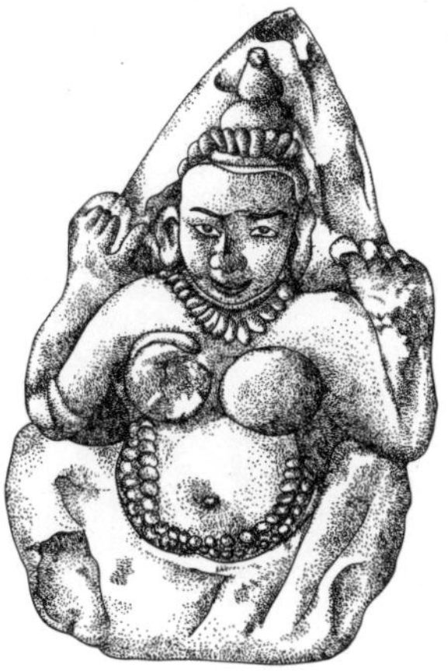

cakras. Some *haṭha yogī*s say, that there are 21 minor *cakras* besides 13 major *cakras* and some other *haṭha yogī*s hold that there are 49 *cakras*, while the ancient *yogī*s taught that there are 144 *cakras*. *Talana cakra* with its 12 red petals is located near the base of the palate and the *manas cakra* with its six petals closely associated with sensations, dreams and astral travelling.

Besides the *cakras mūlādhāra, svādhiṣṭhāna, maṇipūra, anāhata, viśuddha, ājñā, brahmarandhra* and *sahasrāra*, Svāmī Śivānanda[175] mentions of the *lalana cakra* and states:

> *Lalana cakra* is situated at the space just above the *ajñā* and below the *sahasrāra cakra*. 12 *yoga nāḍī*s emanate from this centre. The vibrations that are made by the 12 *nāḍī*s are represented by the Sanskrit letters: *ha, sa, kṣa, ma, la, va, ra, ya, ha, sa, kha* and *phrem*. It has *OṀ* as its *bīja*. At this centre the *yogī* concentrates on the form of his *guru* and obtains all knowledge. This has control over the 12 pairs of nerves that proceed from the brain to different sense organs.

Many yogic compositions have been lost. In the Nātha tradition, the most important literature on *yoga*, which is surviving, is the *Haṭha Yoga Pradīpikā* composed by *yogī* Swātmārāma, a disciple of Gorakhanāth.

In *Haṭha Yoga Pradīpikā*[176] (chapter 4, verse 10), it is mentioned that after *kuṇḍalinī* is roused, *prāṇa* rests in void (*śūnya*). Svāmī Muktibodhānanda Sarasvatī gives an illuminating commentary thus:

> विविधैरासनैः कुंभैर्विचित्रै करणैरपि ।
> प्रबुद्धायां महाशक्तै प्राणः शून्ये प्रलीयते ॥ १० ॥
>
> when the Mahā Śakti is aroused by the various *āsanas*, *prāṇāyāmas* and *mudrās*, the *prāṇa* dissolves into *śūnya*.

---

175. Svāmī Sivananda, *Kuṇḍalinī Yoga*, The Divine Life Society, Sivanandanagar, 1971, pp. 61-62.

176. *HYPBS*, Munger, 1993, p. 432.

Śūnya is void, but it is not a state of nothingness. It is a very deep and dynamic state of consciousness. It is the cause and origin of that which constitutes the manifest universe. It is *bindu* or the nucleus. According to Patañjali's *Yoga Sūtras*, *śūnya* is the step before the final *samādhi*. The word *śūnya* is used generally to describe the unfolding process between *asmita samādhi* and *nirvāṇa*. *Śūnya* also describes the state of *asamprajñāta samādhi* or the negative phase of *samādhi*. Just as the word *samādhi* describes the range of super-consciousness. So *śūnya* describes all the negative phases of *samādhi* in which there is unconscious super-consciousness. Awareness of the object, onlooker and looking are absorbed into one, the symbol shines in the consciousness, but there is no consciousness of it. That awareness is held by the subtle existence of *vāsanā* in the causal body or unconscious mind. The *Vijñānabhairava Tantra* states that: "O Goddess, if one after casting one's gaze on some object, withdraws it slowly and eliminates the knowledge of that object along with the thought and impression of it, he abides in *śūnya* the void." (*dhāraṇā* 95, verse 120) At this point of *samādhi* you become totally helpless.

According to Buddhism there are four types of *śūnya* which are described as: 1. phenomena and *śūnya*, 2. clearness and *śūnya*, 3. bliss and *śūnya*, 4. consciousness and *śūnya*. However, the Mahāyāna Buddhism has categorized *śūnya* into 18 stages: 1. *śūnya* of internal sensory response, 2. *śūnya* of external sensory perception, 3. *śūnya* of both internal and external sensory stimuli, 4. *śūnya* of *śūnya*, 5. the great *śūnya* of space, 6. real *śūnya*, 7. compounded *śūnya*, as of the universe, 8. uncompounded *śūnya* of the unmanifest, 9. infinite *śūnya*, 10. beginningless *śūnya*, 11. remainderless *śūnya*, 12. natural *śūnya*, 13. *śūnya* of phenomena, 14. *śūnya* of prediction, 15. *śūnya* of non-thought, 16. *śūnya* of immateriality, 17. *śūnya* of reality, 18. *śūnya* of non-substantiality of reality. This is a very involved classification compared to the yogic definition in which there are three distinct stages, which intercept and come after *vitarka samādhi*, *vicāra samādhi* and *asmita samādhī*.

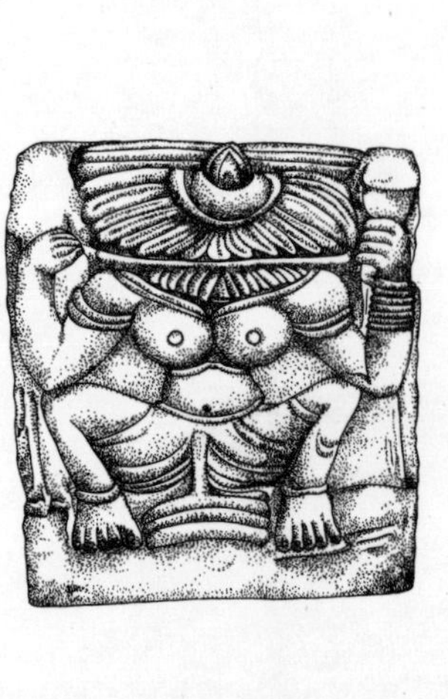

As the *Haṭha Yoga Pradīpikā* is a literature of Nāthism, it can

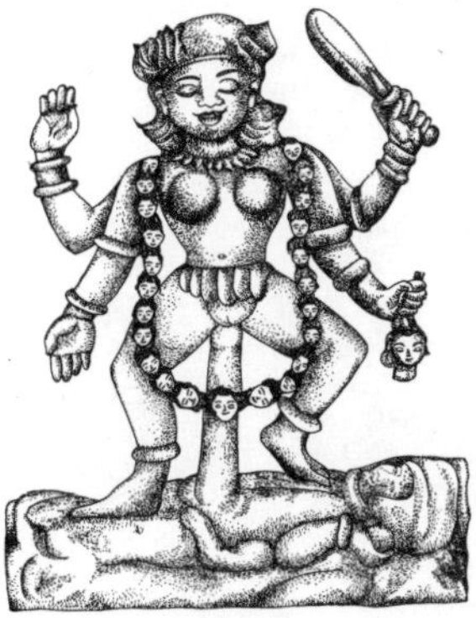

be claimed that the theory of *śūnya* or void had become popular in the yogic Śaiva *tantra*, in the early medieval period, which followed in the Vaiṣaṇva *tantra* later.

Śaivism was popular in the South Kośala region historically from the fourth century AD. An image of Śiva assigned to the fifth century AD is found at Malhār site. One huge *liṅga* inside a temple mound, with a fragmentary inscription of fourth century AD has been discovered in the Maraguḍa valley. The eight-handed Naṭarāja image of Śiva found at Sirpur dates back to the fifth century AD (*Pl.* 25) and an another eight-handed Naṭarāja found at Āsanapaṭ belongs to the sixth century AD (*Pl.* 26). Tāntric Śaivism emerged as a triumphant faith enjoying royal patronage from the time of Mahāśivagupta Bālārjuna for an unbroken period of four centuries in the Mahānadī river valley. Mahāśivagupta Bālārjuna was a great patron of Mattamayūra Śaivism, whose reigning period is assigned within *circa* AD 595-655.[177]

In recent years Malhār plates of Śivagupta, dated year 57 has been traced. Ajay Mitra Shastri[178] informs that Śivagupta built the temple of Bāleśvara-bhaṭṭāraka and for the maintenance of the penance grove (*tapovana*) attached to it, he placed the above-mentioned villages at the disposal of the illustrious revered Bhīmasoma, a pupil of the illustrious Tejasoma and a grand pupil of the illustrious *guru* Rudrasoma. Rudrasoma belonged to the line of teachers who descended from the illustrious Lakulīśanātha who himself was born in the brāhmaṇa family of Somasarman and was initiated with the *mahāvrata*. It is said that 66 incarnations of Śiva appear in various *yugas* for the welfare of the world and that Lakulīśa as an incarnation of Śiva appeared in the *kali* age. There is also a

---

177. S.R. Nema, *Political History of the Somavaṁśī Kings of South Kośala and Orissa*, Oriental Publishers, New Delhi, 1978, p. 135.

178. Ajay Mitra Shastri, *Inscriptions of the Śarabhapuriyas, Pāṇḍuvaṁśīs and Sōmavaṁśīs*, Part II, Motilal Banarsidass, Delhi, 1995, pp. 380-81.

mention of the eight forms of Śiva. A perpetual grant was made to Bhīmasoma to meet the expenses of sacrifices, initiatory rites, preaching and residence of his pupils and grand-pupils (i.e., the line of Śaiva ascetics emanating from him) and of the repairs of the temple.

Images of Lakulīśa are found in the sculptural art of temples at Bhubaneswar. These informations clearly shows that the whole Mahānadī river valley was influenced by Lakulīśa Śaivism and Mattamayūra Śaivism till the late medieval period, when yogic-tāntric Śaivism became popular because of the theory of *śūnya* or void.

XIV

Study on Traditions of Seven Tāntric Maidens and "Sasisena Kāvya"

In the central right valley of the Mahānadī river, tāntric concepts gradually developed in *yoni* worship, the union of male and female principals; and the *yoginī* cult, the esoteric *yoga* of sexual transformation, developed the tradition of seven tāntric maidens; and *Sasisena Kāvya* originated in the Patnagarh and Sonepur regions.

N.K. Sahu[179] states that Patnagarh has been known as Kaunri Patna or Kumari Patna ever since the seven tāntric maidens who lived in this township for sometime had practised the esoteric rites. These maidens were popularly known by their assumed names Gangi Gauduni, Sua Teluni, Jananadei Maluni, Netai Dhobani, Luhukuti Luhuruni, Sukuti Chamaruni and Patrapindhi Saharuni. There are popular tales and traditions in western Orissa, depicting the occult practices and tāntric activities of these maidens. They seem to be the followers of Lakṣmīkara, who propounded Sahajayāna Buddhism in western Orissa in the ninth century AD. As late as the sixteenth century

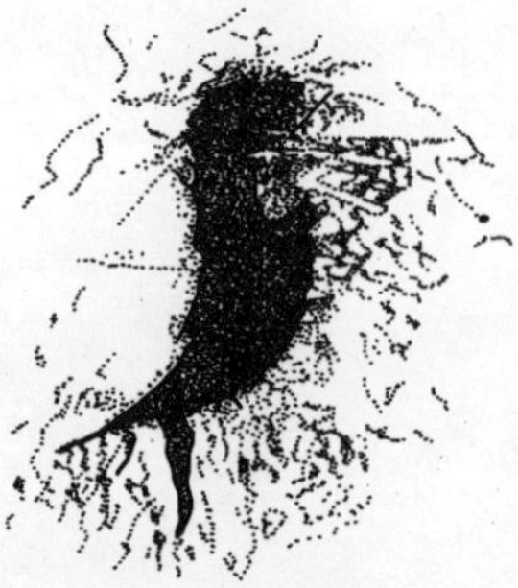

179. N.K. Sahu (State editor), *Gazetteer of India, Orissa, Bolāngīr*, Nilamani Senapati (General editor), Cuttack, 1968, p. 489.

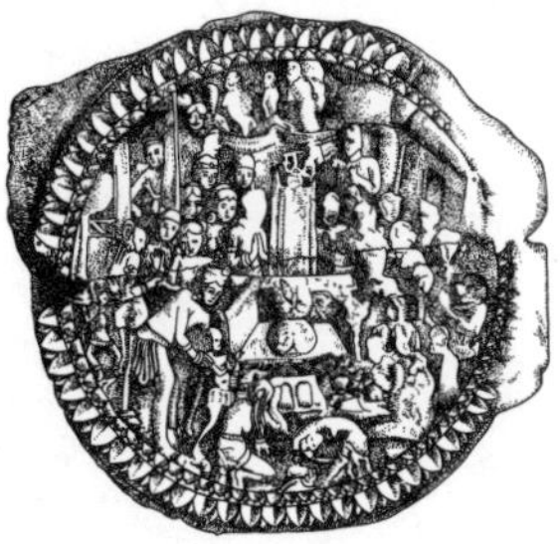

AD the Patna Kingdom was known as Kaunri Patna after the name of the headquarters' town of that name, as known from the *Nirguṇa Māhātmya* of the poet Caitanya Dāsa.

N.K. Sahu considers the famous seven tāntric maidens of Patnagarh area to be the followers of Lakṣmīkara, who propounded Sahajayāna Buddhism. But this is not so as it seems that the seven tāntric maidens of Patnagarh area continued the secret esoteric tāntric rituals of *yoga* of sexual transformation and of the *yoginīs* which had originated earlier in the central right Mahānadī valley. It seems N.K. Sahu is ignorant of the development of the *yoga* of sexual transformation or *yoga* which leads from sex to super-consciousness in this locality and its inclusion in Hinduism or Vedic culture, as expounded in the *Bṛhadāraṇyaka Upaniṣad* (vi, 4.2-3 lines) and the *Śukla Yajurveda*. This *yoga* of sexual transformation became very popular in the early medieval period, as revived by Mattamayūra Śaivism.[180]

Netai Dhobani was the spiritual and tāntric *guru* (master) of the great Gaṅga king Coḍagaṅgadeva of Kaliṅga. This is mentioned in the *Mādalāpāñjī* and its archaeological evidences are the two images of Anantavarma Coḍagaṅgadeva, the Gaṅga Gajapati and Netai Dhobani, in a small miniature temple in Chuḍaṅga Sai of Purī.[181]

P.M. Nayak[182] states that Jagabandhu Singh[183] in the *Pracina Utkala*, tells the story of Coḍagaṅgadeva, who saw Netai Dhobani at Sonepur on his way to coastal Orissa, cooking one of her feet in the burning hearth and her child in the boiling

180. R.P. Mishra, "Mattamayūra Śaivism in Orissa," *Culture and Collections*, ed. Ramprasad Mishra, Punthi Pustak, Kolkata, 1996, pp. 101-39.

181. Anirudha Das, "The Madala Panji," *OHRJ*, vol. XIV, nos. 3 & 4, pp. 6-7 and two sketches of the Images of Chudanga Sai of Puri.

182. P.M. Nayak, "A Fresh look at Sasisena Kavya," *Confluence*, vol. I, ed. P.M. Nayak, Registrar, Sambalpur University, Burla, 1992, passim.

183. Jagabandhu Singh, *Prachina Utkala*, Puri, 1929, p. 101 (Oriya).

cauldron. Even today in Sonepur the washerman worship Netai, the Mālīs worship Madana and the Lohārs worship Sukuti as their tutelary deities. Pandit Gopinath Panigrahi quotes Ramchandra Panigrahi, an old brāhmaṇa of Sonepur, who used to locate the house of Madana and her flower garden, close to the west of the present palace.

N.K. Sahu,[184] while dealing about Sonepur, states:

> A work called *Sasisena* written by Pratap Ray, describes Jnanadei Maluni, one of the seven tāntric maidens, as a resident of Sonepur. Sasisena was the daughter of some feudatory chief of western Orissa, who fell in love with Ahimāṇikya, the son of a *dewan*, when both of them were reading in the school. After their marriage, which was secretly performed with the help of the teacher who officiated as priest, they came and lived at Sonepur, which was also then known by its second name Kamitapura. Jnanadei Maluni, also known as Madana Maluni the tāntric maiden, who was then living in Sonepur, was charmed by the beauty of Ahimāṇikya and so once when he went out alone to the bazar, she induced him to come to her place where he was transformed into a lamb by dint of her esoteric art. This tāntric maiden used to reconvert him into human form in the night, while at day time the unfortunate man remained as a lamb. In the meantime, Sasisena having lost her husband remained in the guise of a man, so that she could not be molested by malevolent persons and could search her husband everywhere in the town. She subsequently got an appointment under the Raja of Sonepur and became a soldier in the army. Very soon she earned reputation for her courage and heroism, particularly when she once killed a man-eater tiger at the risk of her life. The Raja being pleased with Sasisena desired to give his daughter in marriage to her. As Sasisena could not reveal her identity she was forced by circumstances to marry the daughter of the Raja. She, however, described her misfortune to the newly married girl and the latter being full of sympathy for her, did not reveal

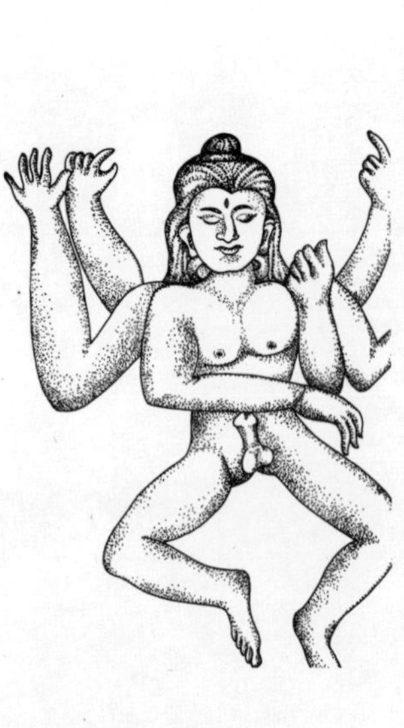

184. N.K. Sahu, *op. cit.*, 1968, pp. 494-95.

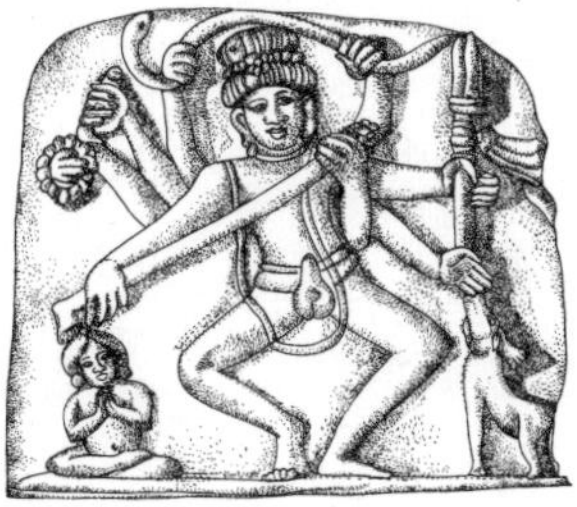

anything about her identity. Both of them searched for Ahimāṇikya by all possible means. They excavated a tank at a place in the west of Sonepur town and constructed four temples on the four sides of the tank. A grand festival took place on the day of consecration of the tank. Jnanadei Maluni came to see the festival at night with Ahimāṇikya who was then in human form. Ahimāṇikya could recognise Sasisena and not being able to contact her, he wrote a few lines on the wall of one of the temples by a piece of chalk informing her that he had been taken captive and transformed as a lamb by the tāntric maiden Jnanadei Maluni. Sasisena came to know everything about her husband from the writing. She told the Raja that she would sacrifice some lambs before the Goddess Bhagavati and that the lamb possessed by Jnanadei Maluni be brought for that purpose. The Raja at her request brought Ahimāṇikya, who was then in the form of lamb, from Jnanadei Maluni. It was then known that the lamb was no other than Ahimāṇikya and by the order of the Raja, Jnanadei Maluni brought him back to human form. Sasisena and Ahimāṇikya met together and on the desire of the Raja both his daughter and Sasisena became the wives of Ahimāṇikya.

This tradition is widely current in Sonepur even to this day. A place on the western part of Sonepur town where the reunion of Sasisena and Ahimāṇikya is believed to have taken place, is now known as Sasisena Tikra. A tank near about is also named as Sasisena Bandha. A temple without any opening has been constructed in the Sasisena Tikra by a former king of Sonepur and has been dedicated to the memory of Sasisena.

On the top of the Sasisena temple in Sonepur, lizards are designed, descending downwards from the *āmalakaśilā* of the temple. Lizard signifies the *nāsikāgra dṛṣṭi*, which is a *haṭha* yogic practice involving gazing at the nose tip. This proves that the esoteric seven tāntric maidens were practising esoteric tāntric *haṭha yoga*. Pratap Rai is the author of *Sasisena Kāvya*. The period of Pratap Rai is uncertain. The stories of seven tāntric maidens and Sasisena, are popular in the folk tales of Assam. P.M.

Nayak[185] asserts that the story of Sasisena is widely prevalent in the eastern States of India. These facts and the discussions shows that the *yoni tantra*, and the *yoga* of sexual transformation had shifted from the central Mahānadī river valley to the eastern States of India and especially to the Kāmākhya and Assam areas.

In-between Ānandapur and Ghaṭagāon Tāriṇī villages of Keoñjhar district, a High School named "Patrasauruni," exists.[186] It seems the occult teaching of "Patrapindhi Sauruni" was popular in Keoñjhar district region, among some followers. The name of "Patrasauruni" High School in Keoñjhar district, seems to be the last remnant of the tradition of the seven tāntric maidens of the central right Mahānadī valley before it went to the Assam region in Eastern India.

XV

Yoga of Sexual Transformation in Jagannātha cult

Purī as the headquarter of the Jagannātha cult has developed as a cosmopolitan, spiritual and yogic religious centre. K.C. Mishra[187] mentions that Jagannātha is worshipped at present not only by the ten-syllabled *mantra, oṁ gopījanavallabhāya svāhā*, but also by the 18-syllabled one, *oṁ klīṁ kṛṣṇāya govindāya gopījanavallabhāya namaḥ*. This *oṁ* or *praṇava* is reminiscent of the Vedic strand: *klīṁ* is indicative of the tāntric one, while the other aspects of the *mantra*s emphasize the Purāṇic and Vaiṣṇavite forms. The sign of co-ordination is noticeable not only in such *mantra*s but also in other characteristic forms of the composite worship.

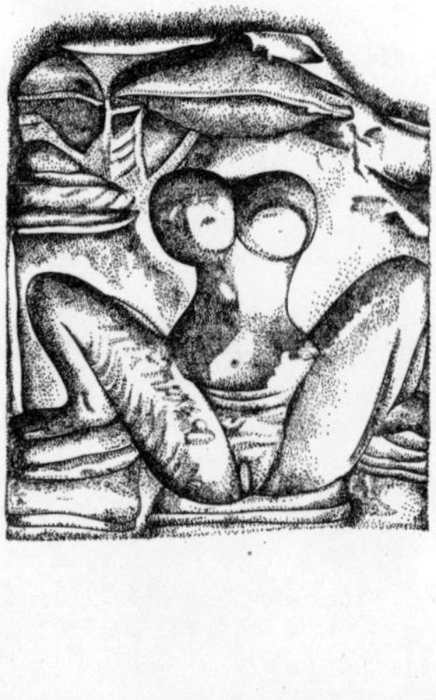

185. P.M. Nayak, "A Fresh look at Sasisena Kavya," *Confluence*, vol. I, ed. P.M. Nayak, Registrar, Sambalpur University, Burla, 1992, pp. 69-76.

186. This information was supplied by Anthropologist Gitanjali Nayak of Puri in AD 2003.

187. K.C. Mishra, *The Cult of Jagannātha*, Firm K.L. Mukhopadhyay, Kolkata, 1971, p. 144.

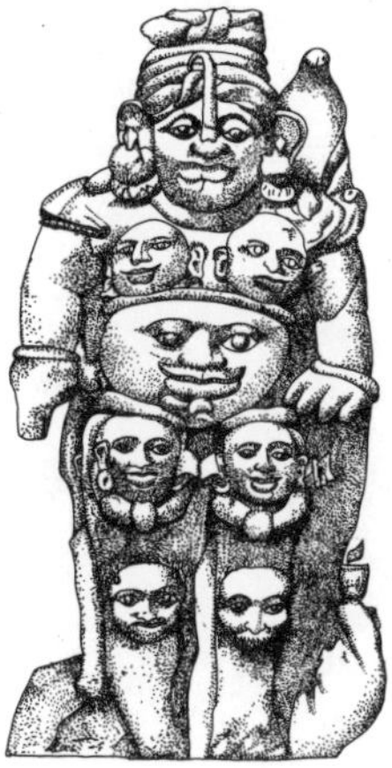

The modes of worship are partly Vedic, partly tāntric and partly Paurāṇic. The Vedic part consists of the veneration paid to the symbol *praṇava* — the symbol of Brahmā. The tāntric tradition evolved various *nyāsas*, such as *Ṣaḍaṅganyāsa*, *Keśavādinyāsa*, *Sṛṣṭistithisaṁhāranyāsa*, *Mātṛ-kānyāsa*, etc., *yantras* such as Śrī and Bhuvaneśvarī, and also *kriyās* (*mudrās*) and *bījamantras*. It is also to be noted that the yogic-tāntric system of impaling the *ṣaṭcakras* (*ṣaṭcakrabheda*) of the body is also given an important part in the mode of worship. The appropriate *dhyānas* and *mantras* propounded by the Paurāṇic tradition explain the form, the nature, the character and the power of the images. The inherent power of the images that are worshipped and meditated upon fulfils the desired object of the devotee according to his deserts.

The conception of Jagannātha, Balabhadra and Subhadra as well as Sudarśana seems to have originated from the yogic-tāntric system and developed into the Purāṇic and Vaiṣṇavite setting. Even though the images are seen in four different forms they are treated as one and the same, and that is why at the time of daily worship three priests simultaneously perform the rites according to the tradition.

About the *mantra* of Kālī, David Frawley[188] mentions:

Kālī's *bīja mantra* or single syllable is *krīṁ*, which is the power of action (*kriyā*). The simple repetition if this *mantra* can be used to worship her. The *mantra klīṁ* is also used in her worship or just simply the repetition of the name Kālī. She also possesses a longer *mantra* of twenty-two syllables.

krīṁ krīṁ krīm hūṁ hūṁ hrīṁ hrīṁ dakṣiṇe
kālike krīṁ krīṁ krīm hūṁ hūṁ hrīṁ hrīṁ svāhā!

Hūṁ is a *mantra* of wrath to ward off negativity. It also serves to enkindle the fire of spiritual knowledge and self-inquiry. *Hrīṁ* is the *mantra* of divine beauty, the descent of grace, purification and transformation. Dakṣiṇa is Kālī as the power of discernment which is both right thought and right action.

188. *TYATWG*, Delhi, 1996, pp. 71-72.

Kālikā is another form of the name Kālī. *Svāhā* is the *mantra* of consecration to the divine, particularly as the inner or spiritual fire of awareness.

Krīṁ is repeated three times followed by *hūṁ* twice and *hrīṁ* twice or a total of seven seed-syllables. *Krīṁ* thus emphasizes inner action, which generates the transformative force of *hūṁ*, which turns into the ecstatic power of *hrīṁ*. These seven syllables can be used by themselves as a *mantra* to Kālī.

The seer of the Kālī *mantra* is Mahākāla, Śiva as the great Lord of time. Only by becoming time can we gain the power of mind necessary to stand the transforming energy of Kālī. Along with the *mantra*, the *kālī yantra* can be used.

Another useful *mantra* for her is the *mantra* for Cāmuṇḍā, the fierce form of Kālī, from the story of the *Devī Māhātmya*.

oṁ aiṁ hrīṁ klīṁ cāmuṇḍāyai vicce svāhā

This *mantra* consists of the supreme word *oṁ* followed by the *mantras* for wisdom, Sarasvatī (*aiṁ*), for purification; Pārvatī (*hrīṁ*) for transformation, Kālī (*klīṁ*), and the *mantra svāhā*, which consummates the offering to Cāmuṇḍā. *Vicce* means cult, in the sense of cutting-off the head of the demon, that cut-off the head of the ego.

Pandit Harisadakarji Sastri[189] had edited the *Śyāma Rahasya Tantra* (Sanskrit) and from this literature, it is known that the *mantra* of Dakṣiṇa Kālī is :

krīṁ krīṁ krīṁ hūṁ hūṁ hūṁ hrīṁ hrīṁ dakṣiṇa kālīke
krīṁ krīṁ krīṁ hūṁ hūṁ hūṁ hrīṁ hrīṁ svāhā.

So, it can be claimed that even in *mantra* worship Lord Jagannātha is Kālī and Dakṣiṇa Kālī. In the iconography of Dakṣina Kālī, she is engaged in *viparītagati* (inverted sexual

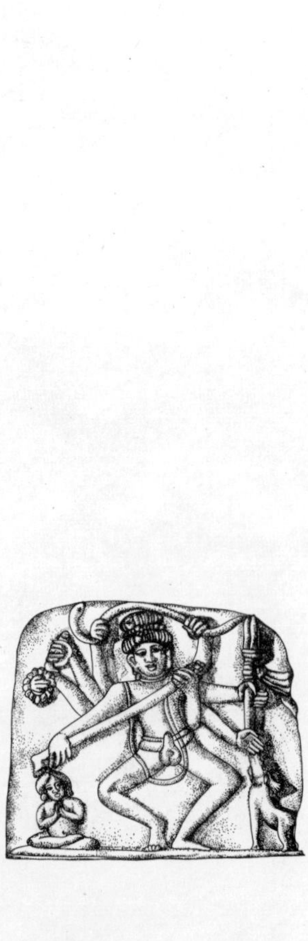

189. Pandit Harisadakarji Sastri (ed.), *Śyāma Rahasya Tantra* (Sanskrit), Sanskrit Pustakalaya, Haridwar, 1911, p. 3.

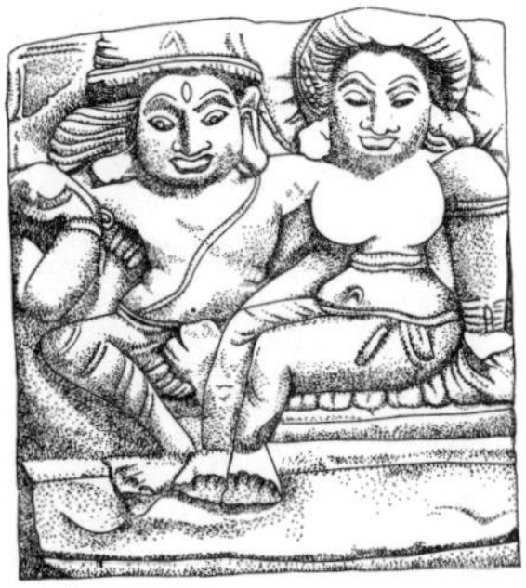

intercourse also called *puriṣāyita*) with Mahākāla (Śiva),[190] which is *haṭha yoga* or *yoga* of sexual transformation. Therefore, it can be claimed that the *haṭha yoga* of sexual transformation is practiced in the Jagannātha cult.

There are *yoginī* images in the Jagannātha temple at Purī. The *yoginī*s are regarded as guardian deities and there are ritual worship also. According to the *Haṭha Yoga Pradīpikā*,[191] a *yoginī* is a woman who practices *vajrolī*.

> If a woman practises *vajroli* and saves her *rajas* and the man's *bindu* by through contraction, she is a *yoginī*.
>
> — *Haṭha Yoga Pradipīkā*, verse 99, chapter 3

190. N.N. Bhattacharyya, *History of the Tāntric Religion*, Manohar, New Delhi, 1987, p. 349.

191. *HYPBS*, Munger, 2nd edn., 1993, p. 362.

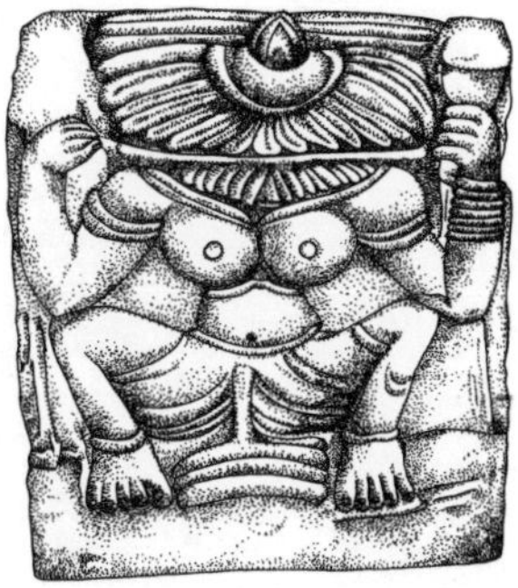

3

Mahānadī Valley was not Bereaved of Lajjā Gaurī Cult

SPIRITUAL yogic art expressions remain a riddle of Indian iconography. Inquiry, search or investigation of their meaning are difficult zetetic. Only through yogic fineness, one can solve the worth or estimation of a spiritual yogic art. One such most sophisticated symbolic image is of Lajjā Gaurī. Two Lajjā Gaurī sculptures discovered in Nuāpāḍā district of Orissa provoked the author to investigate their identity.

I

Carol Radcliffe Bolon[1] has done a comprehensive study of Lajjā Gaurī in Indian Art. She mentions that

> It should be noted that Lajjā Gaurī images were never worshipped throughout all of India; at least they are not known from all areas. They are known from the core area of India, but not from Bihar, Bengal, the far northern States of Punjab, Himachal Pradesh and Kashmir, nor from the southern State of Kerala, and only one odd example is found in Orissa. I suspect this lack of cultural dissemination in at least some of the areas that do not render Lajjā Gaurī images has to do with patterns of ancient population density. . . . The symbolism specific to the Lajjā Gaurī image may have been lost to general comprehension as early as the eleventh century.[2]

---

1. C.R. Bolon, *Forms of the Goddess Lajjā Gaurī in Indian Art*, Motilal Banarsidass, Delhi, 1997, passim.
2. *Ibid.*, 1997, p. 71.

In the upper Mahānadī valley, the Lajjā Gaurī sculptures are found at Malhār (Bilāspur district) which belong to *circa* ninth-tenth century AD, on the Jain temple of Araṅg (Raipur district) and many other sites. The author has discovered one Lajjā Gaurī image from the Kortipadar village area, (*Pl.* 21) which is now kept in his private possession at Khariar. Another Lajjā Gaurī image was discovered from the compound of Panchayet College at Komna, which is now preserved at Dr. N.K. Sahu Museum, of Sambalpur University, at Burla (*Pl.* 22). Both these sites are situated in Nuāpāḍā district.

Lajjā Gaurī cult is concerned with *Tantra*. *Tantra*-wise, the cult of mother attained supremacy among other gods and flourished in many forms under various names. These goddesses are differently named in the *Muṇḍakopaniṣad*, which belongs to the *Atharvaveda*.

R.K. Upadhyaya[3] states that religious scriptures of the Hindus have been traditionally classified into four distinct branches, namely, the Śruti, Smṛti, Purāṇa and Tantra. It is the Śruti from which is derived the authority of the last three varieties of sacred writings. In the event of conflict for supremacy amongst them, it is the Śruti that prevails. To tell the truth, it is the teaching of the Śruti that has been merely elaborated in the succeeding three varieties of religious treatises in order to confirm it for the respective ages (*yugas*). The *tantra* is esteemed as the fifth Veda and is superior to Smṛti and Purāṇa. And all *śāstras* are inferior to the Veda. Yet the religious practices, rites and ceremonies which have been prescribed in the *tantra* supersede the *vaidikācāra* in the present *kali* age. The *tantra* has revealed the heart of the Veda and in fact it is an integral part of it.

A genealogical list found in the *Mahābhārata* shows a number of names of deities like Mārici, Krodha, Kāla, Vinatā, Kadru, Kīrti, Lakṣmī, Dhṛti, Medhā, Puṣṭi, Śraddhā, Krivā, Buddhi, Lajjā, Mati,

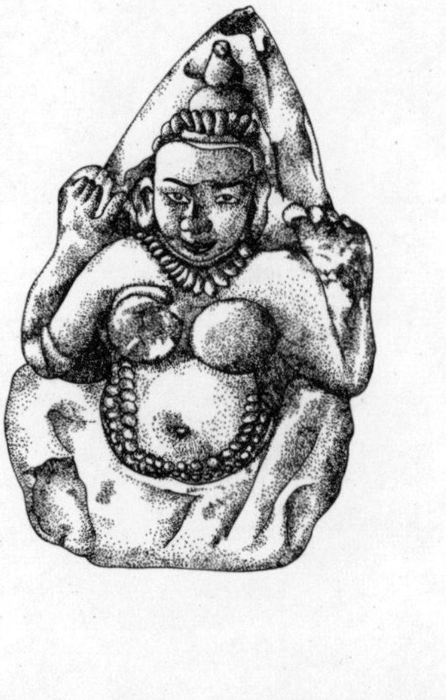

3. R.K. Upadhyaya, *The Concept of God in Śiva Tantra*, Jnananidhi Prakashan, Muzaffarpur, 1984, pp. 27-28.

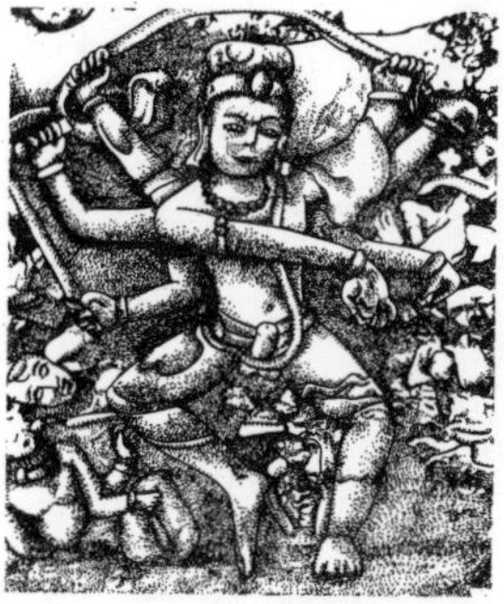

Kālikā, Krodhavaśā, etc.; they are treated as divine mothers giving birth to birds, beasts and human beings.[4]

C.R. Bolon[5] states that the *Viṣṇu Purāṇa* explains that Goddess Lajjā is modesty, personified. As one of Dakṣa's daughter. Lajjā became the wife of Dharma and the mother of a son named Vinaya. Vinaya is the personification of good behaviour. Gaurī means the brilliant one or the golden one, the wife of Śiva or of Varuṇa, the waters, the source of the world, the cosmic cow, the undifferentiated form before creation. The waters, the oceans and the fertilizing rains flow from her; she is the very source of life-giving water and of fertility.[6] The *Viṣṇu Purāṇa* is an early work composed most probably in the last quarter of the third or the first quarter of the fourth century AD.[7]

According to Balaram Srivastava,[8] Śakti, the embodiment of power, wisdom and capacity, thus became the mother *par excellence* who is Mahālakṣmī. She in the form of Durgā killed demons, as Devī revealed knowledge and as Yoganidrā sent all creatures to sleep.

> Śakti is also the embodiment of various virtues and abstract qualities, such as *cetanā* (consciousness), *buddhi* (intelligence), *nidrā* (sleep), *kṣudhā* (hunger), *chāyā* (shadow), *śakti* (energy), *tṛṣṇā* (thirst), *kṣānti* (patience), *jāti* (power of generation), *lajjā* (modesty), *śānti* (peace), *śraddhā* (faith), *kānti* (beauty), *lakṣmī* (prosperity), *vṛtti* (livelihood), *smṛti* (memory), *dayā*

---

4. Sarbeswar Satpathy, *Śakti Iconography in Tāntric Mahāvidyās*, Punthi Pustak, Kolkata, 1991, p. 26.
5. C.R. Bolon, *op. cit.*, Delhi, 1997, p. 64.
6. James Stutley & Margaret Stutley, *Harper's Dictionary of Hinduism*, New York, 1977, p. 96.
7. Rajendra Chandra Hazra, *The Purāṇas, The Cultural Heritage of India*, vol. II, The Ramakrishna Mission, Institute of culture, Kolkata, 1969, p. 257.
8. B. Srivastava, *Iconography of Śakti* (*A Study based on Sritattvanidhi*), Chowkhamba Orientalia, Vārāṇasī, 1978, p. 14.

> (compassion), *tuṣṭi* (contentment), *mātā* (motherhood), *bhrānti* (error, defection), *vyāpti* (all-pervasiveness), *citti* (mind), etc. All these are the metaphysical exposition and manifold manifestations of one energy.[9] This concept of the *Devī Māhātmya* greatly enhanced the prestige of the great mother and established her superiority over other gods and goddessess. In this text the great Goddess has been variously eulogised in the terms of ultimate[10] or universal mother (Jagatmātā or Jananimparā). This supreme mother (Jananimparā) in the *Devī Māhātmya* (I.55.) is no other than the universal nature. She is symbolized as the earth (*Mahiśvararūpa*, XI.4) which represents the great principle of universal motherhood and fertility not only of the visible world, but also as the mother of the whole creation (*Mātarjagatoo-Khilasya*, XI.2), the only support of the world (*Ādhārabhūta jagatstvamekā*, XI.3), etc., Ultimately she has been invoked as one who among all created beings stands firm in the form of mother.

In *Devī Māhātmya*, the reference of Lajjā is found. *Devī Mahātmya*[11] of the *Mārkaṇḍeya Purāṇa*, was composed in the late Gupta period, but certainly not later than AD 600.[12]

The *Kulārṇava Tantra* is one of the most important tāntric works. It was composed probably before AD 1,000.[13] In the thirteenth Ullāsa of the *Kulārṇava Tantra*, bonds of animality are given.[14] Pity, doubt, fear, shame (*lajjā*), disgust, family, disposition and caste, are the bonds; bound by these bonds,

9. *Devī Māhātmya*, V.12-33.
10. *Ibid.*, I.83.
11. J.P. Singh Deo, *Origin of Jagannāth Deity*, Gyan Publishing House, New Delhi, 1991, p. 63.
12. R.C. Hazra, "The Purāṇas," *op. cit.*, 1969, p. 246.
13. N.N. Bhattacharyya, *History of the Tāntric Religion*, Manohar, New Delhi, 1987, p. 72.
14. Ram Kumar Rai, *Kulārṇava Tantra*, Prachya Prakashan, Vārāṇasī, 1983, pp. 242-45.

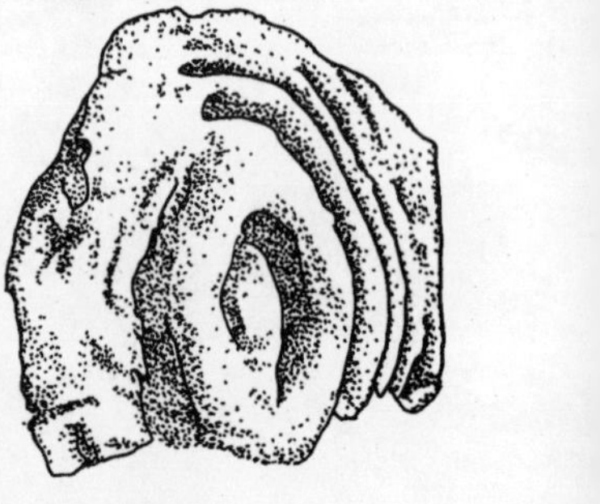

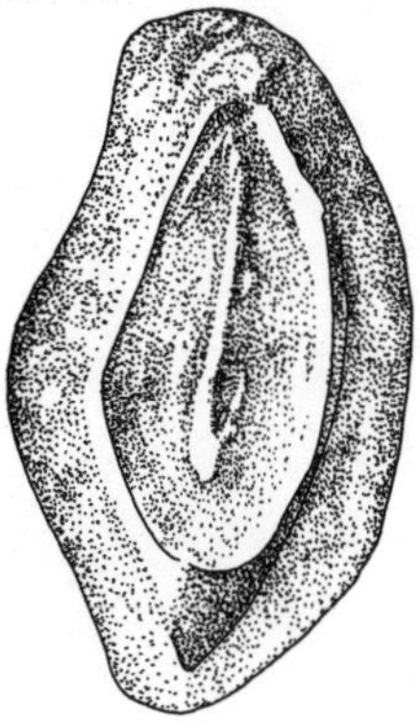

one is a *paśu* (animal). Freed from the bonds one is Śiva; he is the supreme *guru* who removes these bonds.[15]

Sir John Woodroffe[16] states,

> The *Kulārṇava Tantra* mentions eight primary bonds, *dayā* (that is pity as the feeling which binds, as opposed to divine compassion or *karuṇā*, *moha* (ignorance), *lajjā* (shame, which does not mean that a man is to be a shameless sinner but weak, wordly shame of being looked down upon for infringing, conventions and so forth), family (*kula*, which ceases to be a tie), *śīla* (here usage, convention) and *varṇa* (caste); for the enlightened is beyond all its distinctions). When, to take the Svāmī's example, Śrī Kṛṣṇa stole the clothes of the bathing *gopīs* or milkmaids and cowherds and made them approach him naked. He removed the artificial coverings which are imposed on man in the *saṁsāra*. The *gopīs* were eight, as are the bonds, and the errors by which the *jīva* is misled are the clothes which Kṛṣṇa stole. Freed of these the *jīva* is liberated from all bonds arising from his desires, family and society.

Formerly it was sufficient to live in worldly fashion according to the morality governing life in the world. Now a *sādhaka* must go further and transcend the world, or rather seek to do so. He rises by those things which are commonly the cause of fall. When he has completely achieved his purpose and liberated himself from all bonds, he reaches the stage of Śiva (Śivatva).

II

The iconography of Lajjā Gaurī is a problem, because no ancient text describing her image is known. Hindu iconography is well documented in ancient literature, but most of Āgamas and *tantra* literatures are not yet published. C.R. Bolon has studied the

---

15. M.P. Pandit (Readings), *Kulārṇava Tantra*, Motilal Banarsidass, Delhi, 1994, p. 95.

16. Sir John Woodroffe, *Śakti and Śākta* (*Essays and Addresses*), Ganesh & Company, Madras, 1975, p. 101.

different forms of Lajjā Gaurī and has classified them as *Uttānapād* pot form, lotus-headed without arms form, lotus-headed with arms form, anthropomorphic forms and the multifigured plaques. These show the development of Lajjā Gaurī image in Indian iconography art.

The opinion of Svāmī Satyananda Saraswati[17] comes to help, when he states,

> *Tantra* aims to transform every action in life into a ritual, so that an individual performs every action and thought with a feeling of worship and awareness. The action of bathing, dressing, sitting for worship, offering various symbolic sacrifices, sexual relations, stages of development from inception in the womb, birth to marriage, etc., are transformed into worship. The aim of *tantra* is to unleash the cosmic energy in man so that he rises to higher levels of awareness.

The action of life, which has stages of development from the inception in the womb, birth, marriage, etc., comes nearer to the conception of Lajjā Gaurī. The Sanskrit word *lajjā*, is derived from the root *lajjā* meaning to be ashamed. As discussed, the word *lajjā*, means modesty and shame. One who is modest is not decent and is shameless. So, it has to be observed that in what conditions a female remains nude or shameless? It is possible for a female to be shameless during three actions of life, viz., (i) while having bath, (ii) while enjoying sexual pleasure, and (iii) while giving birth.

Lajjā Gaurīs are found sitting in a squatting position. In ancient period, it was prescribed that a female should deliver by giving pressure in squatting position. C.R. Bolon[18] is of opinion that a few Lajjā Gaurī images made to be installed vertically on

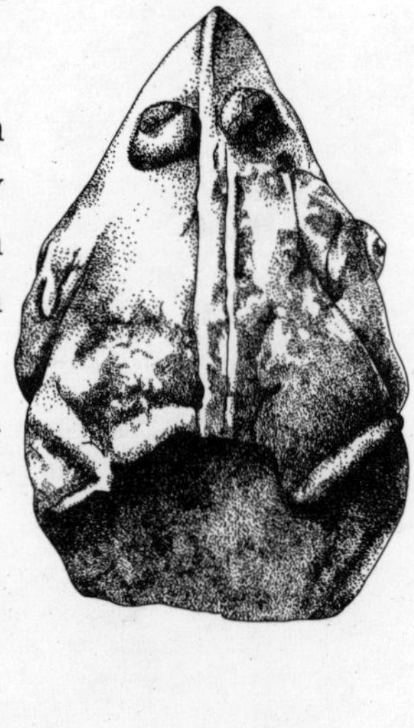

17. Svāmī Satyananda Saraswati, *A Systematic Course in the Ancient Tāntric Techniques of Yoga and Kriya*, Bihar School of Yoga, Munger, 1989, 2nd edn., p. 335.
18. C.R. Bolon, *op. cit.*, Delhi, 1997, p. 6.

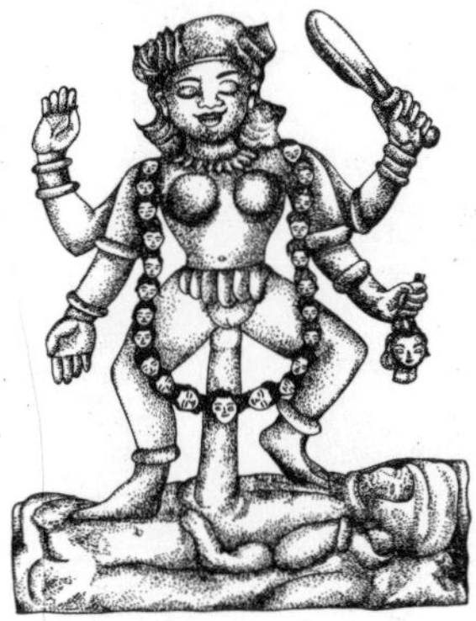

the walls of tanks or similar locations, seem to squat. However, the vast majority of Lajjā Gaurī images are definitely supine, and this position is essential to their meaning. They are not intended to suggest a woman squatting to give birth. The normal birth pose in India is supine.

It is true that the normal birth pose in India is supine nowadays, but that does not mean that squatting pose is no more in practice in giving birth to a child. Most of the tribal females and educated women who follow ancient systems, give birth in squatting position. Though this pose is almost forgotten by the common and general people, it is well known to Āyurvedic doctors and educated individuals who believe in it.

The question arises that if Lajjā Gaurīs are pregnant females, sitting in squatting pose to give birth, then their bulged bellies should have been shown or depicted in the art. It is interesting to point out that in the illustrations given by C.R. Bolon,[19] some Lajjā Gaurīs are depicted as pregnant females with bulging bellies.

It seems the inner yogic secret or esoteric meaning of Lajjā Gaurīs was gradually forgotten or lost and the artists started chiselling Lajjā Gaurīs without bulging bellies, and gave more importance to the *yoni* and lotus like head. The lotus like head of Lajjā Gaurīs are definitely the representation of the *sahasrāra cakra* of the *kuṇḍalinī śakti*. In *tantra*, the *sahasrāra* is the highest point of awareness.[20] The literal meaning of the word *sahasrāra*, is "one thousand." For this reason, it is said to be a lotus with one thousand petals.[21]

The divine mother is shown in various virtues and abstract qualities in *tantra* worship. Lajjā Gaurī is one such forms which depicts the divine mother squatting in a pre-delivery condition

19. C.R. Bolon, *op. cit.*, 1997, Figs. 5, 6, 13, 14 and 18.

20. Svāmī Satyananda Saraswati, *Kuṇḍalinī Tantra*, Bihar School of Yoga, Munger, 1992, p. 205.

21. *Ibid.*, 1992, p. 201.

with a thousand-petalled lotus and holding two *āyudhas* in her two hands, which are weapons, arms, implements of war or a lotus.

In the Lajjā Gaurī found from Kortipadar site and preserved in author's private possession, cloth is worn on the lower portion (*Pl.* 21). It reminds the author of the inclusion of a cloth "woven," between the legs of the Lajjā Gaurī, and left free on each end, as seen in the Nāganātha example (*Fig.* 42) and many others. This could be related to the idea of the goddess as being the "unbounded" or "unfettered."[22]

It is worth knowing the position of *tantra* as dealt by Svāmī Satyananda Sarasvati,[23]

> *Tantra* arose not in order to renounce or escape the world, but to experience the things of the world more fully and at the same time to use the ways of the world to attain higher state of awareness. It is a spiritual system, a psychological system, a psychic system, a science on life — call it what you like. But it is a practical system that produces results and personal experience. It has grown from the experiences and understanding of wise men throughout the ages. *Tantra* is not a stagnant system; it is a system that adapts itself to the needs of the times. In fact, it is a tāntric belief that old texts on *tantra* will fade away and new ones will always be written to replace them. The essence of the texts will be the same, but the expression and relationship to prevalent social conditions will be different. *Tantra* has changed and developed throughout the ages. It has not remained attached to a fixed dogma. It is still growing and adapting itself in the present era and will continue to mould itself to man's needs in the future.

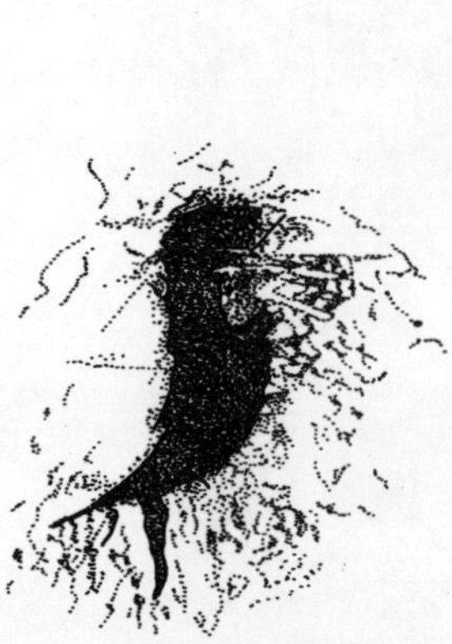

22. C.R. Bolon, *op. cit.*, Delhi, 1997, p. 65. Notes; P. Pal has suggested that the cloth is used by villagers as an aid to birth.
23. Swami Satyananda Saraswati, *A Systematic Course in the Ancient Tantric Techniques of Yoga and Kriya*, Bihar School of Yoga, Munger, 2nd edition, 1989, pp. 323-24.

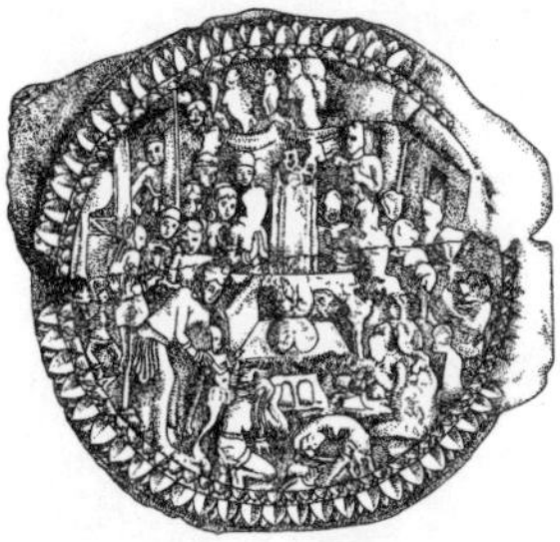

III

Among the anthropomorphic forms of Lajjā Gaurī, C.R. Bolon[24] has cared to study the form which shows her on one side and a frog on the other. She states,

> Condrington[25] suggested that the unique double sided terracotta that bears a form, Lajjā Gaurī on one side and a frog on the other, dates to the Kuṣāṇa period in Mathurā, *circa* second century. His judgement was based on the fact that the Victoria and Albert Museum acquired the piece in a group of Kuṣāṇa objects. Since the damaged piece would be the only example of this form, not dating to the sixth or seventh century, some doubt is cast on Cordrington's ea-ly dating, though due to the damage, its style is difficult to assess and it cannot be dated later with certainty either.

This terracotta is of interest, because here the Lajjā Gaurī is shown in a squatting position with female breasts and head, on one side and on the other side is a frog. The movement of a frog is like a jump, a bounce or it springs suddenly. When a human male has sexual seminal fluid ejaculation, it is like frog's movement. This observation induced the author to peep into the *Muṇḍaka Upaniṣad* because it has already been observed that goddesses are differently named in *Muṇḍaka Upaniṣad*.

Muṇḍaka[26] means barber, head and a branch of the Upaniṣads. *Muṇḍaka Upaniṣad*[27] mentions:

> When the fire is well lighted and the flames flicker, let a man

---

24. C.R. Bolon, *op. cit.*, Delhi, 1997, p. 23, vide : illustration figures 66, 67 and 68.
25. Kenneth de Burgh Codrington, 1935 (May), "Iconography, Classical and Indian," *Man* 35, no. 70, 65-66.
26. Gopal Chandra Praharaj, *Pūrṇacandra Orḍiā Bhāṣākoṣa* (A Lexicon of the Oriyā Language), The Utkal Sahitya Press, Cuttack, vol. V (Consonents Pha — Ma), 1936, p. 6593.
27. Nikhilananda Svāmī, *The Upaniṣads* (Abridged edition), Harper Torch Books, Harper & Row Publishers, New York & Evanston, 1963, pp. 110 & 113.

> offer his oblations in the space between the two portions of melted butter. — I.II.2 Kālī (lit. black), Karāli (terrific), Manojavā (swift as thought), Sulohitā (very red), Sudhūmra *varṇa* (of the colour of bright smoke, purple), Sphūlliṅginī (scintillating) and the luminous, Viśvarūcī (all-gleaming, all formed) — these seven, flickering about, form the seven tongues of fire. — I.II. 4
>
> From him comes the fire (i.e., the heavens) whose fuel is the sun: from the moon comes rain, from rain, the herbs that grow on the earth, from the herbs, the seminal fluid which a man pours into a woman. Thus many living beings are born of the *puruṣa*. — II. I. 6

Puruṣa, here means the universal soul, the divine spirit or essence of the universe.

Though, not directly mentioned, the seminal fluid is seed, germ, origin, source, primary cause, the first or underlying principle, semen virile, vigour, etc.[28] So, seminal fluid is Śakti,[29] which is power, energy, strength, potency, the particular power of a particular deity, the powers of individual deities personified. Where there is *puruṣa*, there is Śakti.

This rare terracotta art of a frog on one side and Lajjā Gaurī on its back, in the collections of Victoria and Albert Museum, Mumbai, seems to identify cosmic or universal seminal fluid and Goddess Lajjā Gaurī. The overall shape is like a drop (*Pls.* 23 & 24). The artist who made this terracotta art seems to have been guided by a *yogī* of repute, who was efficient in tāntric *yoga* practices of the *Kulārṇava Tantra* which is one of the major *tantra*s of the Kaula school and commands great authority, authenticity and respect. It has been profusely quoted by almost all the later tāntric works.

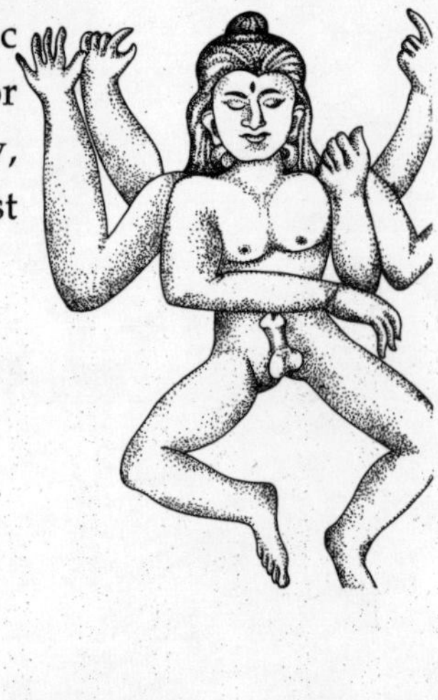

28. Gopal Chandra Praharaj, *op. cit.*, vol. V, Cuttack, 1936, p. 5796.
29. *Ibid.*, 1936, pp. 7494-96.

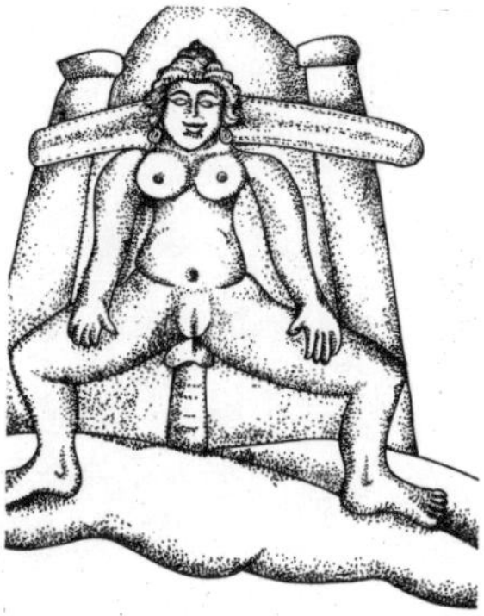

In the *Kulārṇava Tantra*,[30] the ten *mātṛkā-nyāsas* are mentioned thus: (1) *antara-mātṛkā-nyāsa*, (2-4) the three *bahir-mātṛkā-nyāsas*, i.e., *nyāsa* of *sṛṣti*, *sthiti* and *saṁhāra*, (5) *kalā-mātṛkā*, (6) *śrīkaṇṭha-mātṛkā*, (7) *keśava-mātṛkā*, (8) *lajjā bīja-mātṛkā* (9) *ramābīja-mātṛkā* and (10) *kāmabīja-mātṛkā nyāsas*.

Bīja[31] means seminal fluid and *nyāsa*[32] is the feeling of the deity in different parts of the body. *Nyāsa* is an exercise by an aspirant to become God. With this much background, the unique rare terracotta should be identified and named *Lajjā Bīja Mātṛkā*.

By surveying and studying the forms of Goddess Lajjā Gaurī, throughout India, C.R. Bolen[33] very rightly states,

> The variety of iconographic detail of the Lajjā Gaurī figures suggests that the artists followed no text and that the images were quickly adapted to regional or/and other requirements.

It seems Lajjā Gaurī worship was very popular during the early medieval period of Indian history.

IV

Each deity has a specific *mantra*, which is spiritual or empowered speech. The *bīja mantra* or seed syllable of Lajjā Gaurī is *hrīṁ*,[34] which *mantra* by itself can be used to worship her. David Frawley[35] also states:

> The *mantra* for Bhuvaneshvari (one of the Goddess) of *Daśamahāvidyā* or the Goddess of ten wisdom is the single

---

30. Ram Kumar Rai, *Kulārṇava Tantra*, Prachya Prakashan, Vārāṇasī, 1983, p. 68.
31. Gopal Chandra Praharaj, *op. cit.*, vol. V, Cuttack, 1936, p. 5796.
32. N.N. Bhattacharyya, *op. cit.*, Manohar, 1987, p. 454.
33. C.R. Bolon, *op. cit.*, Delhi, 1997, p. 14.
34. Harisadankar Ji Sastri (ed.), *Śyāma Rahasya Tantra*, Sanskrit Pustakalaya, Haridwar, 1911, p. 3.
35. *TYATWG*, Delhi, 1996, p. 101.

> syllable *hrīṁ*. *Hrīṁ* is the most important of all *mantras*. It is called the *Devī Praṇava*, or the equivalent of *oṁ* for the goddess. *Hrīṁ* refers to the heart (*hṛdaya*). It also relates to *hrīṁ*, which is modesty.
>
> The *mantra hrīṁ* is the general *mantra* of Śiva's consort and of Māheśvarī, the supreme Goddess. It can be used for all the ten Goddesses of wisdom and as the main *mantra* of the *śrī cakra* commonly used for *sundarī*. It is a single syllable easy for anyone to use.

The *Devī Gītā* states (XII.28):

> All my worship can be performed with the *mantra hrīṁ*. Of all *mantras*, *hrīṁ* is regarded as the supreme guide.

Hrīṁ is the *mantra* of inner transformation, it gives power to stop things and is the key to controlling thought and speech.

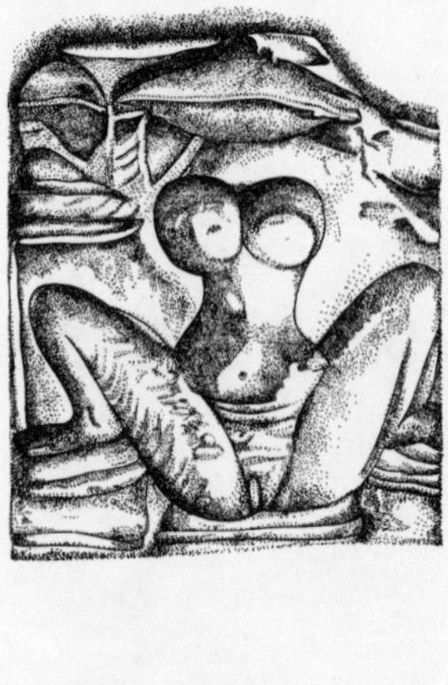

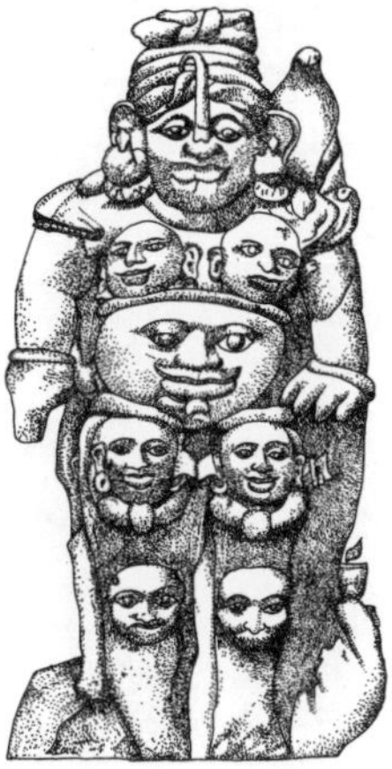

4

Epitomic Haṭha Yogic, Tāntric Sculptural Masterpiece of India

(The Image from Tala is a Composite Tāntric Yogic Figure of Mahākāla and Mahākālī)

I

Two temples known as Devarānī and Jeṭhānī exist at Tala, situated on the bank of the Maniyārī river, near village Amerikanpa in Bilāspur district of Chattisgarh. This area around Tala is significant for the archaeological remains of ancient South Kośala. G.L. Rayakawar and Rahul Kumar Singh of Directorate of Archaeology and Museums of Madhya Pradesh, while working under the supervision of K.K. Chakravarty, discovered one gigantic image of Śiva, near the right door of the Devarānī temple on 11 January 1988.

The image of Śiva from Tala is described by L.S. Nigam in a pamphlet, distributed in 1993 at a Seminar, which reads:

> The image under discussion is about nine feet in height and approximately five tonnes in weight. This two-armed image standing in a *sampada* posture, is massively built with emphasis on muscular strength. It has unusual iconographic features depicting various animals along with human and lion heads as body components. The description of the image is interesting enough as a turban is made of a pair of snakes. The serpent is probably a favourite depiction of the artist. Therefore, the waist band and finger nails are also designed like the snakes. Apart from these, a pair of serpenthood again figures in on either side of the head above the shoulders.

> The snake is also shown entwining the left leg. Among other animals, the peacock is depicted as ornamented ears. Eyebrows and nose are made of a descending lizard. Eyelids may be considered either in the pattern of an open mouth of a frog or as the mouth of a roaring lion. Two figures of fish form the moustaches of the image along with the upper lip, while the lower lip and the chin are shaped like a crab. Both shoulders have the depiction of a *makara* (crocodile). Seven human heads are engraved in various parts of the body, out of which a pair of small heads can be seen on either side of the chest. A bigger face forms the shape of the abdomen. These three faces have the form of moustaches. Each thigh consists of a pair of heads out of which two smiling faces are found on the front side in an *añjalī-baddha* posture while the others can be observed on each side. Two heads of the lion are also depicted on the knees. The *Urdhvamedhva* (erected-penis) is made of the head and the neck of a tortoise. The bell like testicles are designed as forelimbs of the same animal (*Pl.* 27).

The huge and heavy image of Śiva, discovered at Tala, has defied the study, imagination, identification and hypotheses of scholars so far. It has stood as a marvel of its own style and looks cumbersome. Crowded details seem to sit heavily on the composition and it looks as though the structure would fall to pieces by its very weight. Most probably because of this natural tendency, the image had fallen and was lying upside down, till it was discovered by the spade of archaeologists. This was the characteristic of sculptures and images of Vindhya, Madhya Pradesh and Chhattisgarh regions during the early medieval period, as described by Niharranjan Ray.[1]

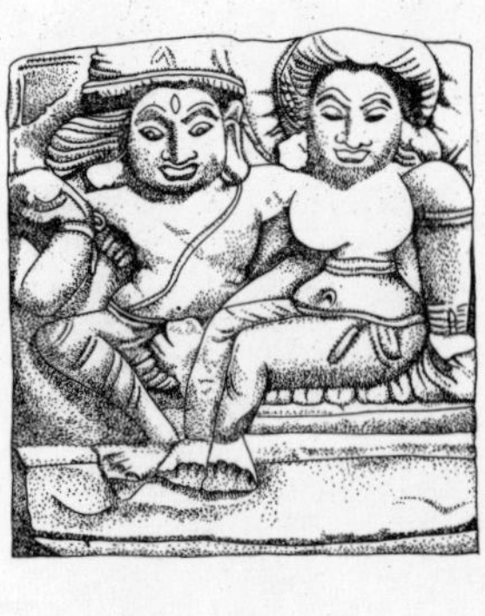

The cult of Śiva had its origin in the pre-Vedic period and his character was formed by the conflation of the attributes of many deities. The phallic emblem of Śiva was first worshipped. Pre-historic rock-shelter painting of Yogīmaṭh Donger (hill) was

1. N.R. Ray, "Sculpture," *THACOTIP*, vol. V, *The Struggle for Empire*, 1966, p. 659.

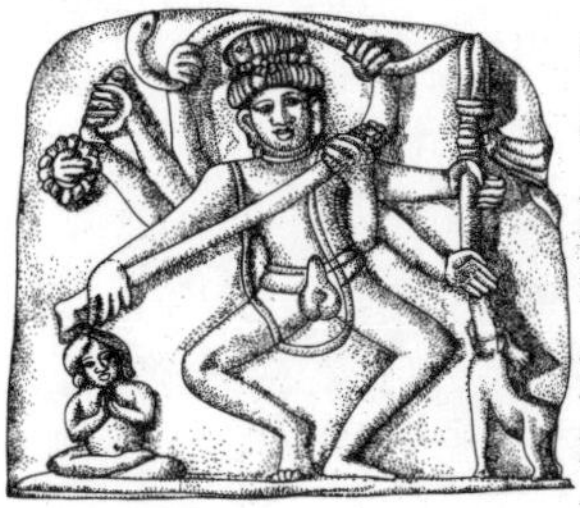

discovered by the author on 21 December, 1970, in the left valley of the Sundar river,[2] within Nuāpāḍā district of Orissa. This painting of bulls, triangles, rings and triple-lines (trinity) is interesting. Belonging to the neolithic period,[3] it speaks of the prevalence of phallism. While surveying the Chaura group of mountains in Nuāpāḍā on 28 March 1995, with Irfan Mohammad of Ranimunda village, the author came across megalithic stone piles and found one pot or port hole stone, within the Podagarh area. Two naturally shaped *Śiva-liṅgas* and one stone with three pronged lines were found, which are *in situ*. At present effort is being made by the local people to construct temples for these *liṅgas*. These are evidences of the Śiva cult and Śākti worship during the megalithic and iron ages in the Mahānadī valley. According to J.N. Banerjea,[4] it is presumable that the human as well as phallic forms of God were at first enshrined in the main sanctum of the Śaiva temples; but later it became a general custom to place the *liṅgas* in it to be the principal object of worship, the human figures of Śiva being present as accessories in the various parts of the temple.

Evolution of Śaiva icons developed gradually and the icons portray a definite sectarian bias, with mythology connected.

Baladeva Upadhyaya[5] rightly states that like the six orthodox systems of Indian philosophy, viz., Yoga, Nyāya, Vaiśeṣika, Sāṁkhya, Mīmāṁsā and Vedānta, *tantra* also have philosophies of their own, which, however, may generally be looked upon largely as modifications of the Sāṁkhya and Vedānta systems. They occupy the fourth position in the order

---

2. J.P. Singh Deo, *Cultural Profile of South Kośala*, Gyan Publishing House, New Delhi, 1987, p. 20.

3. J.P. Singh Deo, "Prehistoric Cave painting of Yogimath Donger," *OHRJ*, vol. XXII, No. 2, pp. 21-22.

4. J.N. Banerjea, "Śaiva Images," *THACOTIP*, vol. II, *The Age of Imperial Unity*, 1968, p. 460.

5. B. Upadhyaya, "Foreword," of R.K. Upadhyaya, *The Concept of God in Śaiva Tantra*, Jnananidhi Prakashan, Muzaffarpur, 1984, passim.

of Hindu scriptures, the preceding three being Śruti, Smṛti and Purāṇas. These sacred scriptures, it is said were revealed in the form of dialogue between Lord Śiva and his sweet consort, Pārvatī. There are two main classes of the *tantras*, viz., Āgama and Nigama. While in the Āgama, Pārvatī is the enquirer and Lord Śiva is the answerer; in the Nigama it is just the reverse.

The authorship of the *tantras* is attributed to Lord Śiva himself though some critics are of the view that Dattātreya, an incarnation of the divine trinity of the Hindus, viz., Brahmā, Viṣṇu and Śiva, is the real author of *tantras*. They are part and parcel of the Vedas and as such, have been accorded equal rank with them. It is said the Vedas emanated from the four mouths of Lord Śiva, while the *tantras* from his fifth mouth. Their designation of Āgama in its own signifies the Vedas. So the three terms, i.e., Vedas, *tantras* and Āgama, are inter-changeable. It is only in respect of the observance of rituals and comparatively unimportant details that there existed divergence in different religious sects. Otherwise, the Vedas and *tantras* are inter-connected and indivisible in their essential character.

Though *tantra* had early origin, yet it was only from about the fifth or sixth century AD that it gradually came into use as a special religious or philosophical concept. The tendency to multiply the variety of Śaiva images was carried to its fullest extent in the early and late medieval periods.

In the words of J.N. Banerjea,[6]

> Among the different types of terrific or *ugra* forms of Śiva, some of which do not seem to illustrate any particular Śaiva mythology, mention may be made of his Bhairava, Aghora, Vīrabhadra and Virūpākṣa-mūrtis.

The image of Śiva from Tala has depiction of animals, birds, reptiles and fishes, which are air-borne, aquatic and land living. Since it signifies the entire species of creation, it might be a

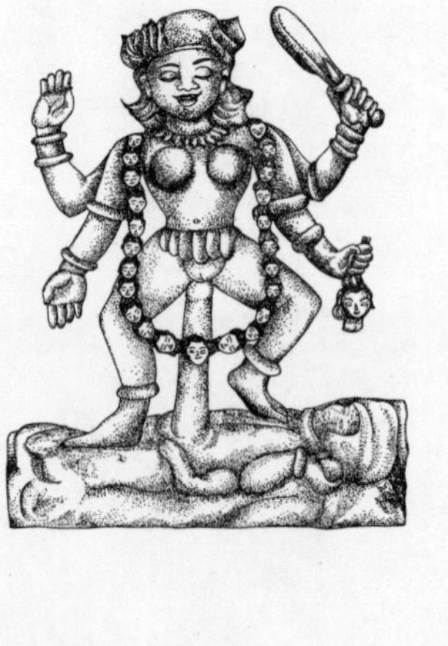

6. J.N. Banerjea, "Iconography," *THACOTIP*, vol. IV, *The Age of Imperial Kanauj*, 1964, p. 308.

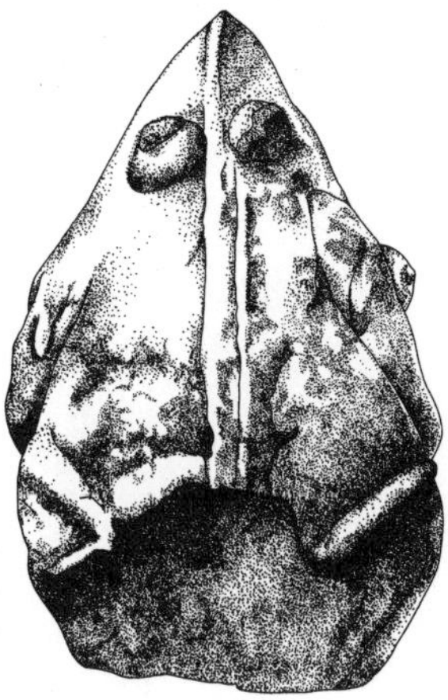

shape of *Virāṭ Puruṣa* or Mahākāla with *tantra* yogic symbols of Śiva.

The techniques of integral *yoga* synthesize all approaches to personal development which leads to the knowledge of the absolute. The turban of the the image is made of a pair of snakes, which is the favourite of Śiva. This symbolizes *kuṇḍalinī*, the serpent power as named by Sir John Woodroffe, of both Śiva and Śakti to have reached the *sahasrāra cakra*.

Eyebrows and nose are made of a descending lizard, which signifies the *nāsikāgara dṛṣṭi* which is a yogic practice that essentially involves gazing at the nose-tip.[7]

The figures of fish form the moustaches of the image along with the upper lip, while the lower lip and the chin are shaped like a crab, which have a yogic meaning. Two figures of fish, which form the moustaches mean the *iḍā* and *piṅgalā nāḍī*s. According to yogic terminology the two nostrils are the Gaṅgā and Yamunā rivers and fish swim in them.

Aghora as a sect or cult of *aghorī* developed among the Śaivas. *Aghorī*s[8] are described as having no feeling of repugnance or abhorrence towards filth, dirt, or dust, etc. The path of *aghora* is an advanced discipline of *tantra*. For an *aghora*, Śiva and Mahākāla are two aspects of the same being. Call Him *ātmā*, *puruṣa*, universal soul, ultimate reality, God the Father or what you will, Śiva is the one, the absolute, without a second, the embodiment of pure consciousness. All duality exists in the manifested universe, and Śiva is beyond all that. Dattātreya was the first *aghorī*.[9]

---

7. Buddhananda Chela, *Moola Bandha The Master Key*, Bihar School of Yoga, Munger, Bihar, 1984, p. 127.
8. G.C. Praharaj (Compiler), *Purnnacandra Ordia Bhasha Kosha* (Oriya Lexicon), vol. I, Cuttack, 1931, pp. 99-101.
9. R.E. Svoboda, *AGHORA* (*At the left hand of God*), Rupa & Co., New Delhi, 1993, p. 85.

For an *aghorī*, the *pañcamakāra* ritual is essential. R.E. Svoboda,[10] an *aghorī* of the U.S.A., has published the autobiography of his *guru* (master) *aghorī* Vimalananda, where it is described thus:

> The ritual in which sex appears, which is known as *pañcamakāra*, is actually of three types depending again upon the class of the celebrant, and in only one type does actual sexual intercourse occur. That version is meant only for tāmasic people, *tamas* being mental inertia or dullness. The intensity of the five (*pañca* means five) articles of worship — meat, fish, parched grain, wine and sex — overwhelms the dullness of the mind with stimulation. If an aspirant has been properly prepared, his increased mental energy can assist his or her spiritual evolution. An ill-prepared aspirant will be overcome by stimulation and will descend into debauchery.
>
> Rājasic people (*rajas* means mental activity) have active minds which must be properly channelled. They need less stimulation and more control, and use ginger, radish, boiled (as opposed to parched) grain, coconut, milk and flowers in their *pañcamakāra* sāttvic people naturally enjoy ample *sattva* (balance of mind and alertness) and do not require external aids to worship. They utilize meat of silence, the fish of breath control, the grain of concentration techniques, the wine of God intoxication, and the coitus of one's ego with the absolute.
>
> The Sanskrit terminology used to describe the *pañcmakāra* hides this meaning beneath its exterior. For example, "fish" stands for breath control, because one's two nostrils are referred to in yogic terminology as rivers: since they are continuously flowing (the right is called Gaṅgā and the left the Yamunā). Just as fish swim in rivers, the breath swims through the nostrils, and holding the breath (*kevala kumbhaka*) is equivalent to "eating the fish."

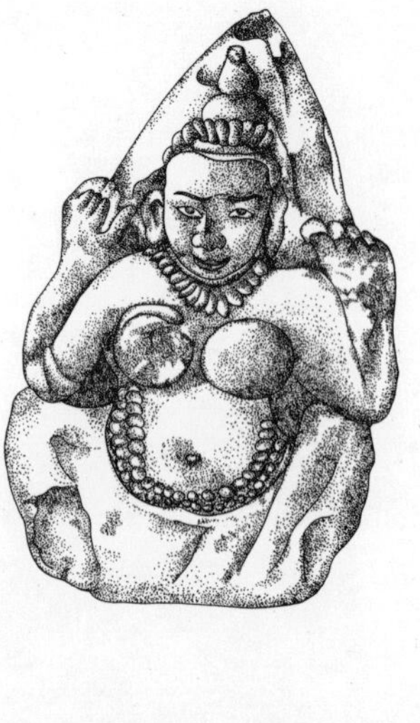

10. R.E. Svoboda, *AGHORA* (*At the left hand of God*), Rupa & Co., New Delhi, 1993, p. 299.

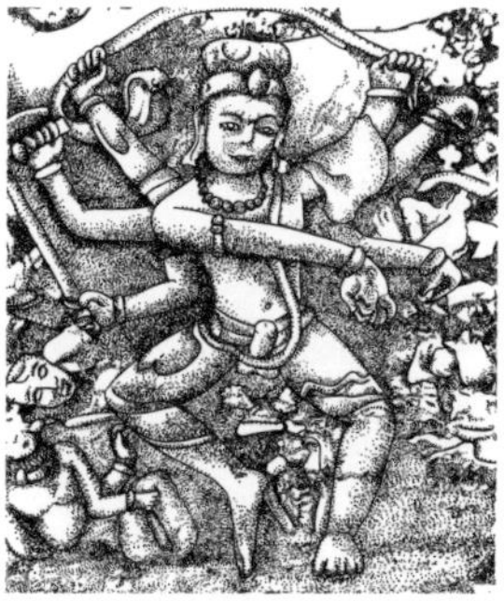

Pañcamakāra is only one of many tāntric rituals but it illustrates well a fundamental tāntric concept: *bhūtaśuddhi*. The physical universe is a permutation of five great elements: earth, water, air, fire and ether, equivalent respectively to the solid, liquid and gaseous states of matter, heat (which transforms matter from one state into another), and the field in which all activity takes place. To achieve universal harmony these five elements must be harmonized. *Pañcamakāra* is a fast, intense way to do this: meat stands for earth, fish for water, wine for fire, grain for air and sex for ether. When one reaches the stage of balance in which these inputs cause no disequilibrium of consciousness or metabolism, it is much less likely that any other fluctuation in the five elements will cause disharmony, and a state of health has been reached, since health is balance and disease is imbalance. This health is infinitely more permanent than ordinary health.

To deal with only five elements, though essential in every tāntric *sādhanā*, would be too mechanistic. Tāntric authorities advocate personification in accompaniment rather than seek to extirpate their emotions entirely as yogic practitioners do. Tāntrics magnify their emotions and transfer them entirely to a deity, a personified cosmic force. All the aspirant's natural propensities can spend themselves in this devotee-deity relationship, avoiding suppression of any desires which might erupt later to disrupt the harmony.

Gaṅgā comes out of the supreme, the matted locks of Lord Śiva and her conveyance is *makara* (crocodile). Therefore, both shoulders of this image have the shape of *makaras*. Two ears are in the shape of peacock, the conveyance of Śiva's son Kārttikeya. Kārttikeya, Skanda or Kumāra is a *brahmacārin*, that is a celibate forever. The implication is that the life-force typified as Kumāra, the youthful hero, present in each individual centre (i.e., *kuṇḍalinī cakras*) controls all life forces that are operating within the body. Being nursed in the six centres of *suṣumṇā* which is symbolized as *agni*, he is conceived of as the six-headed son of fire. Therefore Kārttikeya is the master of six important *cakras* of the *kuṇḍalinī śakti* in each individual, which are the *mūlādhāra, svādhiṣṭhāna, maṇipūra, anāhata, viśuddhi* and *ājñā cakras*. Among the birds, the peacock is the sprinkler of the seed. Since Kārttikeya is a *brahmacārin*, he is fit to use the peacock as his conveyance.

Seven human heads are engraved in various parts of the body. Pair of small heads can be seen on either side of the chest, while a big face forms the shape of the abdomen. Three faces have moustaches and therefore they are male heads. The three male faces can be described as demonic cities, signifying three bodies of gross, astral and causal ego, which were reduced to ashes by the mere laughter of Lord Śiva.

Each thigh consists of a pair of heads; of which two smiling faces are found on the front side in *añjalī-baddha* posture, while the others can be observed on each side. These four faces have no mustaches, therefore can be identified as female faces of Śakti, because her conveyance, the heads of the lion, are also depicted on the knees.

The Supreme Lord is represented as Śiva (the Lord of Yoga, Yogeśvara) and his power is represented as his consort, Śakti. Śakti is the embodiment of power. She is the supporter of the vast cosmos. She is the supreme power by which the creation is upheld. An aspirant does *sādhanā* which helps the union of Śiva and Śakti through the awakening of the forces within his body. One becomes a *siddha* in the *sādhanā* when one is able to awaken *kuṇḍalinī* and pierce the six *cakras*. She is in *mūlādhāra cakra* in our bodies. The Śakti must be awakened by *dhyāṇa*, by *bhāva*, by *japa* and by *mantras śakti*.[11] The four feminine faces found on the thighs depict the four methods of awakening the Śakti.

The three male faces on the chest and abdomen signify the three cities of Tripura Rahasya. The three cities are *āṇava mala*

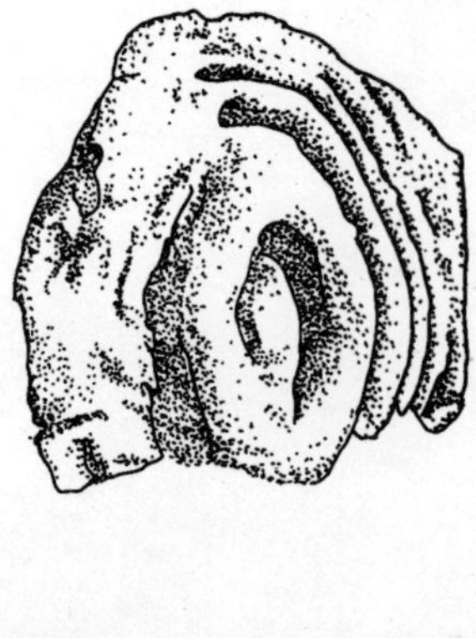

11. Sivananda Swami, *Lord Śiva and His Worship*, The Divine Life Society, Shivanandanagar, 1984, pp. 74-75.

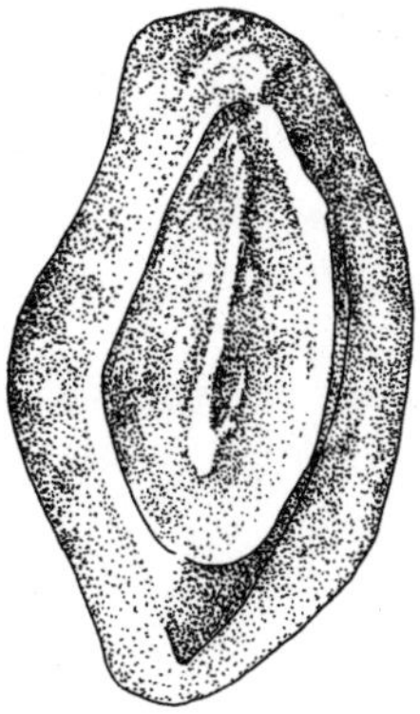

(egoism), *karma* (bondage of *karma*) and *māyā* (the illusory power of Lord Śiva which veils the individual souls). Destroy the first city *āṇava mala* through self-surrender to Lord Śiva and consequent descent of his grace (*anugraha*). Annihilate the second impurity, viz., *karma* through consecrating the fruits of your actions to the Lord and destroying the idea "I am the doer," by developing the *nimitta bhāva*, the feeling that Lord Śiva is working through your various organs and that you are merely an instrument in His hands (*cariyai* and *kṛyai*). You will not be bound by actions. You will attain purity of heart and through it realize Śivānandam or eternal bliss of Śiva. Annihilate the third impurity, viz., *māyā* through recitation of *pañcākṣara*, worship of the *guru*, hearing and reflection of the attributes of the lord and his various *līlā*s and meditation on his form and the *Satchidananda* aspect.[12]

The *ūrdhvamedhra* (penis-erectus) of this image is made of the head and the neck of a tortoise. This symbolizes the *vajrolī mudrā*.[13] Tortoise contracts its head and neck inside its shell. Therefore, the head and the neck of a tortoise, in the shape of the penis-erectus, symbolizes the *vajrolī* practice. In verse 10 chapter 1 of the *Haṭha Yoga Pradīpikā*, it is mentioned,

> For those continually tempered by the heat of *tapa* (the three types of pain — spiritual, environmental and physical) *haṭha* is like the hermitage giving protection from the heat. For those always united in *yoga*, *haṭha* is the basis acting like a tortoise.

The lower lip and the chin of this image are shaped like a crab. A crab has ten legs and they represent *daśamahāvidyā*s of the tāntric Śakti cult.[14] Pushpendra Kumar[15] informs that the Supreme deity

12. Sivananda Swami, *Lord Śiva and His Worship*, The Divine Life Society, Shivanandanagar, 1984, pp. 98-99.
13. (i) Buddhananda Chela, *op. cit.*, 1984, pp. 99-101.
    (ii) R.E. Svoboda, *op. cit.*, 1993, pp. 279-90.
14. Sarbeswar Satpathy, *Śakti Iconography in Tāntric Mahāvidyās*, Punthi Pustak, Kolkata, 1991, pp. 73-89.

→

of *tantras* is known as Śakti, inseparable from Śiva. Śakti and Śiva are not two or double stars, but are ultimately one and the same. These are two[16] modes of the manifestation of the eternal and infinite *Brahmana,* as *puruṣa* and *prakṛti* (but not that of Sāṁkhya, i.e., mother and spirit, whom *tantras* describe as Śiva and Śakti.[17] Two bell like testicles, designed as fore-limbs of the penis-erectus symbolizes ritual.

The *tantras* call Śakti as *parā prakṛti,* i.e., the personified divine energy of the Supreme deity, in other words, Brahmā itself. Without the union of Śakti and Śiva there is no creation. The two are inseparable indeed. Śiva, the pure consciousness, is the silent seer of all experiences while it is Śakti who brings forth the universe, sustains it and destroys it to please Śiva.

Śiva and Śakti are the causal head as Śiva-Śakti *tattvas*. The Supreme Lord is Śiva and his power is his consort, Śakti or Durgā or Kālī. When *kuṇḍalinī* awakens and one is unable to handle it, it is called Kālī. When one can handle it and use the energy for beneficial purposes, it is called Durgā. She is in the *mūlādhāra cakras* in our bodies. Mother *kuṇḍalinī* Śakti unites with Lord in the *sahasrāra cakra* during complete *nirvikalpa samādhi.*[18]

A pair of serpenthood again figures on either side of the head, above the shoulders. These probably symbolizes the *kuṇḍalinī śaktis* of Śiva and Śakti. Śakti *tattva* is really the negative aspect of the Śiva *tattva.* Though they are spoken of separately they are really one. Śakti *tattva* is the will of Śiva. It is said in the very first verse of Kālidāsa's *Raghuvaṁśa* that Śakti and Śiva have the same relationship as the word and its

15. P. Kumar, *Śakti Cult in Ancient India*, Bharatiya Publishing House, Vārāṇasī, 1974, p. 151.

16. Sir J. Woodroffe (ed.), *Mahānirvāṇa Tantram*, 1-16, Gita Press, Gorakhpur, passim.

17. D.N. Bose, Haldar Hiralal, *Tantras: Their Philosophy and Occult Secrets,* Oriental Publishing Co., Kolkata, 1956, p. 74.

18. Sivananda Swami, *Lord Śiva and His Worship*, *op. cit.*, 1984, passim.

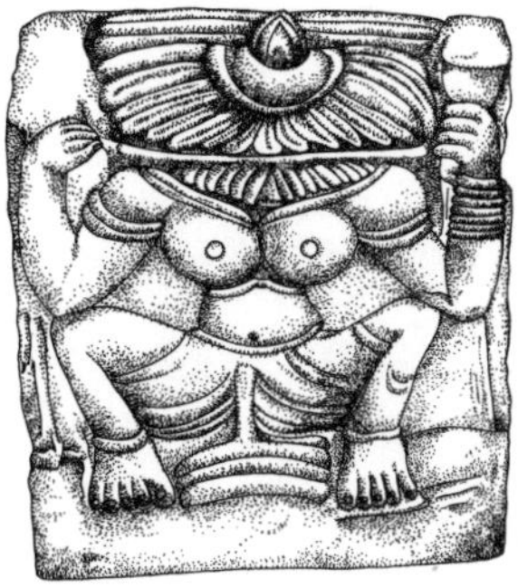

meaning. Just as heat and fire are inseparable, so are Śakti and Śiva. Lord Śiva cannot do anything without Śakti. This is emphasized by Ādi Śaṅkarācārya in the first verse of *Saundarya-Laharī*.[19]

All the informations given above suggests that this image is not a free expression or hypothesis of the sculptor who made it. It seems the sculptor was guided by an advanced tāntric *haṭha yogī*, who was well versed in the tāntric *haṭha yoga* path or was chiselled by the *siddha*. Any literature concerning this image may not be found but it seems to be a composite *haṭha* yogic figure of Mahākāla and Mahākālī, the destroyer of the cosmos, because of its complicated iconographic features.

If any Śaiva and Śākta tāntric literature concerning this image is discovered in future, it should be ever welcomed. The author has done this much of study which would perhaps pave way for further research.

The discovery of this unique image prove the prevalence of the composite Śaiva and Śakta tāntric practices at Tala. It seems the practice of *vajrolī* first developed in the Mahānadī valley because the earliest Naṭarāja images with *ūrdhvaliṅga* (penis-erectus) have been found in this area. According to the *Haṭha* yogic text, man and woman represent Śiva and Śakti. These two *śaktis* are known as *iḍā* and *piṅgalā*. *Iḍā* is Śakti and *piṅgalā* is Śiva. When they unite in the *ājñā cakra* that is the real union. The seat of Śakti is in the *mūlādhāra* and the seat of Śiva is in the *sahasrāra*. When Śakti reaches the *ājñā cakra*, union takes place. The energy created in the *ājñā cakra* moves up to the *sahasrāra cakra*. When Śiva and Śakti unite together, Śiva begins to dance and that is his Naṭarāja aspect of *Ānanda Tāṇḍava*. So, it seems the sexo-yogic system of *vajrolī* was discovered by the Śiva *haṭha* tāntric *yogīs* of the Mahānadī valley quite early period but developed only in the early medieval period. It can be claimed that the best sculptural composite tāntric *haṭha* yogic

19. Sivananda Swami, *Lord Śiva and His Worship*, *op. cit.*, 1984, passim, pp. 85-86.

art, depicting all aspects of Śaiva and Śākti *yoga* in detail is found in the composite Mahākāla and Mahākālī image of Tala. For practical sexo-yogic tāntric practice, there is no difference between the Kāpālika, Kālāmukha, Aghora and Nātha cults of Śaiva, Vaiṣṇava, Śākta, Buddhist and Jaina *tantras*.

The great tradition of India and the Mahānadī valley is Vedic culture, which is the *summum bonum* of spirituality. Source of *tantra* is found in the *Atharvaveda* also. From the Vedic background, it is known that creation is the outcome of divine desire or *kāma* or will (*icchā*). Sarbeswar Satpathy[20] remarks, "Therefore divine is *kāmamayī* or *icchāmayī* in its ultimate consciousness." Tāntric yogic process is the path to conquer *kāma* and *yogīs* and *ṛṣis* of India, i.e., Bhārata had discovered this path to blessedness. Its quintessence is found in the *Śiva Saṁhitā*,[21] *Aṣṭāṅga Yoga* of sage Maharṣi, Patañjali's work *Mahābhāṣya*, *Haṭha Yoga Pradīpikā* of *yogī* Swātmarām,[22] *Gorakṣa Saṁhitā* by *yogī* Gorakhnāth, *Gheraṇḍa Saṁhitā* by sage Gheraṇḍa,[23] *Yogavārttika* of Vijñānabhiksu[24] and many published and unpublished yogic literatures. All the *yogas* are centralized and channellized through discipleship and *guru* (master), whose grace acts like a fortress.

With this background, it can be claimed that the composite image of Mahākāla and Mahākālī at Tala is the final sculptural expression of the *haṭha* yogic-tāntric Śaiva and Śakta cults of the great Mahānadī valley which can be dated within the eleventh-twelfth centuries AD. Therefore about spirituality *tantra*

20. Sarbeswar Satpathy, *op. cit.*, Kolkata, 1991, passim.

21. S.C. Vasu, *Śiva Saṁhitā*, Munshiram Manoharlal, New Delhi, 1979, passim.

22. Panchamsinh, *The Haṭha Yoga Pradīpikā*, Munshiram Manoharlal, New Delhi, 1980, passim.

23. S.C. Vasu, *The Gheraṇḍa Saṁhitā*, Munshiram Manoharlal, New Delhi, 1980, passim.

24. T.S. Rukmani, *Yogavārttika of Vijñānabhikṣu*, Munshiram Manoharlal, New Delhi, vol. I, 1981; vol. II, 1983; vol. III, 1987 and vol. IV, 1989, passim.

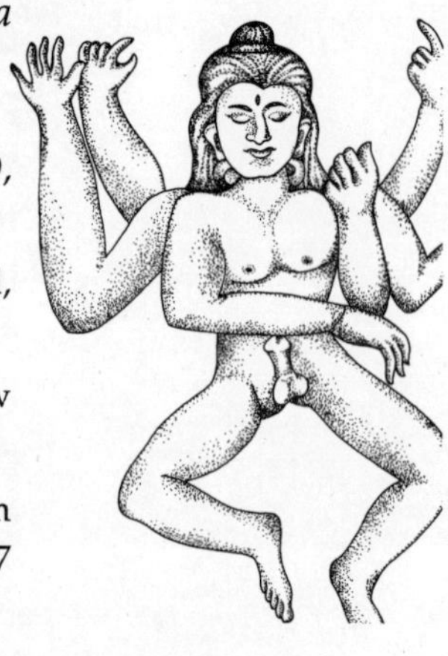

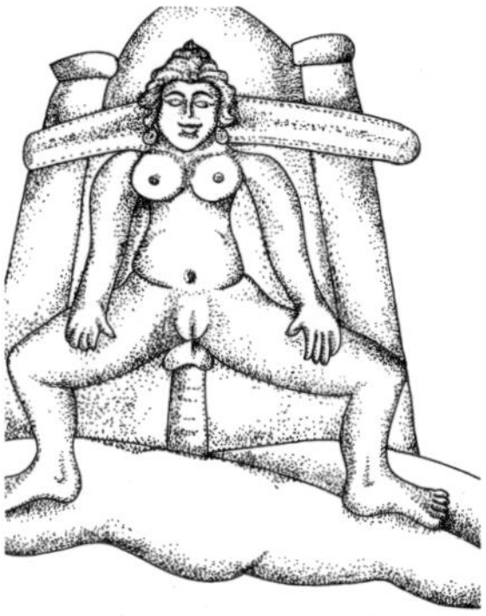

says that to merge with consciousness one must use Śakti as the means. There is a supreme experience where Śiva and Śakti no longer exist as separate entities. Some call it *Brahman*, others call it "not this, not this" to show that it is inexpressible. Others say that it is one without a second. It is the state of *nirvāṇa*, *samādhi*, perfect oneness, and so many other words. This is the stage when Śiva merges so closely with Śakti that they become one. They embrace each other so tightly that they cease to be separate. It depicts the state of being the enraptured embrace where self-identity and separateness disappear. This is the divine embrace.[25]

II

Study on Āgamic Tradition in the Mahānadī Valley

In the history of Vedic or Hinduism, the Āgama cult and its influence occupy a unique place, but this literature which is equally important like the Vedas has been given very little consideration. It is worth knowing about the Āgama.

Āgama[26] means that which has "come down" (*ā-gam* – "to come"); a tradition or spiritual teaching. The term *āgama* is generally applied to the scriptures and theological manuals of the principal Hindu sects written in Sanskrit. They contain mythological, ritualistic and metaphysical matter. The Āgama tradition often run parallel to the Vedic traditions and there has been some criticism against them as to have deviated from the Vedic tradition. Some, on the other hand, hold that the Āgamas are within the Vedic tradition. The Āgamic tradition give prominence to *bhakti* or devotion to the Supreme Being and believe in temple worship and pilgrimages.

---

25. Swami Satyananda Saraswati, *A Systematic Course in the Ancient Tāntric Techniques of Yoga and Kriyā*, Bihar School of Yoga, Munger, 1989, p. 332.

26. Gaṅgā Ram Garg (General editor), *Encyclopaedia of the Hindu World*, vol. I, A - Aj, Concept Publishing Company, New Delhi, 1992, pp. 192-93.

Āgama text consist of four sections dealing with (i) knowledge (*vidyā*) of the Godhead and its relation to the manifest universe, (ii) meditative discipline (*yoga*) or techniques for concentrating on divine images or forms, especially by means of *mantras*, (iii) action (*kriyā*) such as building temples and making and consecrating images and (iv) conduct (*caryā*) or rules for daily worship and festivals, social behaviour, etc. While most of the Āgamas do not, in fact, conform to the above pattern, they are united in their practical concern for external ritual worship of divine images in temples and home shrines and techniques for internal "mental worship" and realization of the divine forms.

These sectarian scriptures and traditions became increasingly influential throughout the first millennium AD with the earliest extant Āgamas generally being placed in the fifth century, although some would prefer to date them several centuries later. In the general historical development of the Hindu religion, the Āgamas came after the *Śruti* and *Smṛti* works. They continue the emphasis on *bhakti* or popular devotional worship of personal deities found in the Purāṇas. Their rise coincides with the growth in importance of temples housing divine images and the Āgamas are essentially the ritual texts that govern the worship (*pūjā*) and other devotional practices (*sādhanā*) associated with these temples and centring on the realization of various Gods and Goddesses enshrined in them.

The Āgama texts are divided into three main divisions — Vaiṣṇava, Śaiva and Śākta. There are several later Upani-ṣads belonging to these Schools (Vaiṣṇava Upaniṣads, Śaiva Upaniṣads and Śākta Upaniṣads).

Vaiṣṇava Āgamas are divided into two sections: Pañcarātra and Vaikhānasa. Pañcarātra literature is very rich, containing more than 200 texts — *Ahirbudhanya-Saṁhitā, Lakṣmī-Tantra, Padmā-Saṁhitā, Pārāśara-Saṁhitā, Sāttvata-Saṁhitā*, etc. The texts belong to a period between AD 600 and 850 and some of them may contain later accretions. The Pañcarātra form of worship is followed in Śrīraṅgam and Kāñcī temples. The

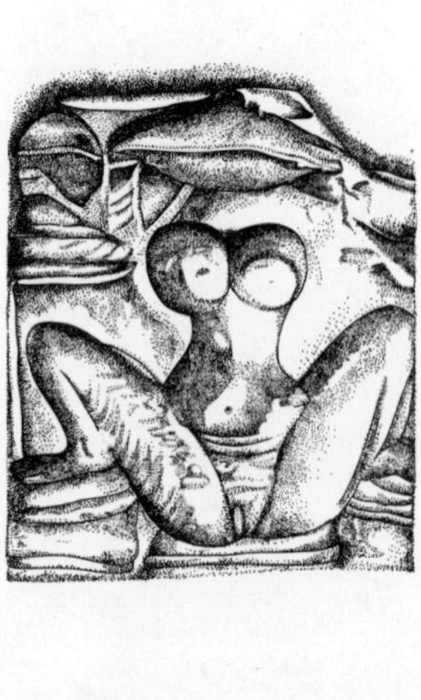

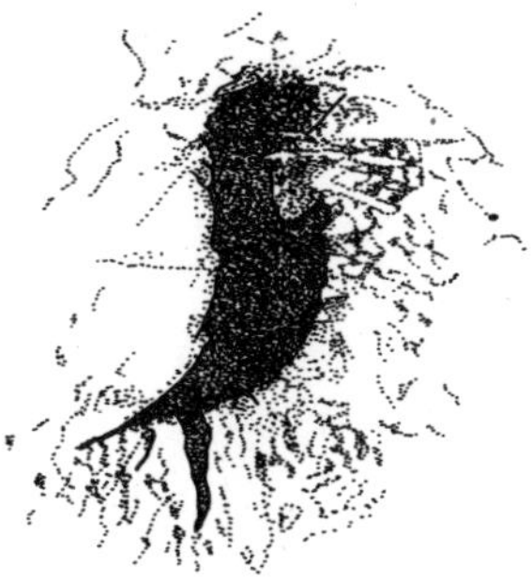

Vaikhānasas belong to the Tamil and Telugu areas. *Atri-Saṁhitā, Kāśyapa-Saṁhitā, Marici-Saṁhitā, Bhṛgu-Saṁhitā*, etc., belong to this school. The rituals and worship at the Tirupati temple are conducted according to the Vaikhānasa tradition.

The Śaiva Āgamas have three sub-divisions: (1) Pāśupata School ascribed to Lakulīśa, (2) Śaiva-Siddhānta School popular in Tamil Nadu which has 28 Āgama texts such as *Kāmikā, Karana Suprabheda* and *Vadhula*, etc., and (3) Pratyabhijñā school of Kaśmir whose authoritative works consist of *Śiva Sūtras* of Vasugupta, *Spandakārikā* of Kallaṭa, *Śiva-dṛṣṭi* of Somānanda and *Pratyabhijñāsūtra* of Utpala (with Abhinavagupta's commentary). Śaivites also sometimes distinguish between those treatises called the Āgama in which Pārvatī asks questions and Śiva answers, and the *nigama*, in which Śiva asks questions and Pārvatī answers. The Āgamas, unlike the Vedas were accessible to women and to the menials of the household. Some early Śaivāgamas were composed in Sanskrit, but in Southern India these were re-written in Tamil, Kannada or other South Indian languages.

The Śāktāgamas are concerned with the worship of Śakti or the world-mother. The Śaktas recognise 77 Āgamas, which are Śāktāgamas or *tantras*, although this figure does not indicate the number of *tantras* actually in existence. Their chief Āgamas are: *Lalitasahasranāma, Saundarya-Laharī, Varivasra-rahasya* of Bhāskararāya, etc.

According to S.P. Sabarathinam,[27]

The two great master-scriptures which deal with the science of space and forms are the Āgamas and the Śilpa-Śāstras, corroborative and corresponding to each other. However, we can deduce an element of difference between these two scriptural streams. While the *śilpa* works set forth the details

27. S.P. Sabarathinam, "Āgamic Treatment of Mahābhūtas in Relation to Maṇḍalas and Arts," *Prakṛti, The Integral Vision*, vol. 3 (*The Āgamic Traditions and the Arts*), K. Vatsyayan (General editor), Indira Gandhi National Centre for the Arts, New Delhi, D.K. Printworld (P) Ltd., New Delhi, 1995, p. 47.

> concerned with structural forms alone, not disowning the concept of mathematical space and time, the Āgamic scriptures copiously deal with both the conceptual and structural forms based on the concepts of space and time.

The genesis of human being is fully experienced and dealt in tāntric Āgamas. The subtle elements are five in number corresponding to the perceivable five gross elements or *mahābhūtas*; space, air, fire, water and earth, which together constitute the perceived gross-world. The order and sequence in which these five subtle elements manifested from *māyā* is explained by Śaṅkara in the *Tattvabodha*.[28]

These *pañcabhūtas* or five subtle elements (or gross elements) are well dealt in the Śaiva ritual, which has special reference to *bhūtaśuddhi*. Therefore, S.S. Janaki[29] says,

> The correspondence between the microcosm and the macrocosm worked out and utilized for esoteric and spiritual purposes is much prevalent in the Śaivite system, as in others.

With this background the *pañcabhūtas* developed in the Śaiva and Āgamic traditions of making of *Śiva-liṅga* in the arts. S.S. Janaki has given the sketch of *tattvas* in *Śiva-liṅga* (vide: plate). This type of *Śiva-liṅgas* made of soft red stones have been discovered on the left of the Indralath brick temple at the Rānīpur-Jharial site, as the presiding deity inside the stone temple at Sereikela village, situated at the confluence of the Tel and Sundar rivers (both in Bolaṅgīr district) and at Paikpāḍā in Raigarh district of Orissa. These three Śiva-Śakti arts prove that there was a strong Āgamic tradition prevalent in the arts of the Mahānadī valley.

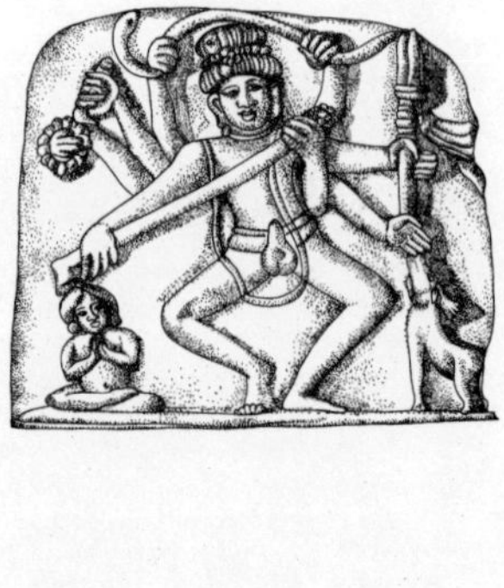

28. Swami Chinmayananda, *Vedānta The Science of Life* (Part One) (*Understanding Human Nature*), Central Chinmaya Mission Trust, Bombay reprint 1983, p. 115.
29. S.S. Janaki, "Pañcabhūtas in Śaiva Ritual with Special reference to Bhūtaśuddhi," *Prakṛti, The Integral Vision*, vol. 3, The *Āgamic Traditions and the Arts*, *op. cit.*, 1995, pp. 37-46.

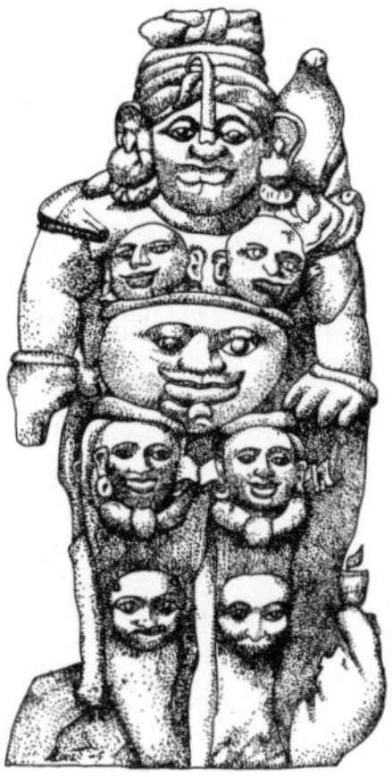

Even the temple architecture of the whole Mahānadī valley is based on the Āgamas, *Vāstuśāstra* and *Śilpa-śāstra*s. Therefore it is needless to mention that temple construction is based on *Vāstumaṇḍala*. The maximum numbers of *Śilpa-śastra*s have been discovered in Orissa than elsewhere in India.[30] The most important among these discoveries is the *śilpa* text, *Saudhikāgama*, which, although unpublished, proves that there was strong Āgamic influence on the art and architecture of sculptures and temples in the whole Mahānadī valley, which can be claimed to be the land of Kāmakalā and the Uḍḍīyāna-*pītha*. In verse 51 of the *Kāma-Kalā-Vilāsa* by Puṇyānanda Nātha,[31] it is stated,

> Śiva the *guru* who abides in the Uḍḍīyāna-*piṭha* did in the *Kṛta-yuga* impart the Vidyā to her, his own Śakti, the Vimarṣa-rūpiṇī Kāmeśvarī.

In view of the importance of the Āgamic tradition, S.P. Sabarathinam[32] concludes thus:

> The way in which the gross elements have been explained and inter-related in the Āgamas seems to be unique and significant. In order to restructure ourselves, we are trained to destructure the gross elements in such a way as to look at them as not invested with inertness but as invested with divinity and as charged with symbols, colours and sounds. All the ritualistic activities have their direct effect on the gross elements. The study of the Āgamas and Śilpa-Śāstras is sure to award the reader with a sound knowledge of the interaction between rituals, images and the elements.

30. R.P. Das, "The Study of Śilpa Śāstra," *Reference Orissa (An Indian State of Eastern Region)*, ed. A.N. Tiwari, Enterprising Publishers, Bhubaneswar, 1999, pp. 174-81.
31. Sir John Woodroffe, *Tantra Rāja Tantra and Kāma-Kalā-Vilāsa*, Ganesh & Co., Madras, 1971, p. 234.
32. S.P. Sabarathinam, "Āgamic treatment of Mahābhūtas in relation to Mandalas and Arts," *Prakṛti*, vol. 3, *op. cit.*, 1995, p. 61.

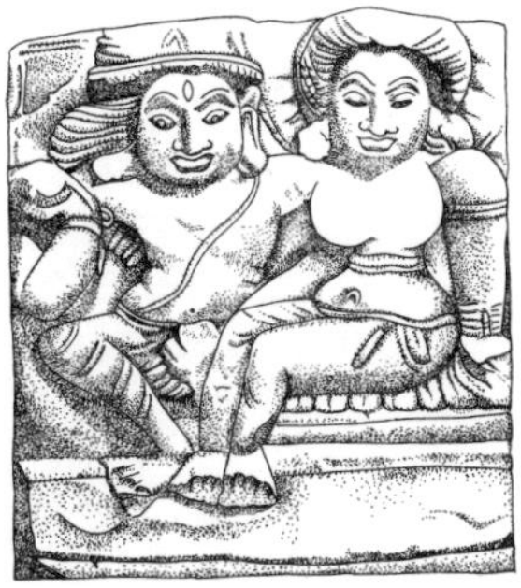

5

From Sex to Salvation

SEX can lead to salvation, but before that it is appropriate to know about knowledge and reality. The knowledge which is acquired from teachers and from books are imitative, repetitive, derivative and educative. Yet another knowledge which is above these types is intuitive. Only intuitive knowledge reaches the reality. Intuition means the power of the mind by which it immediately perceives the truth of things without reasoning or analysis; a truth so perceived, is immediate knowledge in contrast with mediate.

With the rise of *kuṇḍalinī*, a different self-absorption takes place, which is called *samādhi*. The aim of every *yoga* of all religions of the world is to realize the truth through intuitive knowledge.

In intuitive knowledge, an individual attains *samādhi* or self-absorption. *Samādhi* starts with absorption of the self in the duality of structure in consciousness and ends in absorption of the self in identification with the secondless unique self. Self-absorption in the duality of structure in consciousness is called *savikalpa samādhi*. Self-absorption without any sense of duality is called *nirvikalpa samādhi. Savikalpa samādhi* is of four types while the *nirvikalpa samādhi* is of two types, each having three sub-divisions.

Cakra means circle, wheel, *prāṇa* (life), the psychic centre in the subtle body responsible for specific physiological and psychic functions, the conjugating point of *nāḍī*s. There are mainly six *cakra*s of *kuṇḍalinī*: *mūlādhāra, svādhiṣṭhāna, maṇipūra,* *anāhata, viśuddha, ājñā* and *sahasrāra cakra.* Many others *cakras* are also mentioned in tāntric literature, but these six are the main *cakras* for ascent of *kuṇḍalinī.*

Samādhi means culmination of meditation, state of oneness of mind with the object of concentration, supramental consciousness, the stage of *yoga* to be observed in a particular stage of consciousness. With this much information let us study the various definitions on *savikalpa samādhi* and *nirvikalpa samādhi* as given by Sudhir Ranjan Sengupta.[1] These are:

Savikalpa Samādhi

(i) *Savitarka Samādhi* is the Self-absorption in the duality of structure in consciousness with latent sense of controversy in the consciousness.

(ii) *Savicāra Samādhi* is the Self-absorption in the duality of structure in consciousness with a latent sense of discretion in the consciousness.

(iii) *Sānada Samādhi* is the Self-absorption in the duality of structure in consciousness with all absorbing bliss.

(iv) *Sasmita Samādhi* is the Self-absorption in the duality of structure in consciousness with a latest sense of self-existence.

Nirvikalpa Samādhi

(i) *Bhāva Pratyaya Videha Samādhi* consists in the self-absorption without the least trace of duality, in consciousness with complete self-identification with nature of God, without the light of consciousness. This *samādahi* has three sub-divisions, viz., *prakṛti pratyaya, aham pratyaya* and *mahat pratyaya*, i.e., self-consciousness lost in nature, self-consciousness lost in egotism, and in *boddhisattva.*

(ii) *Pūrṇa pratyaya samādhi* means the self-absorption in the

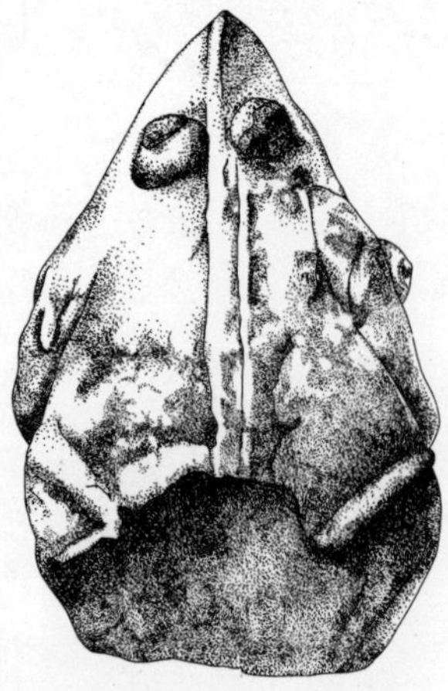

1. S.R. Sengupta, *Mother Cult,* Firma KLM, Kolkata, 1977, pp. 106-7.

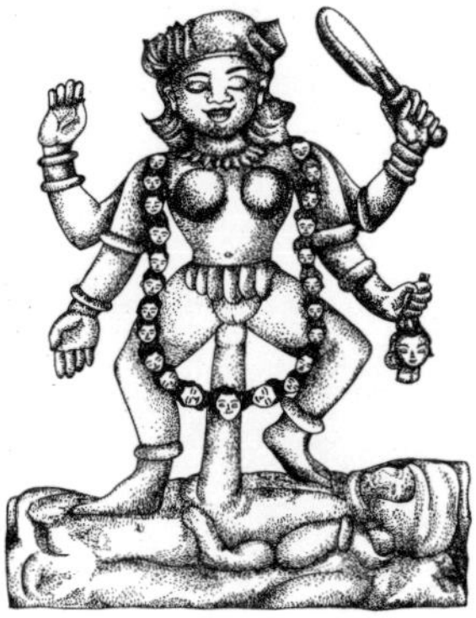

secondless, unique, conscious, absolute self of the Supreme without the least trace of duality. This *samādhi* is possible when the five waves of mind cease to function and the *sādhaka* transcends the basic evolution. *Pūrṇa samādhi,* attained on the realization of the identity of self with the absolute self of God, without the least trace of duality in the self-revealed consciousness, liberates an indiviual soul from the ills of the world and world series as now he knows no other existence except the Supreme Being. The sages say that of these eight varieties of *samādhi, pūrṇa pratyaya videha samādhi* alone can liberate an individual soul.

So yogic paths are the way for intuitive knowledge or *samādhi*s. There are nine types of *yoga*, viz., *bhakti yoga, jñāna yoga, karma yoga, haṭha yoga, rāja yoga, mantra yoga, laya yoga, dhyāna yoga* and esoteric *yoga*.[2] The *yoga* of sexual transformation is concerned with *haṭha yoga*. According to *tantra,* interaction between a man and a woman has three purposes — pleasure, procreation and *samādhi*.

Pleasure

Sex is the whole domain connected with the distinction of male or female in plants and animals. It is the exciting desire (*kāma*). So, there exists sex in plants and animals. It is the human beings who are very skilful in sex. The individual who is more skilful in sex art can give more pleasure to the partner, than an average person.

The subject of *kāma* (desire) was taken up precisely with the same care, seriousness and objectivity as that of *dharma* and *artha* or any other technical topic by the Vedic *ṛṣi*s. Aesthetic consciousness and the principle of enjoyment has been well discussed in Indian literature, which is the inner mind and spirit

2. Niranjanananda Paramahamsa, *Yoga Darshan* (*Vision of the Yoga Upanisads*), Sri Panchdashnam Paramahamsa Alakh Bara, Deoghar, Bihar, 1993, passim.

of India.[3] Auddalāki Śvetaketu, apparently a Vedic sage, first gave an exposition in 500 chapters, which Pāñcāla Bābhravya later condensed it into 150 chapters under seven definite sections (*adhikaraṇas*), namely, general principles (*sādhāraṇa*), sexual union (*sāṁprayogika*), courtship and marriage (*kanyā samprayuktaka*), wife (*bhāryādhikārika*), wife of another person (*pāradārika*), prostitute (*vaiśika*) and secret love of extraneous stimulation (*aupaniṣadika*). Of these topics, Dattaka, at the request of the courtesans of Pāṭaliputra, chose the sixth (*vaiśika*) as his special subject and his example was followed by Cārāyaṇa, Suvarṇanābha, Ghoṭakamukha, Goṇardiya, Goṇikāputra and Kucumāra, each of whom wrote a monograph on one of the remaining subjects in the order given above. In view of the fractional and specialized nature of separate treatises and the difficulty of mastering them, Bābhravya's extensive work the *śāstra* was getting lost and Vātsyāyana's professed object was to write a comprehensive compendium within a reasonable dimension.

Vātsyāyana Mallanāga's *Kāmasūtra* is the oldest Indian literature on sex. In contrast to the ideals of chastity and asceticism, sex is not opposed to the attainment of the higher goal of spiritual development. All the works after Vātsyāyana are just repetitions, with little variations, changes and additions. The sexual morality, physiology and psychology of intercourse remain the same at present, as they were aeons ago.

Dāmodargupta, the author of *Kuṭṭanīmata*, adorned the court of King Jayāpīḍa Vinayāditya of the Karkoṭaka dynasty, who ruled Kashmir *circa* AD 779-810.

Other works on erotic literature may be mentioned serially. The *Rati-Rahasya*, of Kukkoka was composed sometimes before the twelfth century AD. This work is generally known as *Kukkoka* or *Koka-Śāstra*.

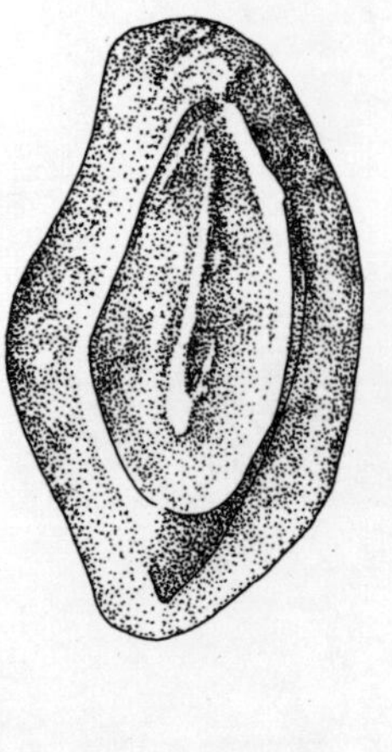

3. N.K. Devaraja, *The Mind and Spirit of India*, Motilal Banarsidass, Delhi, 1967, pp. 36-95.

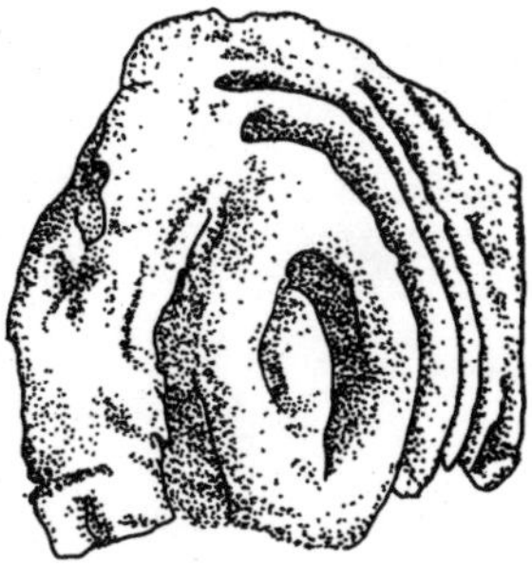

The *Nāgara-sarvasva* by Padmaśrī was written between the tenth and fourteenth centuries AD. The *Pañcasāyaka* by Maithili Jyotirīśvara Kaviśekhara was composed in the beginning of the fourteenth century AD. Mahārāja Praṇḍhadevarāya of Vijayanagara (fifteenth century AD) composed the *Ratiratna-pradīpikā* in seven chapters which is an elaborate treatise on sexual pleasures. The *Kāma-saṁhitā* by Ananta, discussing almost all the aspects of love, was written in AD 1457. *Kandarpacūḍāmaṇi* by King Vīrabhadra of the Vāghelā dynasty was composed in AD 1577. *Anaṅgaraṅga* by Kalyāṇamalla was composed in the sixteenth century AD and the *Rati-Mañjarī* in 60 verses only, by some unknown Jayadeva (different from the author of the *Gīta-Govinda*), are almost entirely with the subject of sexual union (*samprayogika*).[4]

To this galaxy of Indian literature on sex, the Mahānadī valley has also made its contribution. A palm-leaf literature on tāntric hedonism named *Yoga Nirṇaya Tantra* has been discovered from the Śakti Darbar records of former Śakti state, now in Chhattisgarh province. This collection is with Ram Prasad Mishra who is going to edit it soon.

The Pañcaśākhā of Orissa

The *pañcaśākhā* or the five fellow-religionists of Orissa belonged to medieval times. They were all contemporaries of Śrī Caitanya, the great exponent of Gauḍīya Vaiṣṇavism in Bengal, and their religion, both in theory and practice, did much in shaping the society of medieval Orissa, their influence extending to the spheres of ethics, literature and social mores of the area. The *pañcaśākhā* came from different parts of Cuttack and Purī. They were Balarāma Dās, Anata Dās, Jasobanta Dās, Jagannātha Dās and Acyutānanda Dās. Orissa has been a

4. (i) N.N. Bhattacharyya, *History of Indian Erotic Literature*, Munshiram Manoharlal, New Delhi, 1975, passim.

   (ii) Sushil Kumar De, *Ancient Indian Erotics and Erotic Literature*, Firma K.L. Mukhopadhyay, Kolkata, 1969, passim.

meeting ground of almost all the main currents of religious movements of India. The ancient scriptures describe it as a busy place of religious culture. Different kinds of religious thoughts — Brāhmaṇic, Tāntric and Vaiṣṇavite — has been intertwisted here to form a synthesis which has always made its influence felt on all its later religious movements. *Tantra* or *sādhanā* by the mother cult was also once very powerful in Orissa. In *pañcaśākhā* literature *mantra, yantra* and *yoga* find a place. The *pañcaśākhā* have also given the importance to *kuṇḍalinī yoga* or *cakra-bheda*. After *tantra*s, Acyuta has contemplated of a *devatā* on each of the *cakra*s, with his corresponding consort, and with *anādi* and *ādi-mata* in the *ājñā cakra* or the plexus near the forehead. Upon the thousand-petalled lotus is *parama* Brahmā, the ultimate being, who has been equalled with Jagannātha, the presiding Lord of Orissa.[5]

Acyutānanda retorted that the *pañcaśākhā* were all well acquainted with the *śāstra*s and well versed in the ways of *yoga* and the *tantra*s.[6]

There is erotic literature named *Pañcaśāyaka*, in Oriyā language, written by Kavi Samrat Upendra Bhanja of Orissa (vide Appendix).

Upendra Bhañja

Upendra Bhañja is popularly known as the "Kavi Samrāṭ," of Orissa. This epithet literally means "the emperor of poets." In other words, he is the greatest of poets in the Oriyā language. His poetical works have been the centre of severe controversies and scholarly disputations among all sections of readers and writers in Orissa during the past three quarters of a century. To some, Upendra Bhañja is far from being a poet in the sublime sense of the term *kavi*; he is only a "mighty literary acrobat

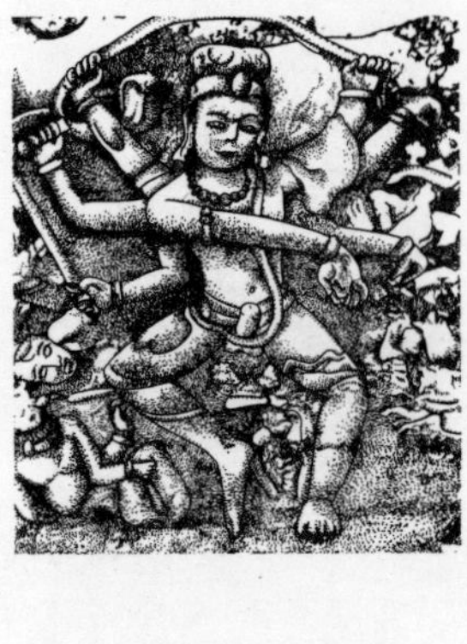

5. Chittaranjan Das, "The Pancha Sakha of Orissa," *Sidelights on History and Culture of Orissa*, Vidyapuri, Cuttack, 1977, pp. 678-91.
6. Chittaranjan Das, *Balarama Das*, Sahitya Akademi, New Delhi, 1982, p. 93.

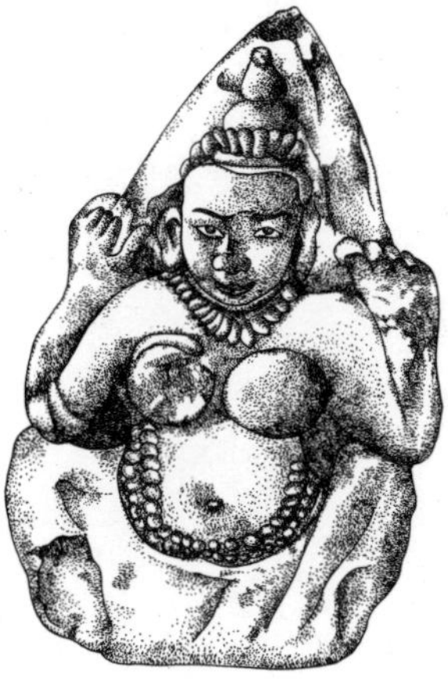

who has shown his greatest skill in verbal jugglery." To others, he is so great a poet that he deserves a place higher than those held by Kālidāsa, Homer, Milton, Rabindranath and the like. Thus, the pendulum of Upendra Bhañja's poetic appreciation oscillates between the two extremities of derogatory denumciations and complimentary commendations. It is needless to point out in this connection that sentimentalism and emotionalism preponderate over all such observations. It is reasonably held that the poet was born between AD 1675 and 1680. Upendra Bhañja was the grandson of Dhanañjaya Bhañja (and the son of Nīlakaṇṭha Bhañja) who ruled over Ghumsur, now part of Gañjam district in south Orissa.[7]

There is a vast innumerable Oriyā literature composed by Upendra Bhañja. It is interesting to find in his writings that he had a deep-seated compassion for the poor or the "have-nots." Oriyā is a unique language with powerful vocabulary and expression of thought. Its alphabets are round, symbolic of cosmic love and union with that of the mother language of original Sanskrit. Oriyā is written as pronounced. Upendra Bhañja's verbal jugglery is unique, wonderful and unsurpassed.

Upendra Bhañja was a *siddha* yogic poet, *siddha* means to be accomplished in mystic formulae, success in *yoga* or penance. He was a devotee of Mother Kālī. *Tantra* gives importance to the motherhood of God and it seems that Upendra Bhañja from his intuitive knowledge could produce a literature named *Pañcaśāyaka* (vide Appendix). The speciality of this literature is that it deals with *candra calana*, medicine, and 64 sex poses, etc.

Candra calana, refers to the erogenous zones of women during different moon days. The moon plays a very important role in women's life. Women are said to be nine times more passionate than men. Different erotic centre in the female body is awakened on each lunar day. If the male concentrates his

7. Somnath Rath, "Upendra Bhanja," *Sidelights on History and Culture of Orissa*, Vidyapuri, Cuttack, 1977, pp. 692-701.

passion on that centre and arouses the female's passion then it will ignite very quickly and the orgasms will be far more intense. A finger feather touch of the clitoris and vaginal opening will be sufficient for a normal woman, to have many oozings. In very rare cases, the erotic zones of a female differs. The art for arousing pleasure and tāntric act are the same.

In Vātsyāyana's *Kāmasūtra*[8] it is mentioned that a female should learn and study the 64 practices of art. There is no mention of sexual poses. The 64 sexual poses are for the first time mentioned by Upendra Bhañja in his *Pañcaśāyaka*. The second author to write on *Causaṭhī rati bandhas* was Gopāla Bhañja whose 19 palm-leaf manuscripts are preserved in the Orissa State Museum, at Bhubaneswar.

So, *candra calana*, "medicine (viagra)," and "64 sex poses," are the unique gifts of Mahānadī valley to the amorous sexual pleasures of human beings, across the globe.

Ancient Indian writers had written much to promote maximum contentment, love and happiness among couples. Sex to them was a provision of God or nature, whichever word we might prefer to use, and was as common to human beings as it was to all animals, birds, reptiles, insects, fish and even vermin.

It was as common and matter-of-fact as were the other instincts of breathing, eating, drinking, sleeping and ejaculating that are essential and inavoidable in all living creatures. Only human beings could make sex act an art. Love-play, art of wooing, kissing, caressing, erotic stroking, coital articulation, embracing, perfect intercourse and attaining the climax with the art of prolonging the coital act should be done. By knowing how to do these acts, one should keep one's sex-life, sex-acts and love-making always fresh.[9] Therefore read the ancient

8. Sir R. Burton & F.F. Arbuthnot (trs), *Vātsyāyana's Kāmasūtra*, Orient Paperback, Delhi, 1982, pp. 30-34.
9. Kenneth Anderson, *Secrets of Sex*, Jaico Publishing House, Bombay, 1973, p. 1 and pp. 14-15 (passim).

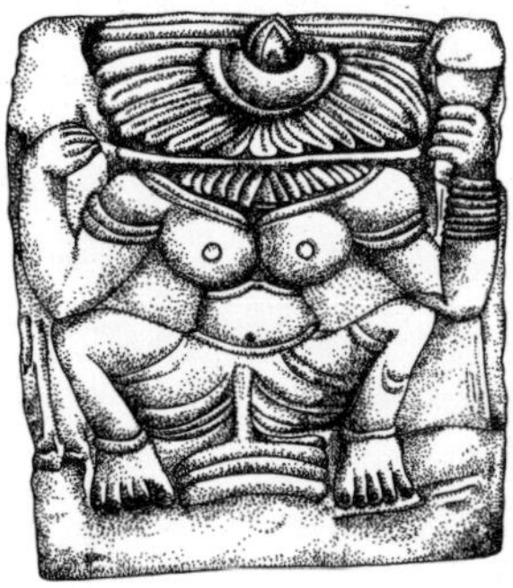

literature and practice their advice. Nothing is dirty in sex or in deriving the maximum pleasure.

Procreation

Procreation is to produce off-spring. When a female becomes pregnant, she delivers an off-spring, but how to get a boy or a girl through yogic and disciplined sex, has been taught in *Bṛhadāraṇyaka Upaniṣad* of the *Śukla Yajurveda*. This yogic science has not yet been properly worked out and popularized. The great task of popularizing this yogic aspect is the responsibility of Vedic *yogīs*, masters and teachers.

Samādhi

Samādhi means culmination of meditation through any *yoga*, state of oneness of mind with the object of concentration, supramental consciousness, the eight stages of *aṣṭāṅga yoga*, as mentioned by Maharṣi Patañjali.[10]

In the tāntric context, the transcendental desire justifies the sexual undertone. Desire creates its objects, as cosmic desire (*kāma*) created the world. Desire multiplies and creates many objects. Withdrawn and being focused on the void of ultimate reality, it becomes a special inner radiance.

For the *yoga* of sexual transformation, i.e., transforming the sexual ejaculation or orgasm of semen or ovum for the rise of *kuṇḍalinī*, a *tāntrika* indulge in sexual intercourse with a female partner as a mechanism for enhancing enjoyment in the direction of ecstasy, and does not conceive it as a quick scurry to orgasm. Control of seminal fluid is thought to entail control of all passions and the achievement of desirelessness. *aghora yogī* Vimalānanda[11] addresses this *yoga* as "Spiritual Erotic Art,"

---

10. Swami Chidananda, *Path to Blessedness (quintessence of the Aṣṭāṅga Yoga of sage Maharṣi Patañjali)*, The Divine Life Society, Shivanandnagar, 1975, passim.

11. R.E. Svoboda, *Aghora — At the left hand of God*, Rupa & Co. New Delhi , 1993, p. 246.

which is known to few people. To practise this *yoga*, some practical experiences of *haṭha yoga* needs to be learned. They are *vajrolī-mudrā*, *sahajolī-mudrā* and *uḍḍīyāna-bandha*. These *mudrā*s and *bandha* are explained by Nātha *yogī* Swātmarāma in his composition *Haṭha-Yoga-Pradīpikā*,[12] and by *aghora yogī* Vimalānanda through his disciple, R.E. Svoboda.

Vajrolī-Mudrā

Vajrolī-mudrā (thunderbolt attitude) is prescribed for men. The practice involves years of preparation which commences with the simple contraction of the urogenital muscles and later the sucking up of liquids. Through this practice of *vajrolī*, the sexual energy, hormones and secretions are reassimilated into the body. Its outcome is the union of the negative and positive poles of energy within one's own body.[13]

While practising *vajrolī*, one can suck one's penis into the body, like a tortoise, which draws its head and legs into its shell. After perfecting the *vajrolī-mudrā*, the practice of *uḍḍīyāna-bandha* becomes easy and one can suck one's sexual ejaculation before it is discharged, into the body, which passes through *iḍā* and *piṅgala nāḍī*s and finally reaches to the *suṣumnā-nāḍī*, the main *nāḍī* in the centre of the spinal cord, which conducts *kuṇḍalinī* Śakti. *Vajrolī-mudra* controls semen.

Sahajolī-Mudrā

Sahajolī-Mudrā is an attitude for spontaneous arousal. In *tantra*, the *vajrolī* is done by men and the same practice when done by women, is called *sahajolī*.

Uḍḍīyāna Bandha

Uḍḍīyāna bandha consists of abdominal retraction lock. *Uḍḍīyāna*

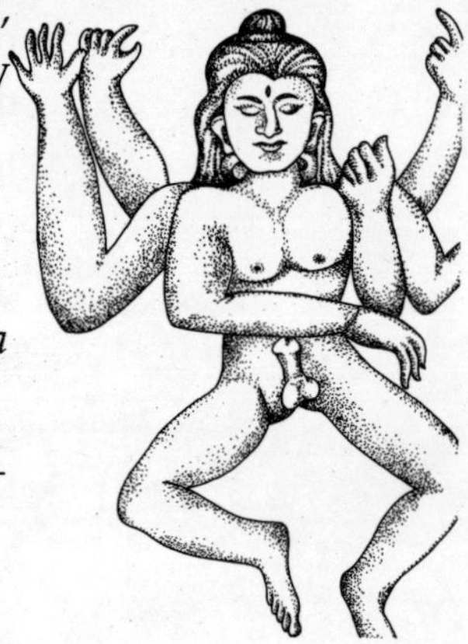

12. Swami Muktibodhananda Saraswati (Commentary), *Haṭha-Yoga-Pradīpikā*, Bihar School of Yoga, Munger, 1993, passim.
13. *Ibid.*, p. 332.

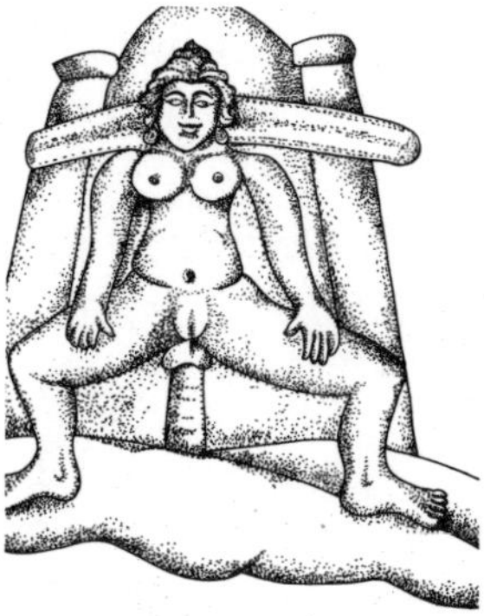

means "to rise up or fly." In the practice of *uḍḍīyāna bandha* the abdomonial organs are pulled up and in, creating a natural upward flow of energy, therefore it is often translated as the stomach lift. *Uḍḍīyāna bandha* changes the course of the downward moving *apāna vāyu* and unites with *prāṇa vāyu* and *samāna vāyu* in the naval centre. When the two opposite energies of *apāna* and *prāṇa* meet in the navel region, there is an explosion of potential force which travels upward through *suṣumṇā nāḍī*. Powered by *udāna vāyu*, it is taken up to the higher centres. Of course, this is a major event in the course of one's *sādhanā* and it does not take place with one or two rounds of practice. It requires a patient and ardent performance in combination with other techniques.[14]

14. Swami Muktibodhananda Saraswati (Commentary), *Haṭha-Yoga-Pradīpikā*, Bihar School of Yoga, Munger, 1993, passim. p. 299.

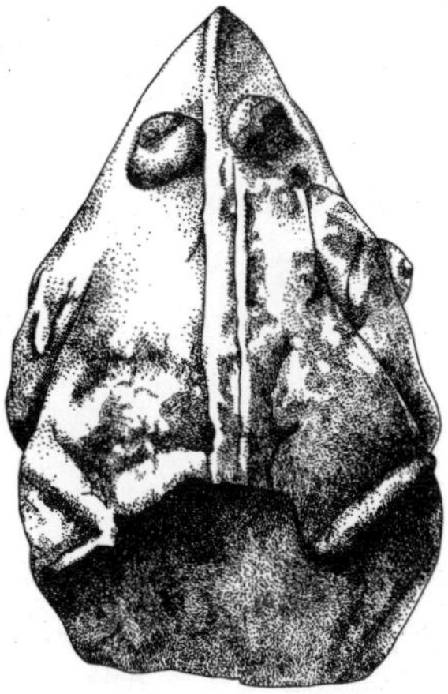

6

Kośalī Style of Temple Architecture

THE art of architecture or *vāstukalā* has a long history in India. K.C. Pandey[1] mentions, "Rasa-Brahma, therefore, is the highest, Nāda-Brahma the lower and Vāstu-Brahma the lowest category of the absolutist Indian philosophy of fine art." The art of temple architecture is therefore divine in Indian tradition.

There is a long narration of temple architecture in India and this can be grouped as (1) pre-Vedic architecture, (2) Vedic architecture, (3) architecture of the post-Vedic age, (4) architecture as described by Pāṇini, (5) architecture of epic age, (6) architecture as mentioned by Viśvakarmā, (7) architecture as described or stated by *maya*, *Purāṇas*, *Āgama*, *tāntric* literatures, Kauṭilya's architecture and Varāhamihira, (8) architecture as described by Bharata, Bhaṭṭa Lollaṭa, Bhaṭṭa Nāyaka and Abhinavagupta.

Besides these, there is a strong Śaiva tradition. According to K.C. Pandey,[2]

> Śaivaism is one of the earliest religions of the world. It seems to be the earliest religion that sprang up on Indian soil as it is evident from the archaeological finds at Harappa and Mohenjodaro. They establish the close relationship between Śaivism and the arts of architecture and sculpture. Therefore, it seems reasonable to suppose that the Śaiva tradition of

1. Kanti Chandra Pandey, *Comparative Aesthetics*, vol. I, Chowkhamba Sanskrit Series, Vārāṇasī, 1995, Chapter XIII, pp. 579-616.
2. *Ibid.*, 1995, pp. 585-87 and p. 616.

architectural and sculptural technique, as recorded in the Śaivāgamas, is the oldest. No doubt, the language of the Śaivāgamas is such that it can be assigned to a period earlier than the classical. But we have to distinguish between the time when the tradition was founded and that when it was recorded. And our assertion is that the record of the tradition is not the oldest, but the tradition itself is the oldest, because the massive architectural works, the ruins of which have been discovered at Harappa and Mohenjodaro together with the remnants of Śaivism such as the phallic emblem of Śiva, presuppose a well recognized technique. The Śaivāgamas, therefore, in our opinion, basically present the original architectural tradition in India, whatever may have been the later interpolations and however late the tradition may have been recorded.

There are 92 Śaivāgamas, a list of which has been given in an earlier work, *Abhinavagupta: A Historical and Philosophical study*. They are generally divided into four parts, *jñāna, yoga, caryā* and *kriyā*. The last part, among other things, deals with architectural and sculptural matters. To mention just a few among them to illustrate the point in land, we may add that the Kāmikāgama deals with architecture and sculpture, in 62 chapters out of the total of 75. In the Karaṇāgama in the beginning there are six chapters from three to eight, dealing with architectural details such as (i) *vāstuvinyāsa-vidhi*, (ii) *ādyoṣṭakā-vidhi*, (iii) *adhiṣṭhāna-vidhi*, (iv) *garbhanyāsa-vidhi*, (v) *prāsādalakṣana-vidhi*, (vi) *prākāralakṣaṇa-vidhi*. And the subsequent six chapters are concerned with sculpture such as *liṅgadakṣvaya-vidhi*, *pratimālakṣaṇa-vidhi*, etc. It talks of different images such as Nṛttamūrti Dakṣiṇāmūrti, Candraśekhara, Ardhanārī, Kālanigraha, Durāri, Caṇḍeśa, Gaurī, Durgā, Lakṣmī, Mohinī, etc. And the Suprabhedāgama has fifteen chapters on architecture and sculpture.

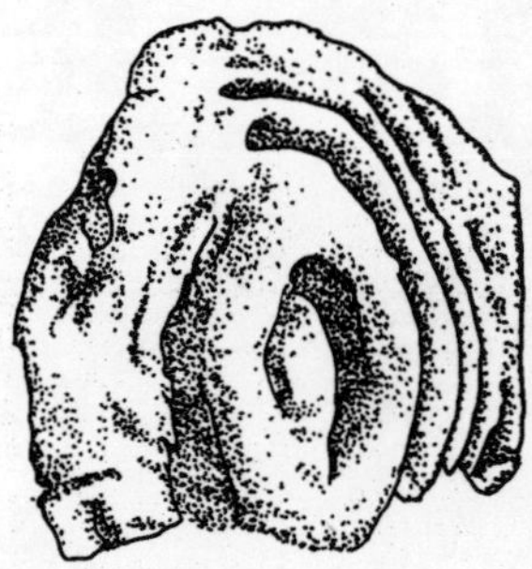

The *Aṁśumadbheda* of Kāśyapa is an important work on architecture. It seems to follow the Śaiva tradition as recorded in the dualistic Śaivāgama, called *Aṁśumān*. Its main contribution is to sculpture to which it devotes as many as 39 chapters, giving the characteristic features of different

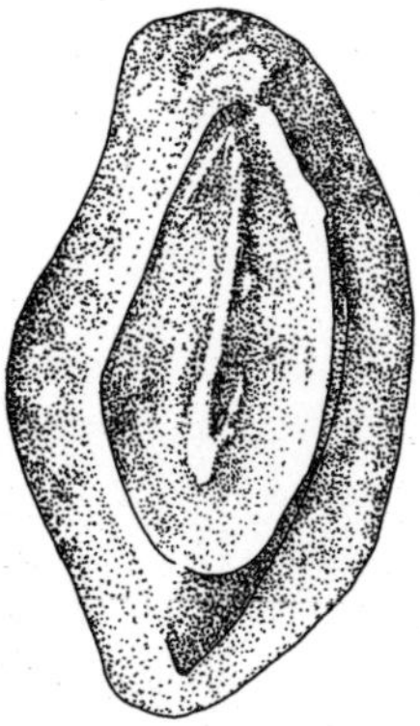

images Śiva such as Candrāśekhara, Ardha-nārīśvara, Gajaha, Paśupata, etc., which represent mythical conceptions of Śiva. It appears that by the time Kaśyapa wrote this work, antagonism between Śaivism and Vaiṣṇavaism had disappeared or at least there was an attempt to reconcile the two as it gives the characteristics of an image of Śiva, half of which was Viṣṇu Haryardha-Hara. In an another available work the sculptural details of many images of Śiva are given.

Agastya is another authority, frequently referred to. From the fragments of the manuscripts (MSS), available in the collection at Madras, it appears that it primarily followed the Śaiva architectural tradition as recorded in the *Aṁśumadbheda* of Kaśyapa. For, in the section on sculpture it is concerned with the characteristics of different images of Śiva such as Candraśekhara, Kalyāṇasundara, Ardhanārīśvara, etc.

The *Tantra Samuccaya* by Nārāyaṇa presents the Śaiva architectural tradition because, according to the author's own statement, the information about architectural matters given therein was collected from the Śaiva Tantras or Āgamas (*so'yaṁ tantramidaṁ vyadhād vahuvidhādudhṛtya tantrārṇavāt*).

With this much of informations on Śaiva tradition in architecture, the opinion of Shiva Shekhar Misra[3] may be stated when he states,

> The Indian temple architecture evolved several forms and features, which indicate the history of Brahmanical worship. Although the Brahmanical worship was in existence long before the beginning of the Christian era, no temple, however, dedicated to Śiva or Viṣṇu seems to have survived that was built before AD 400. An old Brahmanical temple surviving today is at Ramnagar in Bareilly district. The temple is dedicated to Śiva and is said to belong either to the first century BC or the first century AD.

3. Shiva Shekhar Misra, *Fine Arts & Technical Sciences in Indian with special reference to Somesvara's Mānsollāsa*, Krishnadas Academy, Vārāṇasī, 1982, pp. 75-76.

An example of one of earliest forms of the temple is a first rectangular shrine at Sāñcī which dates about AD 400. It is in a very primitive shape and resembles the rock-cut cave temple of the Buddhist period. It is here that we find the nucleus of a Hindu temple, consisting of a *garbhagṛham* with an entrance and the *maṇḍapa*. Looking to the structure of the temple, we find that in a greater part of the country, the sanctuary as a whole is called the *vimāna*. The upper portion of the sanctuary is known as the *śikhara,* i.e., the tower or spire. Inside the *vimāna* there is a small chamber known as the *garbhagṛha* or "womb-house," which is meant for the reception of the divine symbol. The *garbhagṛha* is usually entered through a doorway on its inner or eastern side. In front of the doorway there is a *maṇḍapa* or a "pillared hall." In some of the temples, however, the *maṇḍapa* is a detached building which is isolated from the sanctuary by an open space.

It is by the sixth century AD that three distinctive types of temples were evolved, viz., (1) The *Nāgara,* (2) *Drāviḍa* and (3) *Vesara.*

The main feature of the *nāgara* type is its curvilinear *śikhara* ending with a *kalaśa,* with a pointed spire or *śṛṅga*. This temple is also known as the northern or the Indo-Āryan or Āryāvartta type.

There is a lot of controversy among the scholars[4] regarding the origin of the curvilinear *śikhara* of the *nāgara* style. Simpson expresses the opinion that it is derived from the dome or conical hut of the archaic type, or it is an imitation of some old bamboo processional car. According to Macdonell, it is derived from the *stūpa* or the *caitya*. Rama Prasad Chandā is of the view that it is derived from the archaic *kūṭagāra*.

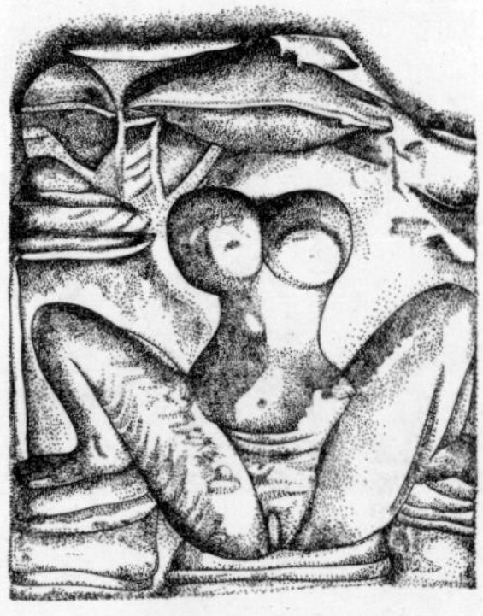

There are much contributions of Āgama and tāntric literatures to the development of temple architecture in India. S.S. Misra[5]

4. G.D. Sarkar, "Notes on the History of the Sikkara Temples," *Rupam*, no. 10, April 1922.
5. S.S. Misra, *op. cit.*, 1982, pp. 69-70.

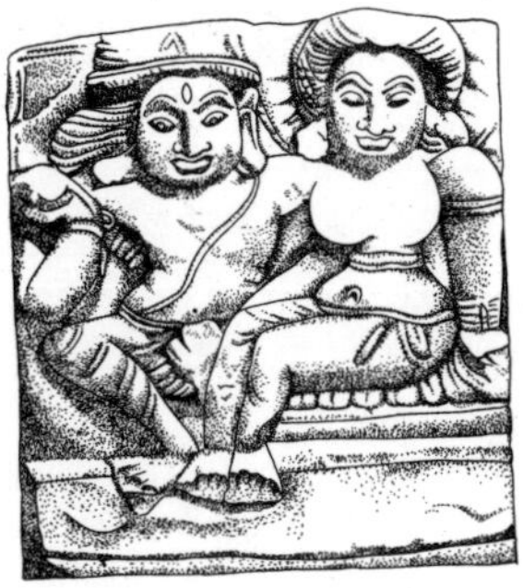

may again be quoted, "The contribution of the vast Āgama literature to the art of architecture is no less remarkable." K.C. Pandey[6] presumes, "that the Śaiva tradition of architectural and sculptural technique, as recorded in the Śaivāgamas is the oldest." As mentioned earlier, the tradition of the Śaivāgamas is very old, yet their language indicates that their period can be assigned earlier than the classical period. The subject-matter of these Āgamas is divided into four parts, viz:, (1) *jñāna*, (2) *yoga*, (3) *caryā*, and (4) *kriyā*.

The architectural technique is found in the *kriyā* portion. The *Kāmikāgama* consists of several chapters on architecture and sculpture, which include the description of *dviśālā*s, *catuśśālā*s, *vardhamāna*, *nandyāvarta*, *svastika-śālā*s and also *pakṣa-śālā*, *hasti-śālā*, etc.

The Karaṇāgama denotes six chapters[7] on architecture dealing with the following:-

1. Vāstuvinyāsa-vidhi
2. Adyeṣṭakā-vidhi
3. Adhiṣthāna-vidhi
4. Garbhanyāsa-vidhi
5. Prāsādalakṣana-vidhi
6. Prākāralakṣaṇa-vidhi

The *Agni Purāṇa* gives a list of 25 tāntric works[8] on the names of their *ācārya*s. Of these Hayaśīrṣa and Garga belong to the northern tradition or *nāgara* school of architecture, while the remaining *ācārya*s belong to the southern or Draviḍian school of architecture.

With reference to the Āgamas, *Mānasāra* and *Mayamata*,

---

6. K.C. Pandey, *Comparative Aesthetics*, vol. I, 2nd edn., Chowkhamba Sanskrit Series, Vārāṇasī, 1959, p. 585.
7. *Karaṇāgama*, Chapters 2 to 8.
8. *Agni Purāṇa*, Chapter 39.

Lalit Kumar Shukla[9] mentions *nāgara, vesara, drāviḍa,* Kośalī and Kaliṅga styles.

The present Orissa which comprises parts of ancient South Kośala, Utkala and Kaliṅga states, had its own *Śilpa-śāstras*. The upper Mahānadī valley, which forms the modern Chhattisgarh province, comprises South Kośala State of ancient and medieval periods. Rajendra Prasad Das[10] mentions of *Bhuvanapradīpa, Pratiṣṭhālakṣaṇa-sāra-samuccaya, Śilpa Prakāśa, Saudhikāgama, Śilpa Sāriṇī, Vāstusūtra Upaniṣad* and *Śilpa-ratnakośa*.

Bhuvanapradīpa[11] is the earliest Śilpa-śāstra of Orissa and it mentions of 36 styles of *rekhā* temples and three varieties of *khākarā* temples. Among these 36 types of *rekhā* temples, Kośalī style is mentioned without details. While describing three types of *khākarā* temples, measurements and descriptions are given and mention is made of Draviḍa *khākarā*, Brarabhi *khākarā* and Kośalī *khākarā*.

In the course of a survey of the Kośalī style of temple architecture, the author surveyed the whole upper Mahānadī river valley, as it comprised the South Kośala state of ancient and medieval periods. While earlier narrating the "Kośalī Style of Temple Architecture," the author[12] was of opinion that *vāstupuruṣa-maṇḍala*, a ritual diagram of 64 small squares, i.e., 8 × 8 = 64 squares forming a large square, was prescribed for

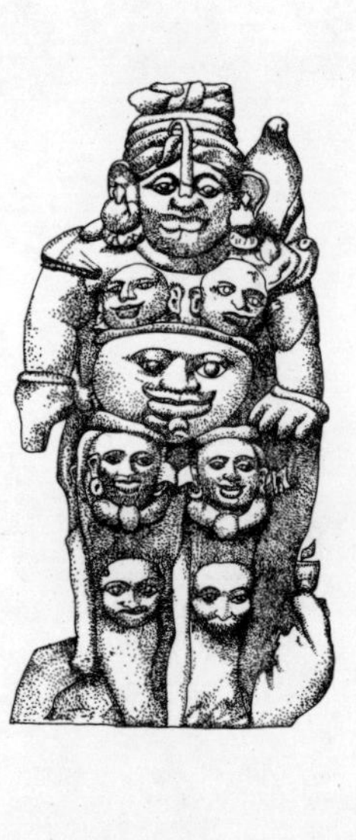

9. L.K. Shukla, *A Study of Hindu Art and Architecture, with special reference to terminology*, Chowkhamba Sanskrit Series Office, Vārāṇasī, 1972, p. 196.

10. R.P. Das, "The Study of Śilpa Śāstras," *Reference Orissa*, ed. A.N. Tiwari, Enterprising Publishers, Bhubaneswar, 1999, pp. 174-81.

11. Nirmal Kumar Bose, *Canons of Orissan Architecture*, Cosmo Publications, New Delhi, 1982, p. 124 and pp. 171-73.

12. J.P. Singh Deo, *Cultural Profile of South Kośala*, Gyan Publishing House, New Delhi, 1987, pp. 329-30.

temples in the *Bṛhat-Saṁhita* by Varāhmihira[13] (*Fig.* 9) who flourished in the sixth century AD. The text originated in north India and how it travelled to far away South Kośala, where most of the temples with the plan of eight by eight squares determining the proportions and placement of parts for the square *nāgara* temples were evolved, is a matter of wonder.

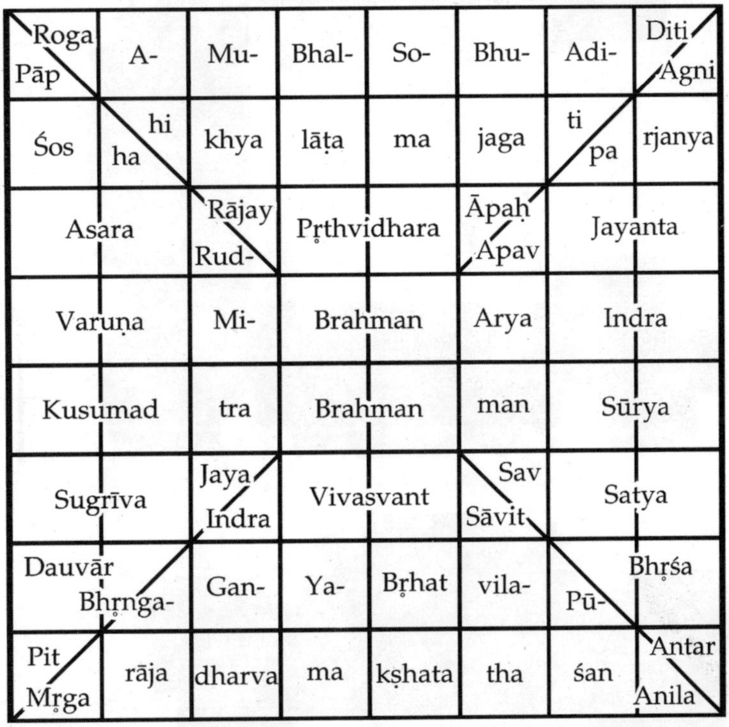

fig. 9.
Vāstupuruśamaṇḍala, 8 x 8 = 64 squares. (Source: Williams, J.G. (ed.), *Kalādarśana — American Studies in the Art of India*, Oxford & IBH Publishing Co. New Delhi, 1981, p. 79).

The stellate plans and the plans of two squares placed diagonally and intersecting each other at 45º angle probably developed by basing on the *vāstupuruṣa-maṇḍala*, in the territory of South Kośala (*Fig.* 6). *Tantra* aims at attaining salvation with the help of mystic diagrams and *mantras*. Therefore, it can definitely be said that the plans of the concerned temples of South Kośala developed with *tantra* influence.

---

13. R.C. Majumdar, "Astronomy," *THACOTIP*, vol. III, The Classical Age, 1970, p. 321.

Rāma temple at Sirpur (*circa* AD 595-605) (*Fig.* 10), the Indal Duel at Kharod (*circa* AD 650-60) (*Fig.* 11), the Siddheśvara

fig. 10.
Plan of the Rāma Temple, Sirpur, Raipur district, Chhattisgarh province. (Source: Williams, J.G. (ed.), *Kalādarśana — American Studies in the Art of India*, 1981, p. 139).

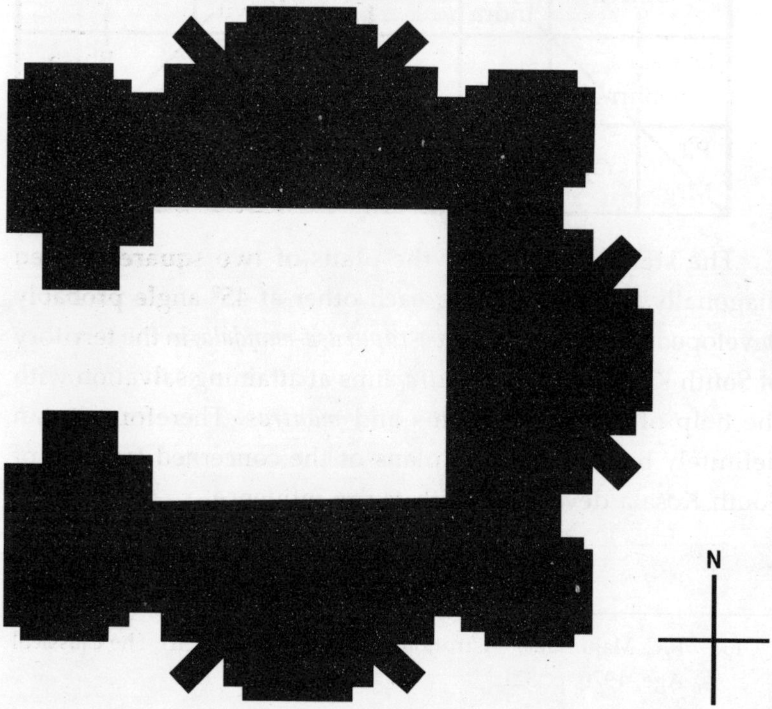

fig. 11.
Plan of Indal Deul, Kharod. (Source: Williams, J.G. (ed.), *Kalādarśana — American Studies in the Art of India*, 1981, p. 141).

temple at Palari (*circa* AD 675-85) and the Śabarī temple at Kharod (*circa* AD 700-10) (*Fig.* 12) have stellate plans.[14] Another

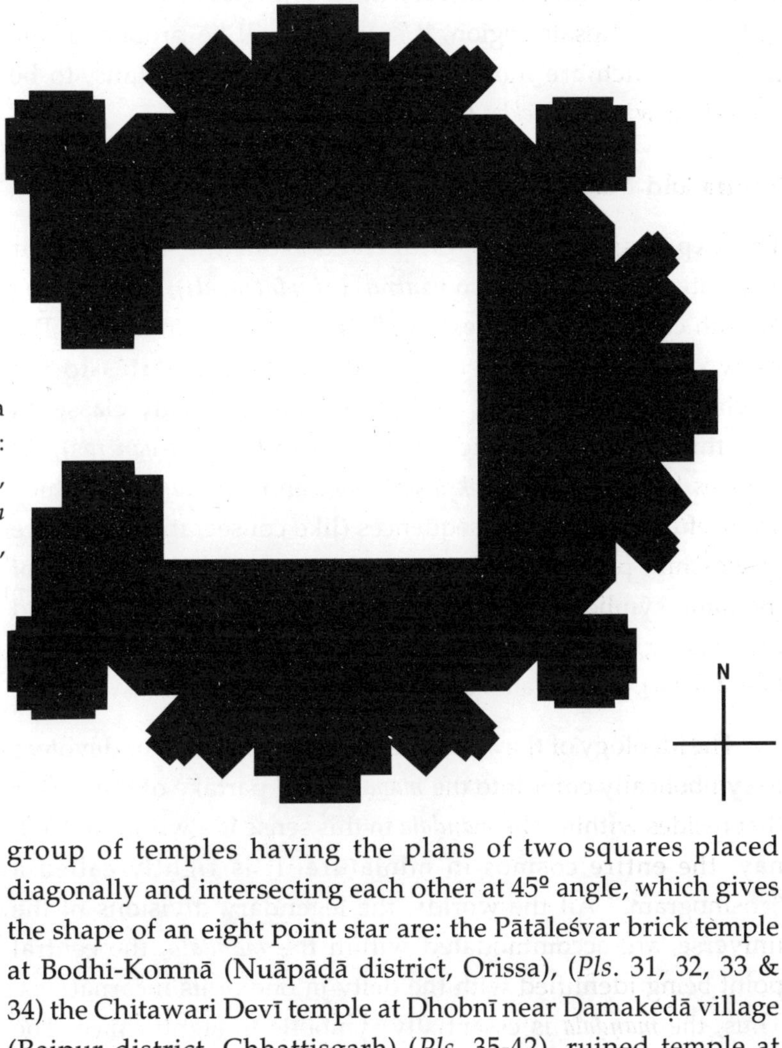

fig. 12.
Plan of the Siddheśvara Temple, Palari. (Source: Williams, J.G. (ed.), *Kalādarśana — American Studies in the Art of India*, 1981, p. 142).

group of temples having the plans of two squares placed diagonally and intersecting each other at 45º angle, which gives the shape of an eight point star are: the Pātāleśvar brick temple at Bodhi-Komnā (Nuāpāḍā district, Orissa), (*Pls.* 31, 32, 33 & 34) the Chitawari Devī temple at Dhobnī near Damakeḍā village (Raipur district, Chhattisgarh) (*Pls.* 35-42), ruined temple at Kansil in the Rānīpur-Jharial complex (Bolaṅgīr district, Orissa) and another ruined temple at Adhabhara village situated about 8 km south of Kharsia (Bilāspur district, Chhattisgarh). As

14. Donald M. Stadtner, "Ancient Kośala and Stellate Plan," *Kalādarśana, American Studies in the Art of India*, ed. G. Williams Joanna, Oxford and IBH. Publishing Co., New Delhi, 1981, p. 137.

single temple with different types of stellate plans are found and four temples with the plans of two squares placed diagonally and intersecting each other at angles of 45º are traced in the South Kośala region, it seems, it will be proper for the temples which are more in number with same plans, to be identified with the *rekhā* type in Kośalī style.

Yantra and Maṇḍala

The expression *yantra*[15] is derived from the root *yam* or alternatively from the form *yantrati* (or *yantrayati*), the meaning in both cases being "to restrain," "to compel" "to bend." The early context in which the word was used relates to the mechanical contrivances. The *yantra*s are generally classified into three types: (1) devices for worship (*puyana-yantra*s), (2) devices for protection (*rakṣā yantra*s), and (3) *maṇḍala*s which are useful in ceremonial sequences (like consecrating the place of worship, placement of the ritual jar or *kalaśa*, placement of the lamp symbolizing God or Goddess, preparing the ground for making food-offerings or *naivedya*) in the initiatory rites (*dīkṣā-vidhi*), and as aids in meditations (*dhyāna*s).

The ideology of the *maṇḍala* allows the aspirants or devotees to symbolically enter into the *maṇḍala* and partake of the power that resides within. The *maṇḍala* in this sense is a world in itself, nay, the entire cosmos in miniature. It is rightly called a "cosmogram." All the worlds, the legendary divisions of the universe, are accommodated within the *maṇḍala*, the central point being identified with the deity in one of its incarnations. Thus, the *maṇḍala* is essentially symbolic in significance. The more elaborate *maṇḍala*s are large in size, sometimes big enough for groups of devotees to sit or move around within their precincts. A *yantra*, contrarily, is always small in size, even when elaborate.

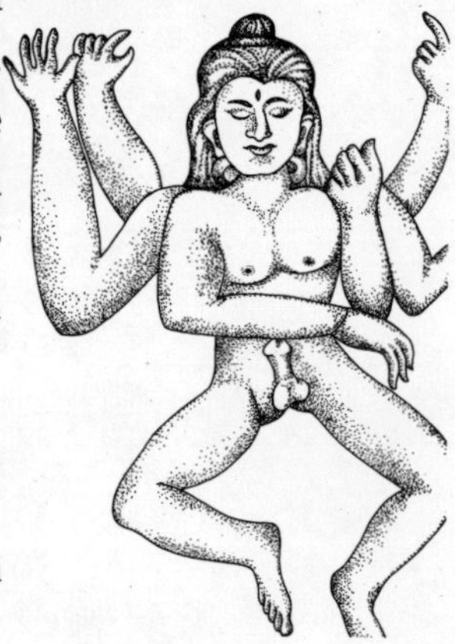

Further Prof. S.K. Ramachandra Rao illustrates that it is

15. Prof. S.K. Ramachandra Rao, *The Yantras*, Sri Satguru Publications, Delhi, 1988, pp. 10, 16 & 18.

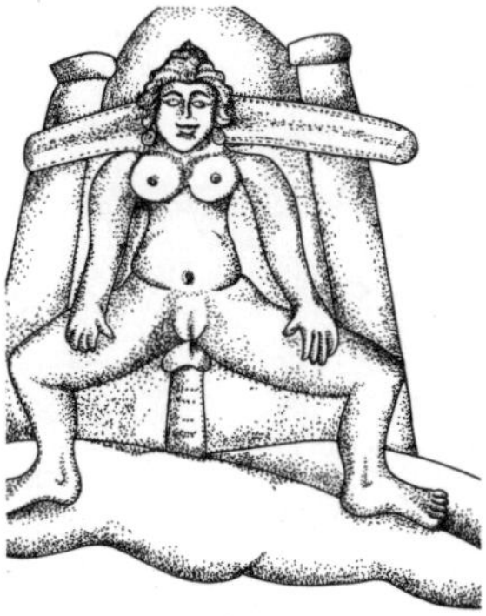

important to remember that the central point is also the undifferentiated but individualized consciousness (*citta*). The modalities like the triangle, the square and the circle are the various emanations from the source which indicate the diffusion of the original power into several diverse forces. The employment of a *maṇḍala* is for the purpose of meditation involved in the gathering up of the forces and focusing consciousness into the central point. Incidental to this is the acquisition of power: the mind that is concentrated is powerful while the mind that is scattered is weak. Thoughts and feelings that are diffuse characterize the normal man. Meditation is a technique of setting them, focusing them into some system.

Maṇḍala in this sense provides the modal for experiencing reality, for reintegration, for self-actualization. It accomodates not only the modalities of the transitional world but even the unconscious processes. The underlying idea is that there is no inherent dichotomy between the external and internal realities, between the physical universe and the psychological world. Things and thoughts are but different modalities of the self-same spirit, whose real nature is undifferentiated consciousness (*citta-mātra*). This is the significance of the tāntric statement that "*saṁsāra* and *mokṣa* are one." The *maṇḍala* is a graphic representation of this idea.

About *yantra*s or mechanical contrivances in ancient India, V. Raghavan[16] states,

> That from ancient times the idea of a *yantra* was very common is proved by two facts, the application of the concept to the esoteric sphere, and the way the *yantra* roused the imagination of the spiritual writers. In esoteric worship the *yantra* was a chart stored up within the confines of spiritual power; drawn on a flat surface or made in relief, it had components or details which had to be strictly conformed to

16. V. Raghavan, *Yantras or Mechanical Contrivances in Ancient India*, (Transaction no. 10), The Indian Institute of Culture, Bangalore, 2nd edn., 1956, p. 2.

and, as an instrument for achieving spiritual power it eminently deserved the same *yantra*. In the minds of the writers, who were essentially men of religious faith and spiritual yearning, the *yantra* or machine always suggested a highly apt analogy for the material universe or the mundane body activated by a god or presided over by a soul.

The word *yantra* is derived from the root *yan*, meaning to control and it has been freely used in ancient India for any contrivance. Some very commonly known simple ones are the water-pulley in the well called *ghaṭiyantra*; an oil-presser was *taila-yantra*, a cane-presser was *ikṣu-yantra*, ploughs, water-lifts and even the weighing balance were referred to as *yantras* (*Arthaśāstra* II, 19; II, 24), and in Tamil even the stone grain-grinder is referred to by the Tamil name "entiram." These should not lead us to think that very complicated mechanisms were not evolved by the ancients.

Svāmī Satyananda Sarasvati[17] illustrates the *maṇḍala* and *yantra* well and states,

> A *maṇḍala* is a magic circle in which one performs tāntric rites. It is a focus of cosmic powers. During worship and other tāntric practices a *maṇḍala* becomes the centre of the universe in a symbolic sense and in a far deeper sense beyond normal comprehension. A tāntric *maṇḍala* is usually laid out according to a fixed. Plan, in fact the making of the *maṇḍala* is a tāntric rite in itself.
>
> As we have already pointed out under the heading "Tantra — The Universal System," everything in the manifest world is in essence a *maṇḍala*. Each and every object is a focal point of consciousness. There is not one thing that is not a *maṇḍala*. Everything is a point of manifestation of Śakti . . . an

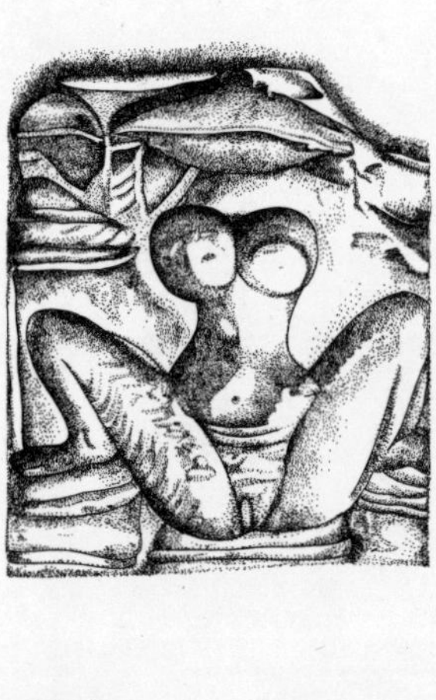

17. Svāmī Satyananda Saraswati, *A Systematic Course in the Ancient Tāntric Techniques of Yoga and Kriyā*, Bihar School of Yoga, Munger, 1981, pp. 335-36.

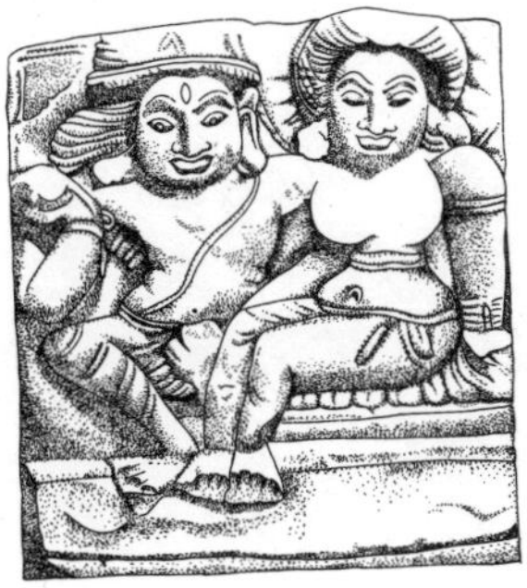

expression of the underlying consciousness. It is for this reason that deep concentration on everything, and we mean anything, can bring about higher awareness and realization of the deeper nature of that object. But almost every person lacks sufficient power of concentration to do this. Instead, the power of the mind is dissipated in all directions. But the power is there to be used when the individual is ready, it only needs to be tapped. It is for this reason that devotion is an important, though not indispensable part of tāntric meditative practices. It increases or super charges the power of concentration. Concentration becomes far more powerful and piercing when it is backed up by emotional feelings or reverence.

Each person is a *maṇḍala*, each thought is a *maṇḍala*, each deity, each *cakra* . . . each and everything. The *guru* (master) too is a *maṇḍala* — a very powerful one in fact. This may be a little far away from the normally accepted meaning of the word *maṇḍala*, but as far as we are concerned the *guru* is indeed a *maṇḍala*. He in a sense, draws down cosmic consciousness, acting as a magnet through which this consciousness expresses itself most obviously and clearly. He, radiates the inner light of consciousness to everyone . . . he glows with it. It is through the *guru* that cosmic powers are unleashed, attracted and transmitted to the disciple. This is the grace of the *guru maṇḍala*.

Sexual union is also a powerful *maṇḍala*. That is why it can be a means to meditation. When a man and a woman make love, they are creating a magic circle, a *maṇḍala*.

The definitions that we have given are wide. For the sake of tradition and simplicity, we will define a *maṇḍala* more specifically as a centre or special place, possibly consecrated by special rites, which is used for tāntric practices. This means, when you are doing your *yoga* practices you are really creating a *maṇḍala*, a magic circle. You are creating a centre and trying to tune in with invoke and harmonize with higher consciousness. Do you realize this? You are really performing a rite when you do *āsanas*, *prāṇāyāma* and other practices. Of course, there is probably no worship involved as such, but it is nevertheless a form of rite. Remember this point if you have a tendency to scoff at rituals.

What is a *yantra*? A *yantra* is a specific form of *maṇḍala* which consists of geometrical shapes and figures, and sometimes diagrams of deities (especially in the Buddhist *tantra* system). This is also a deified form of an aspect of existence, though it is less obvious. A *yantra* is a particularly powerful form of *maṇḍala* and deep concentration on it can lead to higher realization of its nature.

The Sanskrit word *yantra* is a descriptive word perfectly apt for the name of this form of *maṇḍala*. According to the dictionary, it means an instrument, a machine, an apparatus, an implement. And this exactly sums up the mystical diagram in all ways. It is indeed an implement, a machine (though not an electrical or mechanical one) because it acts as an instrument for tuning it with consciousness. It is indeed a machine — a machine to induce the state of meditation. It is a spiritual machine . . . *Maṇḍala* and *yantra*s are an indispensable part of *tantra*, without them *tantra* would not be *tantra*. Without them *tantra* would fail to give the result that it does. We are not asking you to believe in the power of *maṇḍala* and *yantras*, but at least keep an open mind and in the future practice for yourself, so that you can know from your own experiences.

While dealing with the Āgamic tradition and the arts of India, the *yantra* and *maṇḍala* narration cannot be left out. Therefore, S.P. Sabarathinam[18] states,

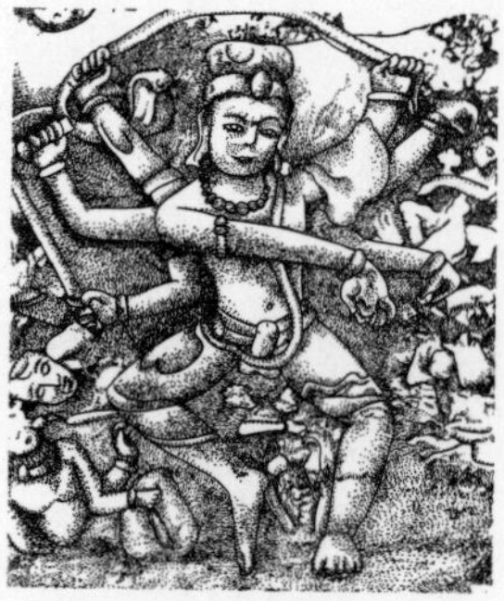

18. S.P. Sabarathinam, "Āgamic treatment of Mahābhūtas in relation to Maṇḍalas and Arts," *Prakṛti — The Integral Vision*, vol. III, K. Vatsyayan (General editor), Indira Gandhi National Centre for the Arts & D.K. Printworld (P) Ltd. New Delhi, 1995, pp. 57 & 58-59.

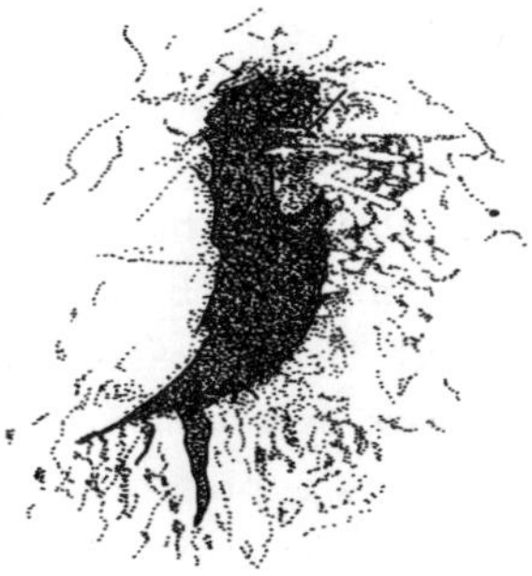

> Every construction is to be strictly based on the *Vāstupuruṣa-maṇḍala.* Longevity, auspiciousness, strength and beauty could be accomplished in any construction only through *Vāstu-maṇḍala.* . . . Needless to mention that temple construction is based on the *Vāstu-maṇḍala.* . . . Being an artistic device, the *maṇḍala* incorporates in itself all the significant aspects of symbols, sounds, colours and divinities, with a stronghold on metaphysical and ontological principles. The Āgamas excel all other scriptures with their elaborate and effective details and descriptions of various *maṇḍalas*. In the Śaivāgamic group, the *Kiraṇāgama* is held in high esteem owing to its copious details and directions on the mechanism of *maṇḍalas*. Besides a separate chapter on the *maṇḍala-vidhi* it prescribes the *Vaktra-maṇḍala* for the worship of Sarasvatī and *kalaśa-maṇḍala* for the worship of Lord Mṛtyuñjaya, the details of which are not to be seen in any other Āgama.
>
> *Maṇḍala* is an aesthetic and mystic design in which the combination and intersection of various forms related to the gross elements and to the deities concerned have their full play. The correspondence of colours, the distribution of letters (*mātṛka-akṣaras*) and the esoteric significance enhance the mystic value of *maṇḍalas*. Each *maṇḍala* has its own principal deity and attendant deities directly or indirectly related to the five gross elements. So the rituals which involve *maṇḍala-pūjā* are highly efficacious in energizing and sanctifying the environment conditioned by the gross elements.

A *maṇḍala* village exists in Belpara Block of Bolaṅgīr district of Orissa and there is also one rare but ruined stellate brick temple structure over a stone plinth within the fort area at Patnagarh in the same district (*Fig.* 13). These prove the vigorous tāntric practices performed in this area in earlier days.

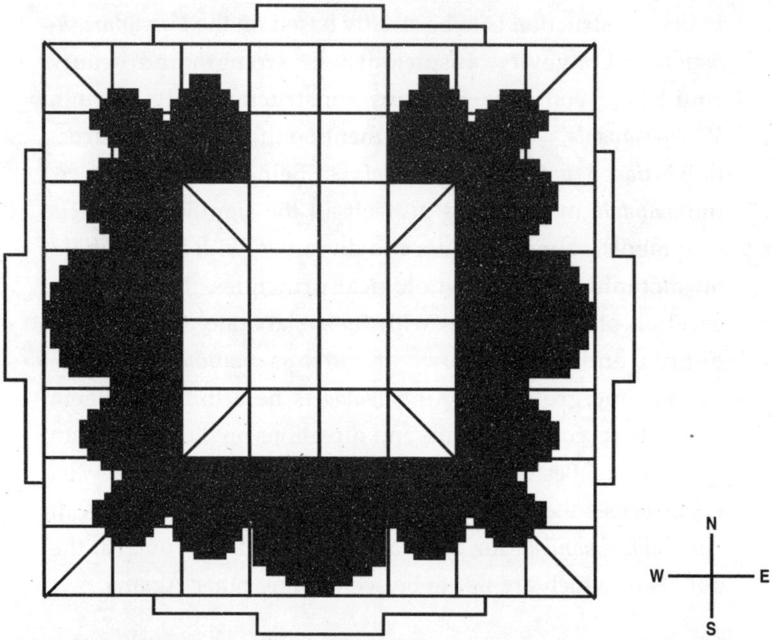

fig. 13.
Plan of the fallen Stellate Brick Temple on the *Pañcaratha* Stone basement at Patnagarh, Bolangīr district, Orissa, based on *Vāstupuruṣamaṇḍala*, 8 × 8 = 64 squares, as prescribed in the sixth century *Bṛhat Saṁhitā*.

Gross Elements

S.P. Sabarathinam[19] states that the individual self, though it is bodily confined to impure *māyā*, is capable of being in touch with the principles of mixed and pure planes only through the grace of Lord Śiva, who manifests himself as Sarva, Bhava, Paśupati, Śāna and Bhīma correspondent to earth, water, fire, air and space respectively.

The gross human body consists of five elements earth, water, fire, air and space, known as *pañcabhūtas* in yogic terminology. According to Svāmī Chinmayananda,[20]

> The gross body so formed is the hutment of experience, the temple of joy or the house of sorrow. The indweller of the body experiences his joys and sorrows only through his physical body. The state in which the ego making use of its physical body comes in contact with the world of objects and

19. S.P. Sabarathinam, "Āgamic treatment of Mahābhūtas in relation to Maṇḍalas and Arts," *Prakṛti — The Integral Vision*, 1995, p. 53.

20. Svāmī Chinmayananda, *Vedanta The Science of Life*, Part I, Central

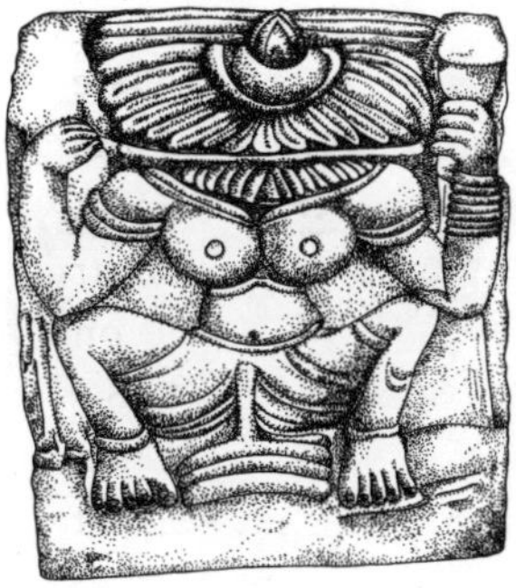

ekes out its joys and sorrows, is the "waking" condition of the *jiva* (living being).

Through ritual and *yoga*, one can achieve the *pañcabhūta-śuddhi*, thereby developing a correspondence between the microcosm and the macrocosm which can be utilized for esoteric and spiritual purposes. In the practice of *pañcabhūta-śuddhi* a master (*guru*) is always needed.

Kośalī Style of Rekhā Temple

The plan of two squares placed diagonally and intersecting each other at 45º angle is traced in the four temples in the South Kośala region, which seems to be based on *yantra*.

The possible *yantra*s are indeed innumerable. The combinations of the primary geometrical forms (triangles, circles and four-sided figures) can be myraid, and the association of *mantra*s with the designs render the number of these combinations really huge. There is a Sanskrit text, comparatively recent, which enumerates as many as 10,000 *yantras* ; The name of this text is *Yantroddhārasarvasva*, and the author (anonymous) claims that he obtained all these *yantra*s from the *Atharvaveda*, however not, explaining how. The largest well-known collection, however, is found as a supplementary section to the *Saundarya-Laharī*, ascribed to the great Śaṅkara: it contains 103 *yantra*s with details concerning their use, known as *prayoga*. Another text the *Yantra-Cintāmaṇi*, contains about 80 *yantras*. The *Mantra-mahodadhi* describes about 70. The *Prapañcasāra-Saṁgraha*, about 60. The *Prayoga-Kaumudī* about 50. The *Mantra-yantra-mahārṇava* about the same number. Other texts like the *Kāma-ratna, Maṇi-mantrakośa, Devatā-pūjana-vidhi, Yantra-prakāśa, Yantra-pratiṣṭhā* and *Yantra-pūjana-prakāra* also contain numerous illustrations of *yantras*.[21]

In the *Śivānandalaharī* (verse 42), Śaṅkarācārya informs that

Chinmaya Mission Trust, Bombay, 1983, p. 130.

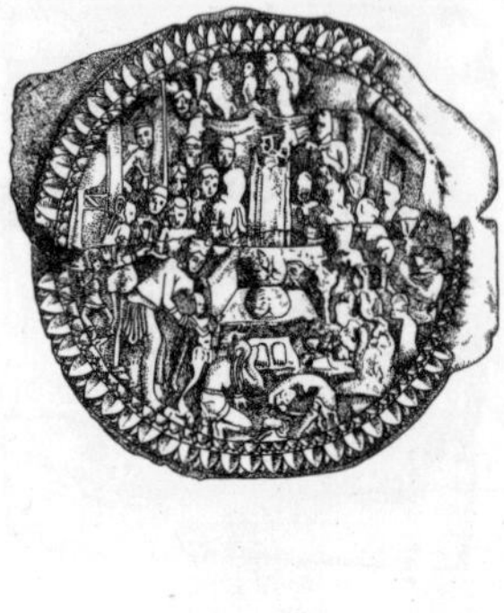

Śiva like to reside in fortresses which are impregnable, well guarded and provided with every convenience.[22]

English Translation of Śivānandalaharī, verse 42

> O God, who art fond of inaccessible fortresses (or Durgā): Do stay always in the fortress of my mind which has magnificences as surrounding moats, great courage as ramparts, high qualities as royal armies and is provided with the gateways of sense organs that are firm in the body and is

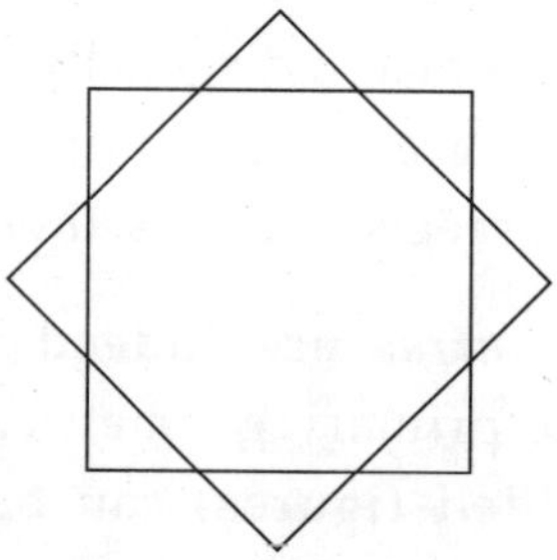

> endowed with a profusion of provisions consisting of knowledge, and thus is complete with all the necessary appurtenances.

The mind is compared here to a fortress, and the Lord is invited to take his residence there. The Lord is fond of fortresses. He may well reside in the fortress of the mind. There is a pun on the word Durgā. It means "fortress," and is also a name of Pārvatī.

The Kośalī style of *rekhā* temple, owes its plan of two squares placed diagonally and intersecting each other at 45º angle, which gives the shape of an eight-point star, to *yantras* of the *mantras* of *Ānanda-Laharī* and *Saundarya-Laharī*, composed by Ādi-Śaṅkarācārya (*Fig*. 14).

---

21. Prof. S.K. Ramachandra Rao, *The Yantras, op. cit.*, 1988, p. 14.
22. T.M.P. Mahadevan, *The Hymns of Śaṅkara*, Motilal Banarsidass,

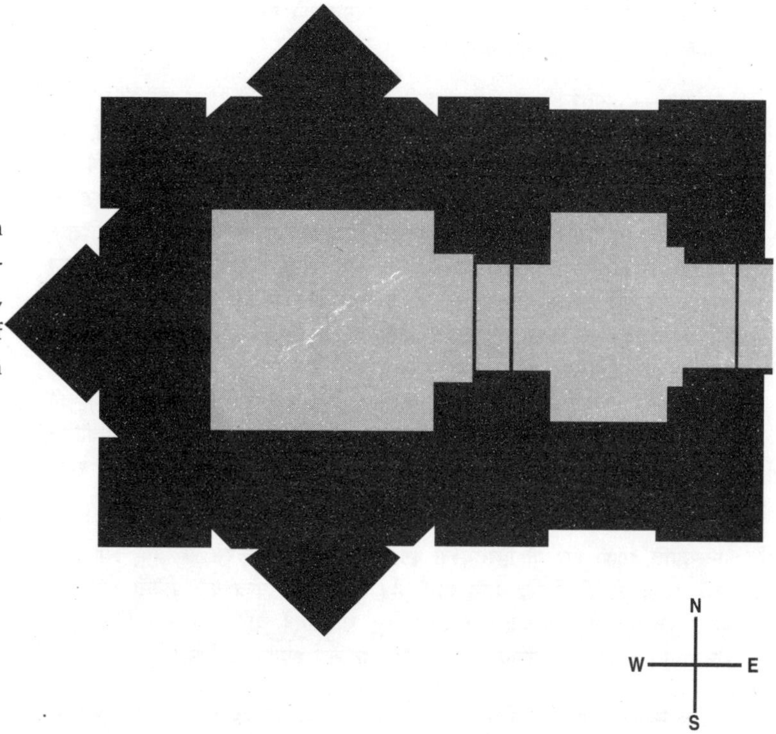

fig. 14.
Plan of the Patalesvara Śiva Brick Temple, Budhi-Komna, Nuapaḍa district, Orissa, which is a plan of Kosali style of Rekha temple.

Svāmī Śivānanda had edited Śaṅkarācārya's *Ānanda-Laharī*, with all its *yantra* diagrams. The author[23] came across the following verse of *Ānanda-Laharī*, whose *yantra* or mystic diagram and explanation is given by Svāmī Śivānanda himself thus:

किरन्तीमङ्गेभ्यः किरणनिकुरुम्बामृतरसं
हृदि त्वामाधत्ते हिमगिरि शिलामूर्तिमिव यः।
स सर्पाणां दर्पं शमयति शकुन्ताधिपइव
ज्वरप्लुष्टंन्दृष्ट्या सुखयति सुधासारसिचया ॥२० ॥

अर्थ — जो अपने हृदय में तुझ पर इस प्रकार ध्यान करता है कि तेरे शरीर के सारे अंगों से किरण के रूप में अमृत प्रवाहित हो रहा है, तथा तू चन्द्रकांतमणि से निर्मित मूर्ति के समान विभासित है, वह भक्त सर्पों के दर्प को हर लेता है। जिस प्रकार पक्षियों के राजा गरुड़ सर्पों के दर्प को हरते हैं तथा

Delhi, 1986, pp. 81 and 121-22.

23. (i) The author is indebted to Sri Sashi Bhushan Mishra, for kindly supplying the above mentioned datas of "*Ānanda-Laharī* of Śaṅkarācārya," ed. Svāmī Śivānanda, on 31st July 1983.

वह अपनी दृष्टिमात्र से, जिससे शीतल अमृत की वर्षा होती है, ज्वर संतप्त व्यक्तियों के ज्वर को दूर कर देता है।

व्याख्या — अमृतेश्वरी के रूप में देवी का ध्यान करने से जिस फल की प्राप्ति होती है, उसका वर्णन इस श्लोक में किया गया है। अमृतेश्वरी के रूप में देवी पर ध्यान करने से विशेष प्रकार की शक्ति प्राप्त होती है। ऐसे व्यक्ति से सर्प भय खाता है। सर्प उसको देखते ही भाग जाते हैं। ऐसा भक्त सर्पों को गरुड़ के समान दिखाई देता है। एलौपैथिक, हौम्योपैथिक डॉक्टर तथा आयुर्वेदिक कविराज औषधि के द्वारा रोगियों का उपचार करते हैं। परन्तु देवी की कृपा से देवी का भक्त दृष्टिमात्र से ही रोगियों को सर्पदंश से बचा सकता है। उसकी दृष्टि में सर्प-विष को हरण करने की शक्ति होती है। इसके अतिरिक्त दृष्टिमात्र से वह सारे प्रकार के ज्वरों का अपहरण कर सकता है। उसकी दृष्टि से जो शीतल अमृत की वर्षा होती है उससे सारे प्रकार के ज्वर छूट जाते हैं। यह भी देवी की कृपा का फल है। योगीजन अमृत का पान करते हैं जो अमृत-नाड़ी से प्रवाहित होता है। वह आनन्द तथा भावातिरेक से पूर्ण हो जाता है। अमृत-नाड़ी सारी नाड़ियों को अमृत से परिप्लावित कर देती है।

नित्यप्रति 1000 बार के हिसाब से 45 दिनों तक जप करने से विष तथा ज्वर को दूर करने की सिद्धि प्राप्त होती है। विभूति पर यन्त्र को अंकित कीजिये। जल का कलश रखिये। क्षीर तथा मधु चढ़ाइये। यदि आप 45 दिनों तक नित्यप्रति 2000 बार उसका जप करेंगे तो सर्प आपके वशीभूत हो जायेंगे।

This *yantra* is also found at two places in verse 20 and verse 42 of the *Saundarya-Laharī* of Ādi Śaṅkarācārya[24] with their *yantras*.

Trans.: He who meditates on you in the form of a moon-stone statue, exuding nectar from the myriad rays emanating from your limbs, destroys the arrogance of serpents like the kind of bird, Garuḍa, and cures the fever-ridden with a glance, shedding as it were panaceal nectar.

— *Saundarya-Laharī*, 20

Trans.: O Daughter of the snowy mountains! he who describes your golden crown studded with gem-like sun would mistake the crescent moon rendering many splendour by the lustre of precious stones in the golden crown, as the bow of Indra.

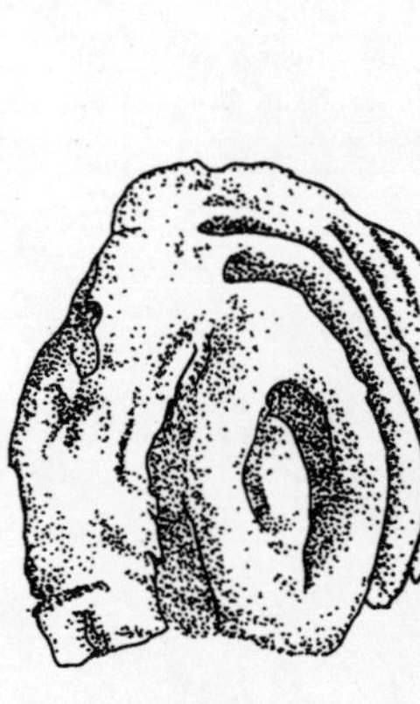

(ii) *Ānanda-Laharī of Śaṅkarācārya*, ed. D. Ghosh, Sanskrit Book Depot (P.) Ltd., Kolkata, 1985, Verse 20, p. 29.

Notes : In the 50 verses commencing from the 42nd, the poet describes the physical form of the Supreme power from the crown to the feet.

— *Saundarya-Laharī*, 42

Madhu Khanna[25] also portrays the *kāmakalā yantra*, which has the plan of two squares placed diagonally and intersecting each other at 45º angle, as mentioned in *Śilpa Prakāśa*, a manuscript of Orissa on *śilpa śāstra* (*Fig.* 15).

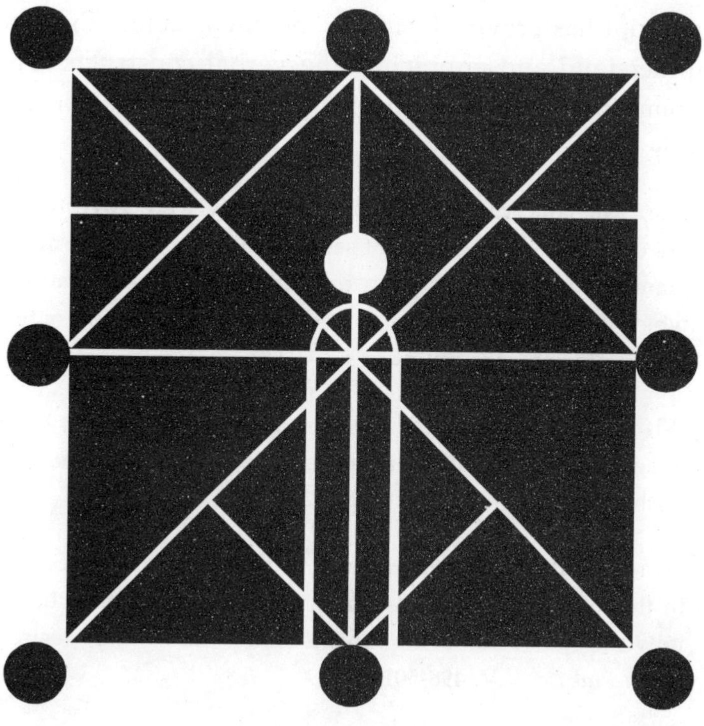

fig. 15.
Kāmakalā Yantra, symbol of the unity of Śiva and Śakti as shown in *Śilpa Prakāśa* Orissa manuscript, 9th-12th centuries AD (Source: Madhu Khanna, *Yantra: The Tāntric Symbol of Cosmic Unity*, Thames and Hudson, London, 1994, p. 144).

Śilpa Prakāśa,[26] is an important *śilpa śāstra* of Orissa. Its author was Rāmacandra Kaulācārya, hailing from a Udgata brāhmaṇa family of a village on the banks of the Musali river

24. *Saundarya-Laharī of Śaṅkarācārya*, ed. V.K. Subramanian, Motilal Banarsidass, Delhi, 1986, verses 20 and 42, pp. 23 & 77. Vide the *Yantras*, pp. 66 and 77. For verse 20, vide, pp. 11-12.

25. (i) Madhu Khanna, *Yantra The Yāntric Symbol of Cosmic Unity*, Thames and Hudson, London, 1994, p. 144.

(ii) A Boner & S.R. Sarma (eds.), *Śilpa Prakāśa of Ramachandra* (present Musanai between Purī and Koṇārka), then a part of the Dhauni *maṇḍala.* The date of composition is not found in the text but the editors date it between the tenth and twelfth centuries AD. Rāmacandra was a practising *śilpī,* who wrote the book as an instructions to his disciples only under the "command and influence" of his *Sadguru* Mādhava Bhaṭṭa who was conversant with many *śilpa*s. . . . It is a detailed description of the construction of the various compositional diagrams called *yantra*s for the sculptures. The illustrator of the *Mañjuṣā* manuscript has provided *yantra*s, thereby enabling the reader to understand and appreciate the verbal constructs. These diagrams furnished the textual support which Alice Boner was looking for.

> The basic conception of a spiritual reality were governing not only the subject-matter of sacred sculpture but were also manifested in a plastic form through geometrical patterns which is revealed in the application of the *kāmakalā yantra* to specific *kāmabandha* sculptures.
>
> Without Śiva and Śakti, creation would be nothing but imagination. Without the action of *kāma* there would be no birth or death.
>
> Śiva himself is visibly manifested as the *mahāliṅga* and Śakti in the form of the *bhaga* (womb). By their union the whole universe comes into being. This is called the work of desire (*Śilpa Prakāśa*, V.V. 498-501).
>
> Proceeding from this basic conception, the *Śilpa Prakāśa* lays down that a place (temple) without love images is known as a "place to be shunned" (*tyakta maṇḍala*); continuing further it says that according to Kaulācāras, it is to be shunned like the den of death and that without offering *pūjā* to the *kāmakalā yantra*, the Śakti *pūjā* and the *sādhanā* become useless as the bath of an elephant. Having said so the *Śilpa Prakāśa* proceeds to explain the construction of the *kāmakalā yantra*, its presiding deity, her associates and attendants and the *dhyānas* of Mahākāmakāleśvarī and Śiva Kāmakāleśvara.

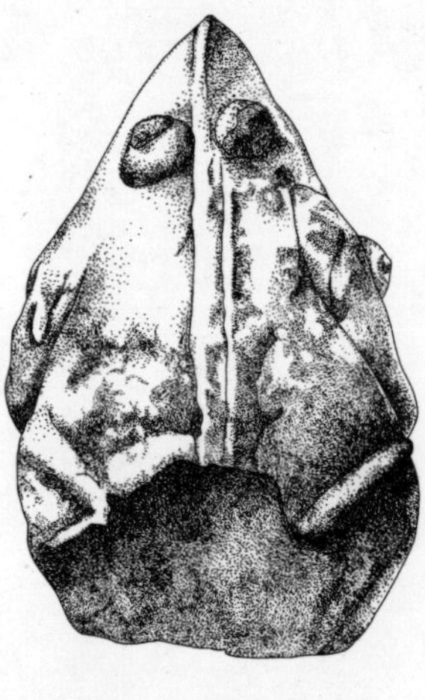

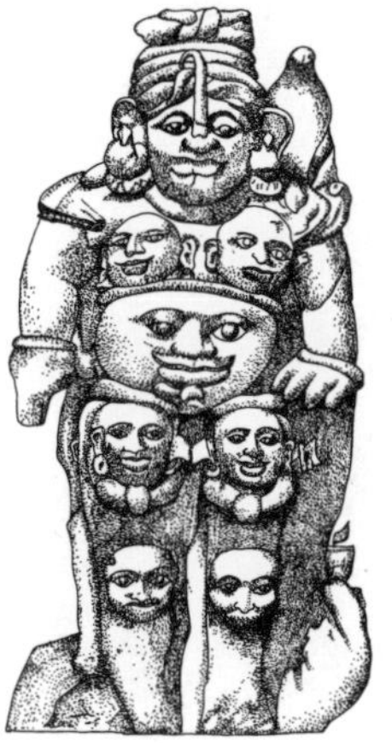

This *yantra* is extolled as the giver of protection to all (including obviously the temple), as the giver of power (*pratyakṣa-śaktidāḥ*) and as the manifest bestower of all perfections (*siddhis*). Placed in a temple it ensures the monument to stand forever. Through this not only all obstacles and fears are destroyed, but even the ghosts (*bhūtas*), departed spirits (*pretas*), goblins (*piśācas*), fearful demons (*kaunapas*) and other hideous creatures (*vikaṭas*) flee away at its mere sight.

This utterly secret *yantra* is to be placed in temples dedicated to Śakti and Rudra. Since this is utterly secret, it is not to be known to everyone. For this reason a love scene (*mithuna-mūrti*) is to be carved on the lines of the *yantra*. The *kāmabandha* is placed there to give delight to the people.

The fact that the practice of carving *mithuna* sculptures along the lines of the *kāmakalā yantra* was not confined to Orissa but also followed elsewhere in India has been revealed by the renowned dedicated Scholar Devangana Desai's study *Religious Imagery of Khajuraho*.[27] She found that the famous "head-down" *mithuna* sculpture at the juncture of the *vimāna* and *śāla* of the Kandarīya Mahādeva and Viśvanātha temples there, has been carved along the lines of the *kāmakalā yantra* of the *Śilpa Prakāśa*.

This proves that the Kośalī style of the *rekhā* temple architecture developed on the plan based on the *kāmakalā yantra* and it influenced the development of temple architecture and sculpture particularly in Orissa and in all directions of India as well.[28]

Without observing the entire course of evolution of the temples in the Mahānadī valley, A.N. Parida[29] states,

27. D. Desai, *The Religious Imagery of Khajuraho*, Project for Indian Cultural Studies Publication IV, Mumbai, 1996, p. 195, plate 203.

28. J.P. Singh Deo, "Kośalī Style of Temple Architecture," *OHRJ*, vol. XXIV, XXV & XXVI, pp. 175-76.

29. A.N. Parida, *Early Temples of Orissa* (*From the sixth century* AD *to* →

> Temples situated in western districts of Orissa basically belong to the Bhubaneswar type, but the geographical position of the area coupled with the historical development of a particular period had brought them under the Central India influence. The influence was so profound that the temples are easily distinguishable from the dominant Bhubaneswar style. Thereby these temples constitute a sub-group of the Bhubaneswar style. The changes that occurred in the temples of western districts include the change in the silhouette of the *gaṇḍī*, the star-shaped ground plan of the Bauḍ temples, indentations on the inner walls, balconied windows of the *mukhaśālā*s, raised platforms and decorated pillars inside the *mukhaśālā* of the temples in undivided Bolaṅgīr district, haloes with the beaded outlines, and demi-medallion-like canopies over the heads of the images. Most of the above features failed to penetrate into the coastal belt. The Bhubaneswar temple-style was so deep-rooted that the developments in the western districts could not prevail over it.

A.N. Parida seems to have no vision of the gradual temple development based on the *kāmakalā yantra*, in the long history of temples of Mahānadī valley and is inclined to observe all the developments of temple architecture in a capsule form at Bhubaneswar. His study shows that he has no knowledge of tāntric influence of the *yantra*s, in development of plans and other sections of temples. Therefore his complete work, *Early Temples of Orissa*, seems to be a drawing-room writing with very narrow, hurried and hasty observations, not fit to be accepted. A.N. Parida writes impiously and profanely, hence his remarks are not acceptable.

In a recent work Bettina Baumer and Rajendra Prasad Das[30]

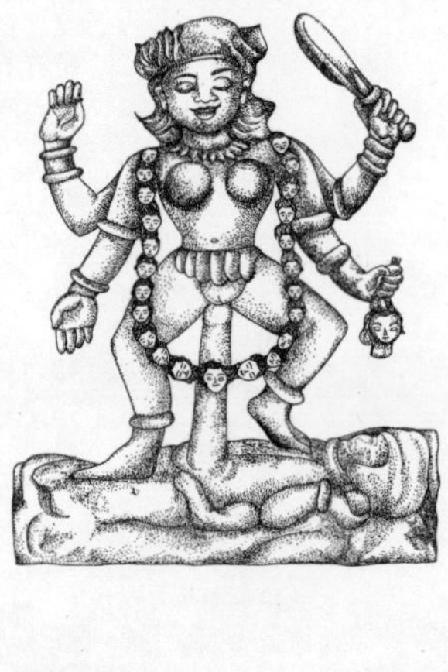

→ *the end of Somavamsi Rule*), Commonwealth Publisher, New Delhi, 1999, p. 157.

30. B. Baumer & R.P. Das, *Śilparatnakośa* (*A Glossary of Orissan Temple Architecture*), Indira Gandhi National Centre for the Arts, New Delhi & Motilal Banarsidass, Delhi, 1994, fig. 52, p. 147, fig. 53, p. 148, fig. 54, p. 151 and figs. 55 & 56, p. 152.

have shown that the ground plan of the Rājarānī temple at Bhubaneswar is based upon the *śrī cakra* or the *śri yantra*. *Śrī yantra* is a diagrammatic embodiment of the creative sexual activity of the universe.[31] The observations prove that the *kāmakalā* (desire fulfilling) is the undertone of the Mahānadī river valley civilization and spiritual culture.

Later variation of the plan of Kōśali style of Rekhā temple plan, can be seen on the ground plan of Viṣṇu temple at Janjgir (*Fig*. 16) and ground plans of Nilkaṇṭheśvara temple at Dādpur and Nakshapali (*Fig*. 17 and *Pl*. 30).

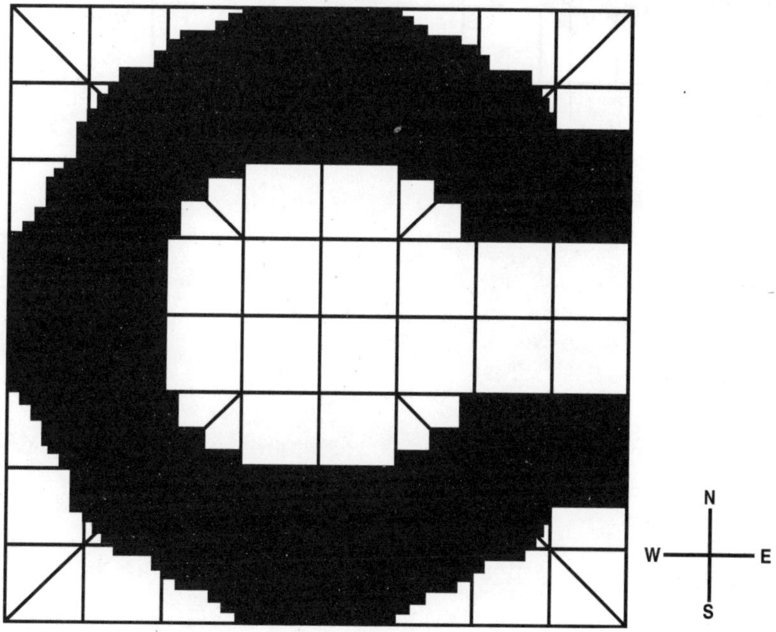

fig. 16.
Ground plan of the Viṣṇu Temple at Janjgir, Dist. Bilāspur, Chhattisgarh. Later variation of the plan of the Kośali style of Rekhā Temple plan.

31. Pranab Bandyopadhyay, *The Goddess of Tantra*, Punthi Pustak, Kolkata, 1987, p. 48.

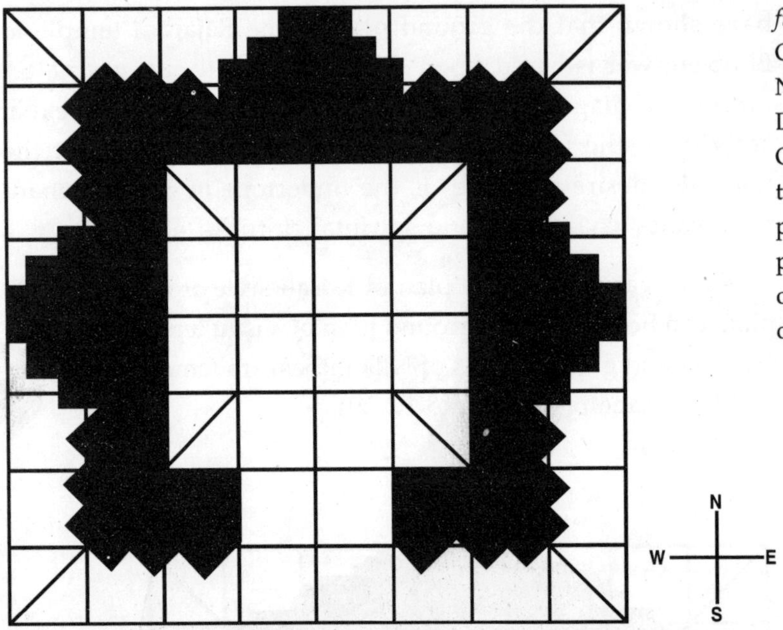

fig. 17.
Ground plan of the Nīlakaṇṭheśwara Temple at Dadpur, Kālāhāṇḍi Dist., Orissa. Such a planned temple stands at Nakshapali village, Dist. Sambalpur, Orissa. Later variation of the plan of Kośali style of the Rekhā Temple plan.

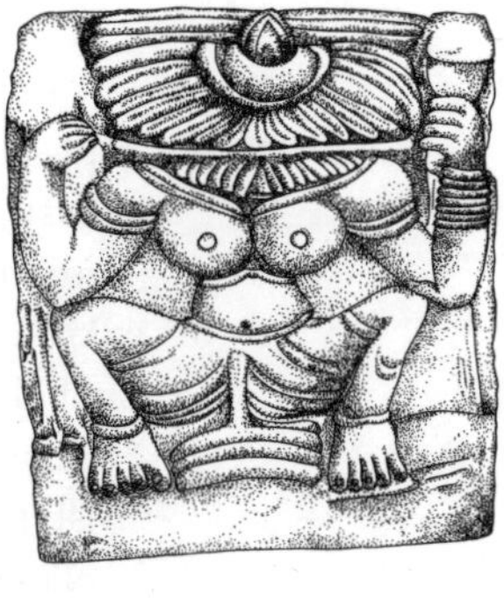

7

Significance of Three Tāntric Temples at Bauḍ

BAUḌ is located in the central Orissa province, on the right bank of the Mahānadī river. It was an important Buddhist centre in the ninth century AD. It is likely that the very name Bauḍ had been derived from Buddhism. There is a colossal image of the Buddha in the earth-touching position near the local palace. The remains of a quadrangular monastery have been recently unearthed near the Buddha image.[1]

According to Gazetteer[2] Bauḍ was a great Buddhist centre in Orissa.[3] It is suggested by some scholars that there once existed two Buddhist *vihāras*.[4] Two remarkable Buddhist statues found in Bauḍ are indicative of the fact that it was once a centre of Buddhist culture. Of the two statues one is without head while another is found in full form. Referring to this Buddhist statue situated in front of the palace of the former *rājā* of Bauḍ, R.D. Banerjee[5] says the great Buddha at Bauḍ is the best example of the second renaissance in Buddhist sculpture in the tenth century AD. The image is still *in situ*.

The total height of this image is 6' 9", of which the seated

1. A.N. Parida, "Archaeological Sites and Monuments of Orissa," *Sidelights on History and Culture of Orissa*, ed. M.N. Das, Vidyapuri, Cuttack, 1977, p. 492.
2. D.C. Kuanr (State ed.), *Orissa District Gazetteers, Bauḍh-Khondmals*, N. Senapati (Chief ed.), Cuttack, 1983, p. 32.
3. *Ibid.*, R.D. Banerjee, *History of Orissa*, vol. II, (?), p. 393.
4. *Ibid.*, Bisi Prahallad, *Collection* (MSS.), p. 3.
5. *Ibid.*, R.D. Banerjee, *History of Orissa*, vol. II, (?), p. 390.

> figure measure 4' 3" in height and 3' 10" from knee to knee. It is seated in the *bhūmisparśa-mudrā* on a lotus throne 1' 2" in height placed on a pedastal, 11" in height and 4' 6" in breadth. Like the great Buddha at Udayagiri in Cuttack district, the whole image is built up in sections with separately carved stones. The only attendant figures are two *gandharva*s flying with garlands in their hands on the side of the head. On the whole the colossus of Bauḍ compares favourably with the similar colossal at Udayagiri and Lalitgiri in Cuttack district. The image is uninscribed and beneath the pedestal is the ancient stone pavement of the original shrine.[6]

In the declining period of Buddhism, this region was influenced by what is called tāntric Buddhism. This is evident from the worship of Bhairavī, a tāntric deity in many villages in the area. Later Śaivism and Vaiṣṇavism emerged to be popular.

While dealing with Mahāyānic and tāntric Art in Orissa, N.K. Sahu[7] gives a fastidious description of Bauḍ and states,

> The Bauḍ region was a great centre of Mahāyānic and Tāntric Buddhism in the medieval period and Prof. R.D. Banerji is of the opinion that Buddhism lingered longer in Bauḍ than in other parts of Orissa. The most important Buddhist antiquity in Bauḍ is the colossal image of Buddha seated in on earth-touching posture in front of the palace of the Raja Saheb. The image is built in sections like the colossal of Khadipadā and Udayagiri, but it is larger in size than either of them. The plastic treatment, however, is more crude and warrants a somewhat later date than the eighth century AD. The image is seated on a stone altar, in front of which the stone pavement of the ancient temple may be traced and scattered remains of Buddhist images are also found in the neighbourhood. This image plays an important role in the religious life of the people of Bauḍ even in the present days, and on all auspicious occasions it is worshipped by them as "Buḍhārāja" which is but a variant form of Buddharāja. Buddhist figures, both Mahāyānic and

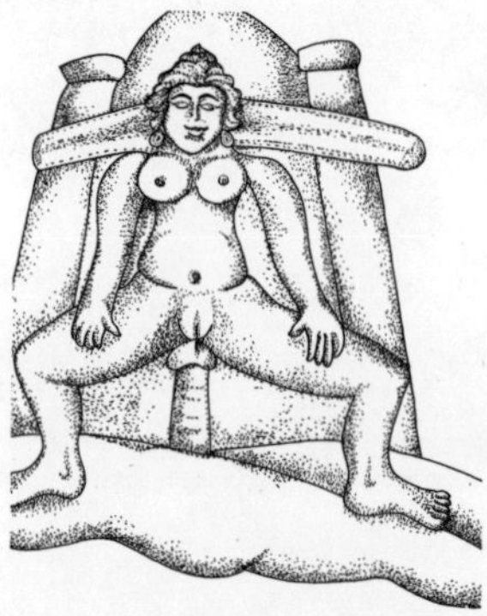

6. R.D. Banerjee, *History of Orissa*,
7. N.K. Sahu, *Buddhism in Orissa*, Utkal University, 1958, pp. 203-04.

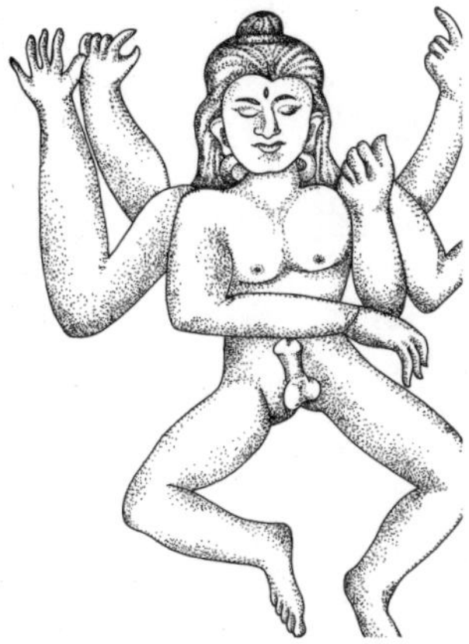

Tāntric, are found in large numbers within the compound of the Rāmeśvara temple but many of them are either broken or covered with thick layers of vermilion. The Rāmeśavara group of images are all regarded at present as Hindu deities, although a number of them carry the usual Buddhist creed *ye dharma hetu*. . . etc. One among them, a seated image of remarkable grace and beauty, which is now worshipped as Ugra Tārā, is identified by Prof. R.D. Banerji with Mahattari Tārā, and the same scholar also points out that the big image leaning against the back wall of the Rāmeśvara temple is that of "the Lokeśvara class."[8]

We have found two exquisite bronze images from Bauḍ, which probably belonged to the ninth century AD. One of them is a richly ornamental figure of two armed Maitreya seated gracefully in Lalita pose on the throne, holding in the left hand a bunch of Nāgakesara flowers and in the right the nectar vase. The other image is that of a variety of Lokeśvara and is in better state of preservation. Although in Lalita attitude, it sits erect on a lotus throne and places its right foot on a foot-stool (*pāda pīṭha*). It is four armed and one faced, and is richly ornamental, while the modelling of the body conveys the impression of roundness and volume. It carries in the upper right hand a conch-shell and in the upper left hand a lotus, while the lower right hand is in *varada* pose and the lower left is placed on the throne. Such a variety of Lokeśvara is however rarely found and we are disposed to identify it as Śaṅkhanātha Lokeśvara,[9] although this God is stated to have only two arms with a conch in the right and a lotus in the left hand.

These antiquities indicate that the place was a popular centre of Buddhism in the medieval times, and the name "Bauḍ" carries with it today the reminiscences of the Buddhistic heritage of the past.

With construction of three tāntric Śiva temples at Bauḍ, the

8. *JBROS*, 1909, p. 69.

9. B. Bhattacharya, *JBORS*, 1928, Pt. LXVIII, fig. 101.

Buddhistic site was converted into a Hindu site. The origin of *tantra* is lost in antiquity and the Vedas had accepted or included the tāntric path. David Frawley[10] states that there has also been a tendency among scholars to derive the ritualistic tāntric tradition from the philosophic Vedāntic tradition and to make the former pre-Āryan and the latter Āryan. Yet the chief features of *tantra* are also those of the Veda, which is highly ritualistic. These include the importance of *mantra*, myth, the fire-sacrifice and the worship of terrible forms of the divine. All tāntric *mantras* are based on Sanskrit and many derive from Vedic verses. For example, the great *mantra HUṀ*, used in both Hinduism and Buddhism is the *bīja mantra* or seed syllable for *agni*. *Agni* is called *hotar*, from the root meaning "the invoker." The Vedic Gods are usually invoked with verbal forms of the root *HU*.

> Tāntric rituals are fire and are patterned after Vedic fire rituals. Tāntric deities with their power and sometimes violence are much like the Vedic. In fact, more of the outer side of the Vedic religion can be found in *tantra* than in the philosophical texts. The Vedic horse-sacrifice resembles some strange tāntric ritual more than the Vedānt philosophy, though if we look deeply, we see its connection with the latter as well. In fact, the oldest and longest Upaniṣad, the *Bṛhadāraṇyaka*, begins with the tāntric-like image of the horse sacrifice, not with a philosophical dialogue.
>
> In tāntric philosophy, the Vedic gods like Agni, Soma and Sūrya appear as powers of *yoga* and are related to different *cakras* of the subtle body, as we have noted. Kashmir Śaivism, the most exalted of Tāntric philosophies wherein perhaps the *mantra* achieved its greatest power and articulation, came from a famous homeland of the Vedic chants.

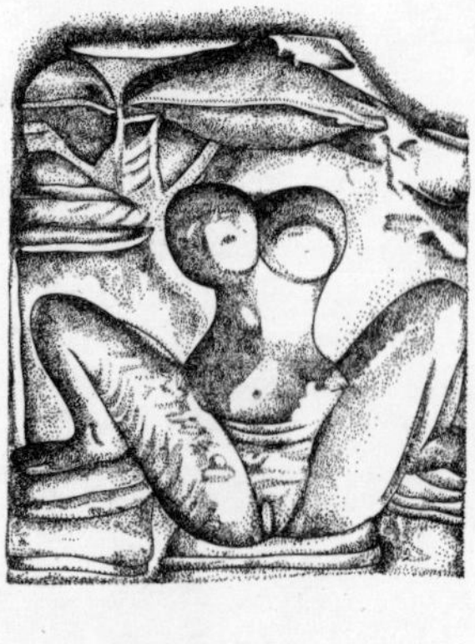

The *tantra* tradition is also mentioned in the *Rāmāyaṇa* and

10. D. Frawley, *Gods, Sages and Kings* (*Vedic Secrets of Ancient Civilization*), Motilal Banarasidass, Delhi, 1995, pp. 228-29.

Mahābhārata also.[11] In the words of H.D. Bhattacharyya,[12]

> In its present widely accepted sense *tantra* means a literature which spreads knowledge and particularly knowledge of profound things with the aid of mystic diagrams (*yantra*) and words possessing esoteric meanings (*mantra*), and helps the attainment of salvation . . . it is only in later literature, from about the fifth or sixth century AD that *tantra* as a special religious or philosophical concept gradually came into use.

From the early Christian centuries, Mattamayūra Tāntric Śaivism became popular in the whole Mahānadī river valley.[13] Among the early Somavaṁśī kings of the upper Mahānadī valley, i.e., South Kośala, it was Mahāśivagupta Bālārjuna, whose reigning period is assigned within *circa* AD 595-655 by S.R. Nema,[14] who being a great devotee of Śiva, enjoyed the epithet *Paramamāheśvara* in his charters and also had the Śaivite emblem of the bull on his seal. . . . We know from the Senakapat inscription[15] that Durgarakṣita, the son of Devarakṣita, was a bee at the feet, i.e., a servant of Mahāśivagupta Bālārjuna. He, being a worshipper of Śambhu, constructed a temple of Śiva at the village (modern Senakapāt) and made it over to an ascetic, Sadāśivācārya who was probably the spiritual successor of Sadyahśivācārya, hailing from the penance grove, entitled Amaradaka. In Lodhiā plates, as seen above, the donee Śūlapāṇi was a disciple of Pramathācārya who is said to be an inhabitant

11. R.K. Upadhyaya, *The Concept of God in Śaiva Tantra*, Jnananidhi Prakashan, Muzaffarpur, 1984, pp. 30-31.
12. H.D. Bhattacharyya, "Tāntric Religion," *THACOTIP*, vol. IV, *The Age of Imperial Kanauj*, 1964, pp. 315-16.
13. Mishra Ram Prasad, "Mattamayūra Śaivism in Orissa," *Culture and Collections*, R.P. Mishra (ed.), Punthi Pustak, Kolkata, 1996, pp. 101-39.
14. S.R. Nema, *Political History of the Somavaṁśī Kings of South Kośāla and Orissa*, Oriental Publishers, New Delhi, 1978, pp. 128 and 135.
15. *EI*, vol. XXXI, pp. 30-33.

of Pāñcayajña-tapovana is Dvaitavana. Here it is sufficient to say that these Śaiva *ācāryas*, probably belonged to a sect of tāntric Śaivism which later came to be called Mattamayūra and as such, it may be assumed that Mahāśivagupta may have accepted the doctrine of the Pāśupata *dharma*.[16]

With this tāntric Śaiva background, it seems the stellate plan of two squares placed diagonally and intersecting each other at 45º angle, which gives the shape of an eight point star developed in the South Kośala region where it can be seen in (1) the Pātāleśwar Śiva temple at Bodhi-Komna (Nuāpāḍā district), (2) Citawari Devī temple at Dhobni near Damakeda village (Raipur district). Originally it was a Śiva temple. The *śiva-liṅga* is painted red by vermillion by vandalism and worshipped as Citawari Devī. The original Śakti of the Śiva-Śakti is removed and kept resting at the back wall inside the *garbhagṛha* (sanctum), (3) Temple in ruins at Kansil village area in the Rānīpur-Jharial complex (Bolaṅgīr district) and (4) A ruined temple at Abhabhara village situated roughly 8 km south of Kharsia (Bilaspur district).[17]

Bhuvanapradīpa,[18] the earliest or ancient architectural text of Orissa, mentions 36 types of *rekhā* temples and among these, one specification of Kośalī *rekhā* temple is found. As single temples with different types of stellate plans are found and as four temples with the plans of two squares placed diagonally and intersecting each other at angles of 45º are traced in the South Kośala region, it seems, it will be proper for the temples which are more in number with the same plan to be identified with the Kośalī *rekhā* style of temple architecture.

So, it is definite that with the tāntric *yantra* influence, the

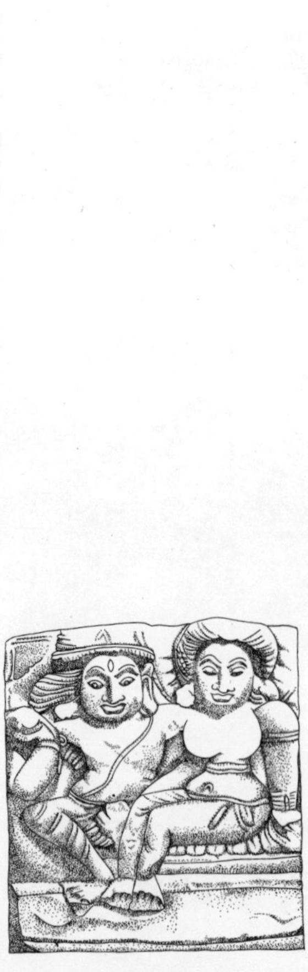

16. *Inscriptions of Orissa*, vol. IV, pp. 349-50.
17. J.P. Singh Deo, *Cultural Profile of South Kośala*, Gyan Publishing House, New Delhi, 1987, pp. 329-30.
18. N.K. Bose, *Canons of Orissan Architecture*, Cosmo Publications, New Delhi, 1982, p. 124.

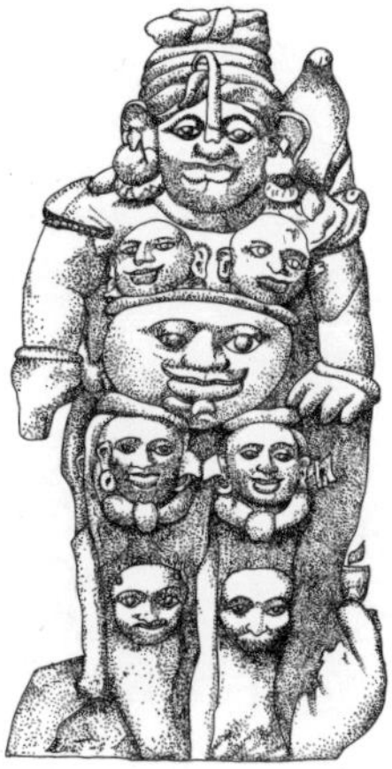

Kośalī style of *rekhā* temple had developed[19] within the seventh-eighth centuries AD and had influenced the development of temple architectures in all directions.

Gazetteer[20] mentions that a group of three temples of Śiva at Bauḍ called the Rāmeśwar or Rāmanātha temples, dating back to the ninth century AD are reputed for their special features. In the words of R.D. Banerjee:

> The decorative motifs and the plastic art of the three temples at Bauḍ are certainly superior to and older than the great Liṅgarāja, Ananta Vasudeva group . . . one particular feature of the Bauḍ temples is worth particular attention. Their plan is quite different from that of any other temples. . . . In plan these three temples are eight-rayed stars and the Argha-pattas of the *liṅga*s are also similar.

The construction of Rāmeśwar temple at Bauḍ was started by the last ruling Chief Rājā Nārāyaṇa Prasad Deva of Bauḍ, but it remained uncomplete because of the Second World War of the twentieth century AD. Even though the three tāntric temples of Bauḍ are standing in a triangular pattern inside the modern compound of Rāmeśwar temple, they have no modern construction.

About these three tāntric temples of Bauḍ, Karuna Sagar Behera[21] narrates:

> At Bauḍ town there are three small temples, within the compound of the Rāmeśwar temple, which have great significances from the architectural point of view. Of these temples, one faces west and the other two with the same architectural and sculptural features face the east.

---

19. (i) J.P. Singh Deo, "Kośalī Style of Temple Architecture," *OHRJ*, vol. XXIV, XXV and XXVI, pp. 169-76.

    (ii) J.P. Singh Deo, "Two Varieties of Kośalī Style of Temple Architecture," *OHRJ*, vol. XXX, No. 1, pp. 91-95.

20. *Orissa District Gazetteers, Bauḍh-Khondmals*, Cuttack, 1983, p. 33.

21. K.S. Behera, *Temples of Orissa*, Orissa Sahitya Akademi, Bhubaneswar, 1993, pp. 35-36.

J.D. Beglar who visited the place in 1874-75 has left a concise account of the temple. Each of these temples stands by itself on a raised platform and each consists of a cell and an attached portico. The plan show the minute recesses and angularities which produce a charming effect on the variety of light and shade and confer an appearance of greater height from the continued cluster of vertical lines they really possess.[22] With these recesses and angularities the ground plan is in the shape of an eight-rayed star. The plan has been obtained on the principle of intersecting squares, but obviously this unique ground plan was due to the tāntric necessity for not only the ground plan of the temple but also the Śakti of the *Śiva-liṅga* is star-shaped.

On the temples we find Navagraha slabs which are common in later temples. These are so profusely ornamented that Beglar remarked "though small they are gems of art in their own humble way." The clear-cut interlacing of *caitya*-windows of the *śikhara* is arresting and similar designs are seen on the *anurathapaga* of the deula of the Mukteswar temple at Bhubaneswar. These two temples, as Dr. K.C. Panigrahi points out, possess many decorative elements in common,[23] and therefore may not have been far removed from each other in time. In shape and style of decorative treatment they differ considerably from the temples of the earlier period, but at the same time they do not possess the characteristics of temples like the Brahmeśwar at Bhubaneswar, which was erected by the mother of the Somavaṁśī King Uddyotkesarī. Therefore we may assign them to the early period of the Somavaṁśī rule in Orissa.[24]

The triangular placing of the three Śaiva tāntric temples at

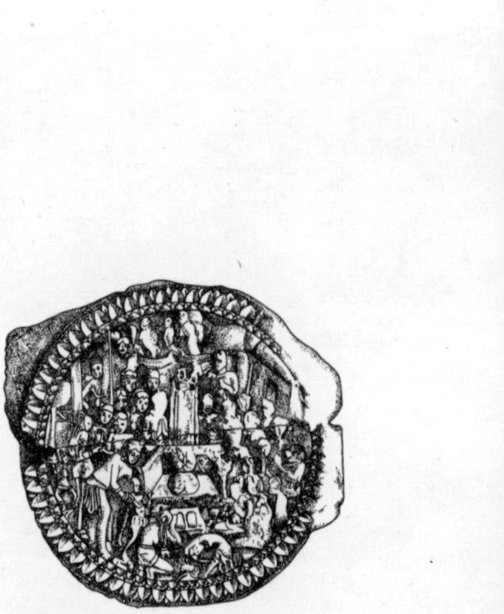

22. Cunningham's *Archaeological Survey of India*, vol. XIII, (?), pp. 118-19.
23. K.C. Panigrahi, *Archaeological Remains in Bhubaneswar*, Orient Longmans, New Delhi, 1961, pp. 158-59.
24. *Ibid.*, p. 159.

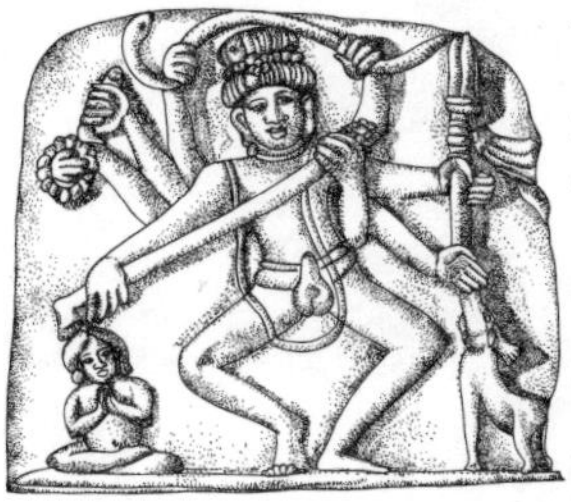

Bauḍ, is of interest. The single temple in the east, facing west, is named Paścima Somanātha and has a *cakra* as *dhvaja*. The Vaiṣṇava *dhvaja* of *cakra* on a Śaiva tāntric temple shows synchronization of Śaivism and Vaiṣṇavism. Digambara Jaina images are found on the *gaṇḍī* of this temple. To the north is the Kapileśwar temple, (*Fig*. 18 & *Pl*. 43) towards the south is Bhubaneswar and both face east. All of them are dedicated to Śiva and in each shrine, a *liṅga* is installed. Buddha images are found on the *gaṇḍī*s (bodies) of the Kapileśwar and Bhubaneswar temples. The Śaktis (*arghya*) of these three Śaiva tāntric temples are in the plan of the temples, which is a *yantra*. All these prove that a great religious synchronization, synthesis and syncretism of Jainism, Buddhism, Śaivism and Vaiṣṇavism was going on there, through the tāntric ritual practice and tāntric *yoga*, during the construction of these temples. These there temples have a tāntric *yantra* plan, which developed with the influence of the Kośalī *rekhā* style of temple architecture.

fig. 18.
Plan of the Kapileśwara Temple, Bauḍ, Dist.

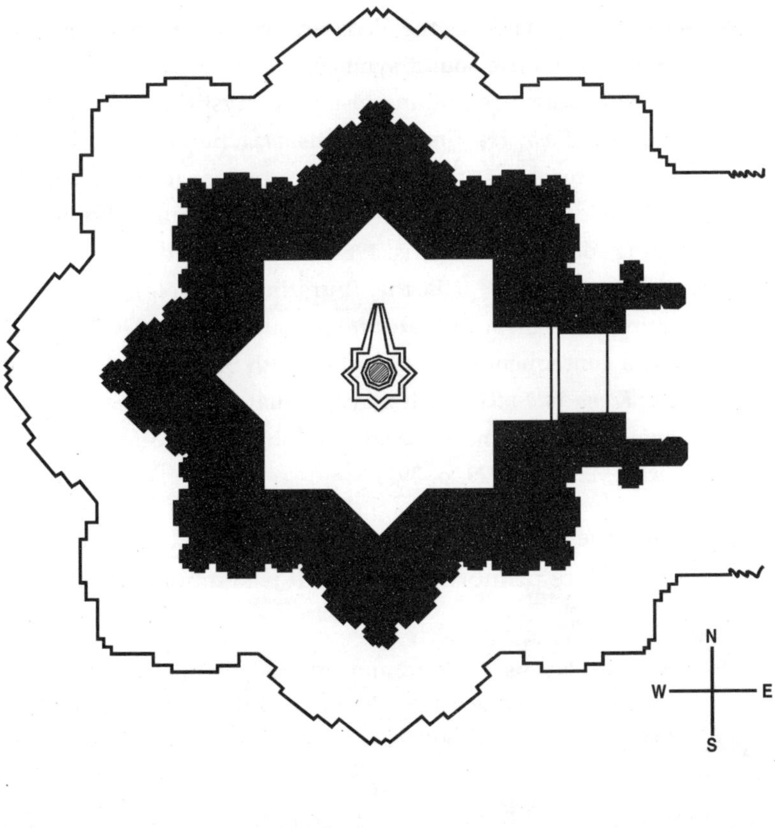

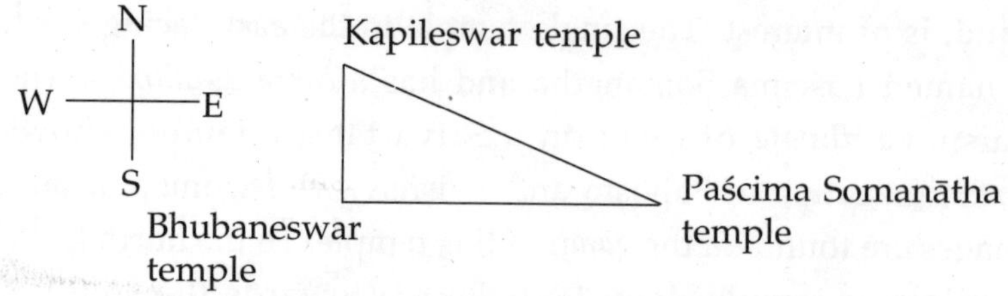

As these temples stand in a triangular formation (*Pl.* 44), it can be supposed that the *trikoṇa* consists of *icchā*, *jñāna* and *kriyā* Śaktis. In the *Śāradātilaka* I, 78, it is recorded that from *saguṇa* Śiva rise Śakti, *nāda* and *bindu*. This *bindu* is threefold: (a) *bindu* (Śiva), (b) *bīja* (Śakti) and (c) *nāda* (Śiva-Śakti).

About Phonic Emanation, Dirk Jan Hoens[25] states thus:

> One of the most essential traits of tantrism is its conception of a phonic plane of existence parallel to, and even basic to, the objective world. It is a leading factor in cosmic evolution. The theory of sound and meaning probably originated in the speculation on the sacred syllables, particularly *oṁ*, which, as we saw, originated in the Veda and continues to be the main focus of tāntric sound symbolism. The first stages of phonic emanation are nothing else than mystic primordial constituents of *oṁ*. The first of them is *nāda*, paraphrased by Padoux (in French) as "first sonorous resonance (of the Parā Vāc, see below) an extremely subtle state of pure phonic energy" (Padoux, *Parole*, Paris, 1964, p. 51). According to the *Netratantra* 21, 62 f., it is the "bursting" (*sphota*) sound emanating from Śiva. But later texts usually derive it from Śakti as a consequence of her contact with Śiva (*Netratantra* 21, 62 f.: *Kāma-kalā-vilāsa* 9). It may be equated with *kuṇḍalinī*; it is symbolized by the crescent (Sir John Woodroffe, *Śakti and Śakta*, Madras, 1929, p. 397).

Then comes the *bindu*, an extremely concentrated embrosial "drop" of the pure primordial speech. It is symbolized by a dot

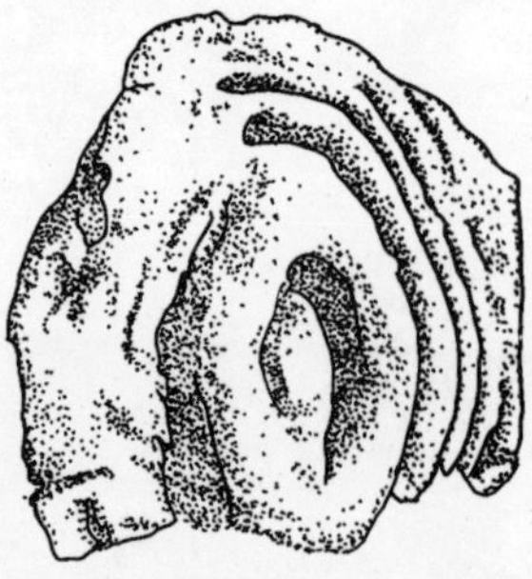

25. Dirk Jan Hoens, "Tantra and other Constituents of Tāntric Practice, "Handbuch Der Orientalistik-II, ABT., IV. Band, 2. ABSCHN," *Hindu Tantrism*, Leiden/Koln, E.J. Brill, 1979, pp. 93-95.

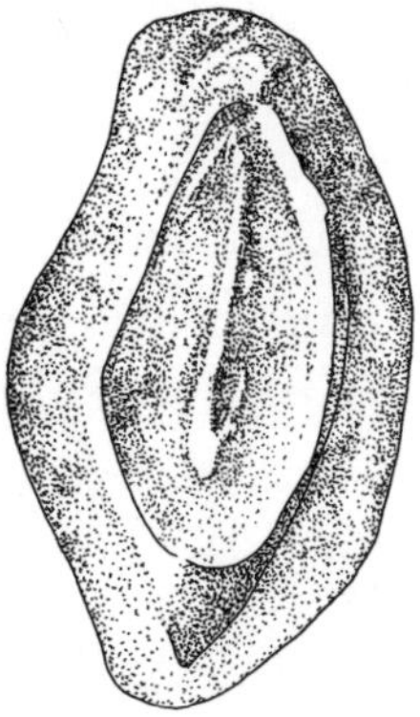

or the full moon. *Bindu* and *nāda* are usually treated in combination as a decisive factor in the evolution of speech and reality. The subject is intensely complicated because of the differences in thought and presentation found in the sources as well as with modern authors. In a short survey it seems that the best way is to take the system presented by the very influential (*Śāradātilaka* 1, 7 ff.), as a base. Its author assumes an initial triad which consists of Śiva (the *bindu*) Śakti (the *bīja*) and their union (not mentioned by name, but its effect or product is called the *nāda*). This triad is called a "three fold *bindu*," identical with the Supreme Śakti. In the first stage, it causes to emanate triads of Śaktis and male deities:

Śiva (*bindu*)	Śakti (*bīja*)	Their union (*nāda*)
Raudri	Vāmā	Jyeṣṭhā
Icchā	Kriyā	Jñāna
Rudra	Brahmā	Viṣṇu
Agni (fire)	Soma (Moon)	Sūrya (Sun)

In addition to this evolutionary series, there is a second one according to which the division of the supreme *bindu* produce *rava* "sound" which is *śabda-Brahman*, "phonic (aspect of) *Brahman*," i.e., the principle of intelligence in audible form. In the human microcosm, it is manifested as *kuṇḍalinī*. A third "mythological," series originating from Śiva-*bindu* is: Sadāśiva-Īśvara-Rudra-Viṣṇu-Brahmā.

The word *bindu* can thus stand for different things. Its extreme versatility is ably discussed by Padoux (*A Parole*, Paris, 1964, p. 93 ff.; cf., also G. Kaviraj, *Śāktadṛṣti*, Patna, 1963 (in Hindi, p. 77). For instance in the tāntric code language, *bindu* can also be used for *amṛta* "fluid of immortality" and for sperms. When the *Yoginī-hṛdaya-tantra* (1.10 f.) described *bindu* as "of the nature of the void, being the supreme essence of illumination" etc., it obviously meant the Śiva. Amṛtānanda, declares this to be the case, but adds the remark that there is a second *bindu* which is of the nature of Soma and Agni, the Ravi (Sun) called *kāma*, the nature of which is the blissful union, (*sāmarasya*) of Śiva and Śakti. This what the *Yoginī-hṛdaya-tantra* itself (1.12) styles the Baindava *cakra* "the orbit of the *bindu*" which forms the central triangle (with its point downwards) of the *śrīcakra*. It is also called Baindavāsana "the seat of the *bindu*" i.e., Śiva and Śakti united on the dead body of Sadāśiva (the inactive category of Sadāśiva) as a couch (*Yoginī-hṛdaya-tantra* 1.14 and comm.). The name Ravi may have been prompted by two factors: (a) The Vedic triad Agni-Soma-Sūrya (fire, fluid, sun), (b) the term *rava* "sound" used in a comparable position as a synonym for *nāda* in the *Śāradātilaka* 1.7 ff.

A further step is that the two-fold *bindu*, Śakti-Śiva, is characterized by both Amṛtānanda and Rāghavabhaṭṭa in the mentioned passages of the *Yoginī-hṛdaya-tantra* and the *Śāradātilaka*, by white and red colours suggestive of semen and menstrual flux, the two factors of reproduction in Hindu (including Tāntric) embryology. The triad *Śiva-Śakti-Nāda* obtained the name *Kāmakalā*, the divine particle (manifesting itself as) desire, personified as Tripurasundarī (*Jñānārṇava-tantra* 10.8). In this context, Śiva and Śakti are called Kāmeśvara and Kāmeśvarī. The *kāmakalā* symbolizes the creative union of the primeval parental pair, a pulsating cosmic atom with two nuclei graphically represented by a white and red dot which automatically produce a third point of gravity. This situation is often represented graphically as a triangle. This can be done in two ways, with the point upwards or downwards. The second variety which expresses the initial cosmic dynamism would look like this:

Śiva
Kāmeśvara
(White Agni)

Śakti Kāmeśvarī
(Red; Soma)

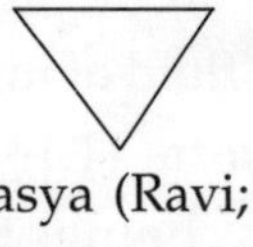

Sāmarasya (Ravi;
Kāma)

In this tāntric background, it can be claimed that the three Śaiva tāntric temples of Bauḍ, standing in a triangular shape were planned and built by advanced tāntric formulae.

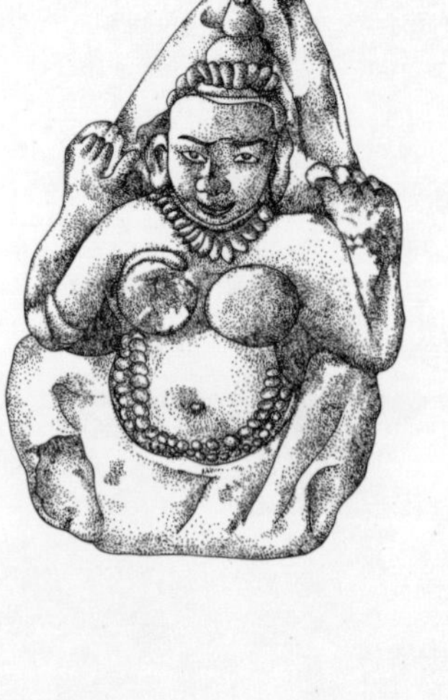

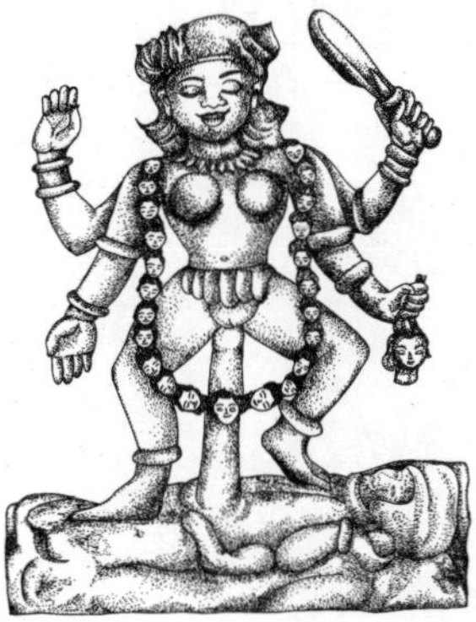

This tāntric formulae seems to have been carried to coastal Orissa by the Somavaṁśīs. Jaipur is famous for its Virāja site. Leaving the temple of Virāja, one finds shrines of Śiva scattered all over the town and its vicinity, of which the most important are those of Akhaṇḍaleśwar, Aṅgeśwar and Trilocaneśwar. The Virāja *kṣetra* is triangular. In each corner, there is one *Śiva-liṅga* almost at equal distance from one another. These three Śiva-*liṅgas* are Bileswar, Khilateśwar and Baruṇeśwar.[26]

This Śaiva tāntric formulae of Śiva-Kāmeśvara, Śakti-Kāmeśvarī and Sāmarasya had extended its influence to Gañjam district also, as at the centre of Asikā is seen a Śiva temple named Tribidheśvara. Three *liṅgas* are found on the single Śakti deity of this temple. The local people have a belief that it was the abode of the holy trinity, Brahmā, Viṣṇu and Maheśvara.[27] In spiritual sense, the deity of this temple of Asikā signifies the tāntric formulae of Śiva-Kāmeśvara, Śakti-Kāmeśvari and Sāmarasya. The three *liṅgas* in a single Śakti are drawn inside like a tortoise head which symbolizes the *vajrolī haṭha yogic mudrā*, i.e., the *yoga* of sexual transformation (*Pls.* 45 & 46).

---

26. N.C. Behuria (Chief ed.), *Gazetteer of India, Orissa State*, vol. II, Cuttack, 1991, p. 315.

27. A.K. Rath, *Studies on Some Aspects of the History and Culture of Orissa*, Punthi Pustak, Kolkata, 1987, p. 209.

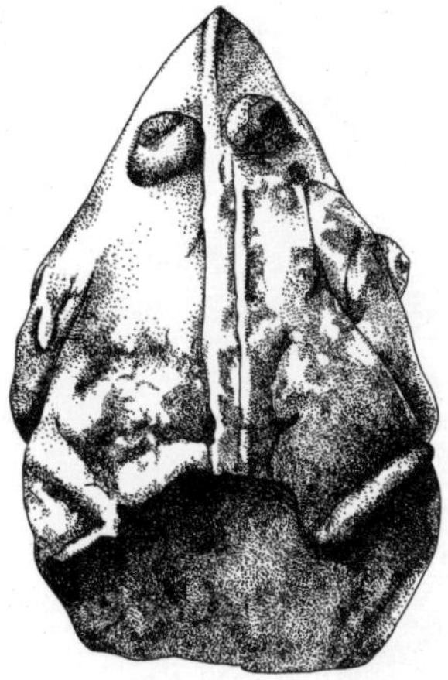

8

Tāntric Influence on Temple Architecture of Mahānadī Valley

THERE are several important river systems in peninsular India. In the eastern Deccan, the Mahānadī river originates from the Sihawa mountain of Raipur district of Chhattisgarh and flows into the Bay of Bengal, thereby forming the major river of Chhattisgarh and Orissa provinces. Orissa as it is today consists of portions of three ancient regions, Kaliṅga, Utkala and Kośala which in due course of centuries under the political, social and economic pressure, joined together in the twelfth century AD and developed to form a distinct Oriyā society in the realm of India.[1] Though Tantra has pre-historic origin, it came into use only from the post-Gupta period as a special religious or philosophical concept and the construction of Brāhmaṇical or Hindu temples in the Mahānadī valley also developed between the sixth to sixteenth centuries AD.

The early temples in the Mahānadī valley were in the shape of simple square temples. The construction of a square using gnomon and cord is described in the *Śulva Sūtra*s of the Veda, for the first time.[2] The square grid reflected the Vedic cosmology, which saw the world as square. The square was later developed to *vāstu-puruṣa maṇḍala* of 64 squares, a ritual diagram prescribed in the *Bṛhat-Saṁhitā*[3] for temples in the

---

1. H.K. Mahatab, "Culture of Orissa," *OHRJ*, vol. XXX, nos. 2, 3 & 4, p. 1.
2. B. Dhatta, *The Science of Sulba*, Kolkata, 1932, passim.
3. M.W. Meister, "Muṇḍeśvarī: Ambiguity and certainty in the analysis of a temple plan," *Kalādarśana*, American Studies in the →

sixth-century (*Fig.* 9). The *Īśānaśivagumdeva-paddhati*, mention that a *vāstu* of 64 squares is for worship by brāhmaṇas and those of the 81 squares for worship by kings.

The Hindu temple is believed to represent a human body. This reflects the universal doctrine of basic correspondence between man and cosmos — man as microcosmos and cosmos as macroanthrope, which found expression both in theoretical as well as in practical application in tāntric *yoga*. A popular Sanskrit saying *kṣetram śarīra prastaram*, also conveys that temples were made in the form of a human body.

Simple square temples were first built throughout the Mahānadī valley. The Māṭharas[4] ruled coastal southern Orissa during the fourth and fifth centuries AD and the Nalas[5] ruled the upper Mahānadī valley during the third to fifth centuries AD. It can be claimed that these two ruling dynasties were responsible for building square temple with *triratha* plan throughout the Mahānadī valley. C.B. Patel wrongly assigns all the standing temples of the upper Mahānadī valley to the Nala period.

About the evolution of temple architecture in Orissa, K.S. Behera[6] states the Orissan temple style was in full vigour in the wake of the vast religious and cultural resurgence that took place when the Śailodbhava kings ruled from the middle of the sixth century till the first quarter of the eighth century. The temple building activities gained momentum under the Bhaumakaras (AD 736-950), the Somavaṁśīs (AD 950-1112), and reached the climax during the Gaṅga period (AD 1112-1435). The

→ Art of India, ed. G.W. Joanna, Oxford & I.B.H. Publishing Co. New Delhi, 1981, p. 79.

4. K.C. Panigrahi, *History of Orissa*, Kitab Mahal, Cuttack, 1981, p. 46.

5. C.B. Patel, *Dynastic History of Nalas*, Punthi Pustak, Kolkata, 1990, pp. 229-57.

6. K.S. Behera, "Brahmanical Temples of Orissa," *Orissa Review* (Monument Special), January 1976, Bhubaneswar, p. 58.

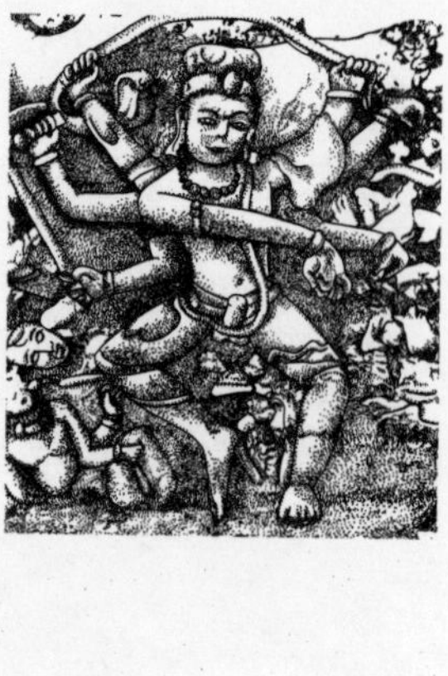

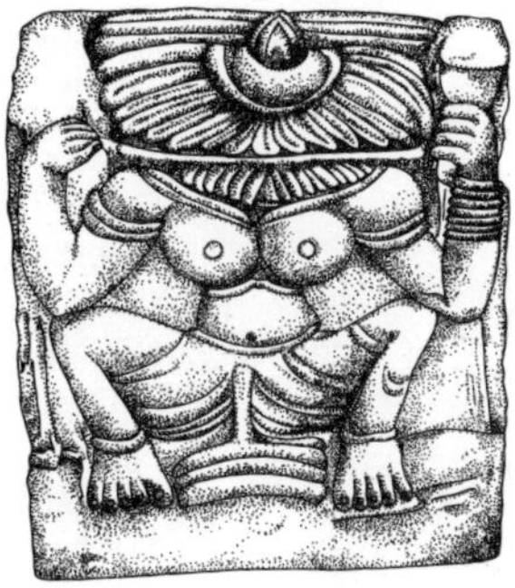

activity continued even under the Sūryavaṁśī Gajapatis (AD 1435-1542), though on a very small scale.

The temples of the Mahānadī valley are in *nāgara* style. In the South Kośala portion, comprising the upper Mahānadī valley, the Kośalī Style of *rekhā* and *khākharā* temples are found. From literatures like Āgama, *Mayamata*, *Mānasara* and *Bhuvanapradīpa*, these two varieties of Kośalī Styles of temple architecture are known.

The regional style with all its modification and transformation that it underwent in course of evolution has beautified the Orissan temples to such an extent that it came to be known as "Kaliṅga Style." An inscription dated AD 1235 on the capital of a pillar in the *mukha-maṇḍapa* of Amṛteśvar temple at Holal of Bellary district in Karnataka, mentions the "Kaliṅga Style" along with *nāgara*, *drāviḍa* and *vesara* styles.

Orissa had its own canons of architecture. The *Bhuvanapradīpa* seems to be the earliest whose exact period is not known. The date of composition of the *Śilpa Prakāśa*, is also not found in the text, but its editors Alice Boner and Sadasiva Rath Sharma date it between the tenth and twelfth centuries AD. According to Rajendra Prasad Das,[7]

> Proceeding from the basic conception, the *Śilpa Prakāśa* lays down that a place (temple) without love images is known as a "place to be shunned" (*tyakta maṇḍala*). Continuing further it says that according to Kaulācāras, that which is shunned like the den of death and without offering *pūjā* to *kāmakalā yantra*, the Śakti *pūjā* and the *sādhanā* become useless as the bath of an elephant. Having said this the *Śilpa Prakāśa*, proceeds to explain the construction of the *kāmakalā yantra*, its presiding deity, her associates and attendants and the *dhyāna*s of Mahākāma-kāleśvarī and Śiva Kāmakāleśvara.

The discussion shows that *kāmakalā yantra* borrowed from the

---

7. R.P. Das, "The Study of Śilpa Śāstras," *Reference Orissa*, ed. A.N. Tiwari, Enterprising Publishers, Bhubaneswar, 1999, p. 178.

"Kośalī style of temple architecture," was brought to coastal Orissa, where the *pañcaratha* planned temple architecture and full-fledgedly developed and which ultimately became the matured form of Kaliṅga style. In the inner sanctum, *garbhagṛha*, the plan is square. According to the *Śilpa Prakāśa*, an intersecting square on the square plan has to be imagined, which forms *kāmakalā yantra* (*Fig.* 15).

The *śilpa* texts of Orissa mention three types of temples — *rekhā*, *pīḍhā* and *khākharā*. The *rekhā* and *pīḍhā* form two component parts of one architecture set up. *Rekhā* temple forms the main sanctum while the porch having a pyramidal roof in front of the sanctum is made of *pīḍhā*. The *khākharā* order is noted for its surmounting semi-cylindrical roof and such temples were meant for tāntric Śakti worship.

Till the Bhaumakara period, the *rekhā* temples of Orissa were of the *tri-ratha* plan and were having *aṣṭagraha* images. Meanwhile, during the post-Gupta period in the upper Mahānadī valley, which comprised South Kośala state, a lot of experimentation of stellate plan temple construction was going on. Of the few standing and surviving stellate planned temples of the upper Mahānadī valley, mention can be made of Rāma temple of Sirpur (*Fig.* 10), Indal Deul of Kharod (*Fig.* 11), Siddheśvara temple of Palari (*Fig.* 12), Śabari temple of Kharod, Pātāleśwar temple of Bodhi-Komna, Chellia temple of Rānīpur-Jharial complex, Citawari Devī temple of Dhobni and the stone foundation of Adhabhara.[8] One ruined stellate plane brick temple on a stone platform is found in the fort area of Patnagarh (vide the plan).

Among all the stellate plans, emphasis should be given to those with two squares placed diagonally and inter-secting each other at 45º angle (*Fig.* 14), thereby making an eight-point star

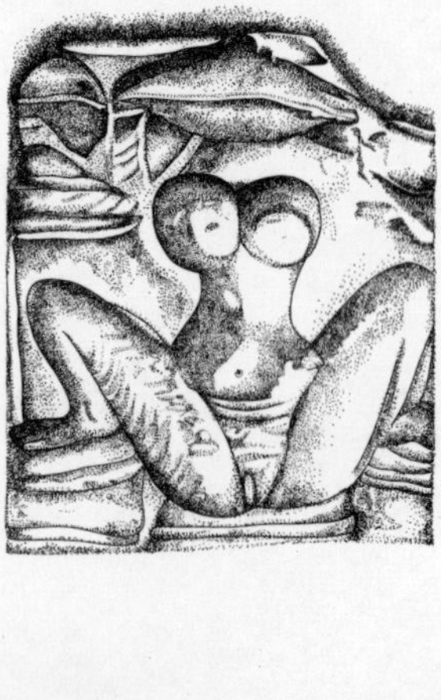

8. M.W. Meister, *op. cit.*, 1981, pp. 137-45.

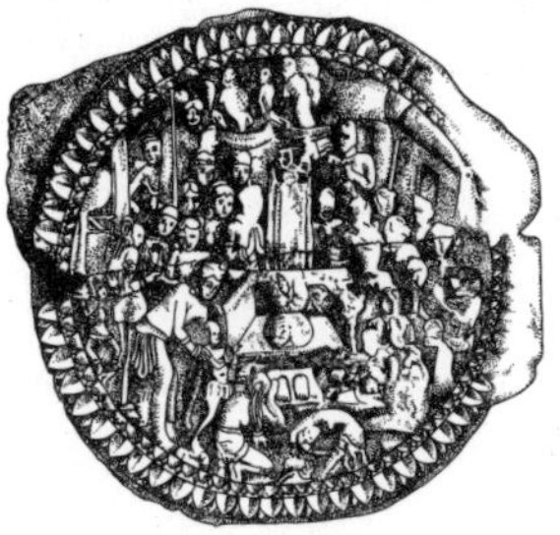

which is a *Yantra*[9], as described in the *Ānanda-Laharī*,[10] *Saundarya-Laharī*,[11] and many tāntric texts both published and unpublished. This *yantra* is considered to be the *kāmakalā yantra*.[12] The four Śiva temples namely, the Pātāleśwar Śiva temple of Bodhi-Komna; Nuāpāḍā district, Orissa; the Chellia temple of Rānīpur-Jharial complex, Bolaṅgīr district, Orissa; the Citawari Devi temple of Dhobni, Raipur district, Chhattisgarh; and the stone foundation of Adhabhara, Bilāspur district, Chhattisgarh; have plans of two squares placed diagonally and inter-secting each other at angles of 45º. So, these temples are in Kośalī *rekhā* style.[13]

From about the fourth century AD the Mahānadī valley was influenced by the Mattamayūra Tāntric Śaivism.[14] It will be suffice to mention that Mahāśivagupta Bālārjuna, the Pāṇḍuvaṁśī king of South Kośala, whose reigning period is assigned to *circa*. AD 595-655, was a follower of Mattamayūra Śaivism[15] and it was during his period that the *rekhā* Śiva temples in Kośalī style were built throughout his dominion.

---

9. S.K. Ramachandra Rao, *Yantras*, Sri Satguru Publications, Delhi, 1988, p. 51, vide fig. 21.
10. D. Ghosh, *Āananda-Laharī — Śaṅkarācārya*, Sanskrit Book Depot, Kolkata, 1986, Sloka 20, pp. 29-30.
11. V.K. Subramanian, *Saundarya-Laharī of Śaṅkarācārya*, Motilal Banarsidass, Delhi, 1977, verse no., 20, p. 66, verse no. 42, p. 77 and verse no. 80, p. 96.
12. The author is indebted to Sri Sashi Bhushan Mishra for supplying the *yantra* of śloka 20 of *Ānanda-Laharī*, as edited by Svami Sivananda, on 31st July 1983, at Bhubaneswar.
13. J.P. Singh Deo, *Cultural Profile of South Kosala*, Gyan Publishing House, New Delhi, 1987, p. 330.
14. R.P. Mishra, "Mattamayūra Śaivism in Orissa," *Culture and Collection*, ed. R.P. Mishra, Punthi Pustak, Kolkata, 1996, pp. 103-39.
15. S.R. Nema, *Political History of the Somavaṁśī Kings of South Kośala and Orissa*, Oriental Publishers, New Delhi, 1978, pp. 129-39.

Among the *rekhā* temples, the *Bhuvanapradīpa*[16] mentions the Kośalī *rekhā* and Kośalī *khākharā* temples.[17] Lalit Kumar Shukla[18] mention *nāgara, vesara, drāviḍa,* Kośalī, Kaliṅga, Pāñcāli, Māgadhī, Śaurasenī, Vaṅgī, Vyantara, Bhūmija, Lāṭa, Vāvāta, Vṛkṣājāti, etc., styles of temple architecture.

Ealier *tri-ratha* temples were built in the entire Mahānadī valley, including coastal Orissa and it seems the Kośalī style of *rekhā* temple architecture influenced the development of star-shaped temples, the plan of intersecting squares and *pancaratha* plans, which later developed into *saptaratha* and *navaratha* plans, throughout the country.[19]

The Kośalī style of *rekhā* temple had influenced the three Śaiva tāntric temples standing in a triangular formation inside the compound of modern uncomplete Rāmanātha temple at Bauḍ, on the right bank of the Mahānadī river (*Pl.* 44). About these three tāntric temples at Bauḍ, K.S. Behera[20] states that of these temples, one faces west while the other two having the same architectural and sculptural features, faces the east.

Of the three tāntric temples at Bauḍ, the Kapileśwar (*Pl.* 43) and Bhubaneswar temples face east while the Paścima Somanātha temple towards west, facing directly the Bhubaneswar temple. These three tāntric Śiva temples are the Śiva-Kāmeśvara, Śakti-Kāmeśvarī and Sāmarasya as described

---

16. N.K. Bose, *Canons of Orissan Architecture*, Cosmo Publications, New Delhi, 1982, p. 124.
17. N.K. Bose, *Canons of Orissan Architecture*, Cosmo Publications, New Delhi, 1982, pp. 172-73.
18. L.K. Shukla, *A Study of Hindu Art and Architecture*, Chowkhamba Sanskrit Series Office, Varanasi, 1972, p. 196.
19. J.P. Singh Deo, "Kośalī Style of Temple Architecture," *OHRJ*, vol. XXIV, XXV & XXVI, pp. 160-79.
20. K.S. Behera, *Temple of Orissa*, Orissa Sahitya Academi, Bhubaneswar, 1993, pp. 35-36.

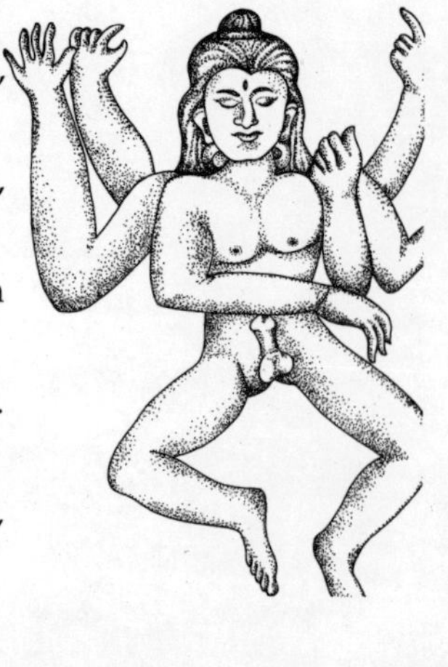

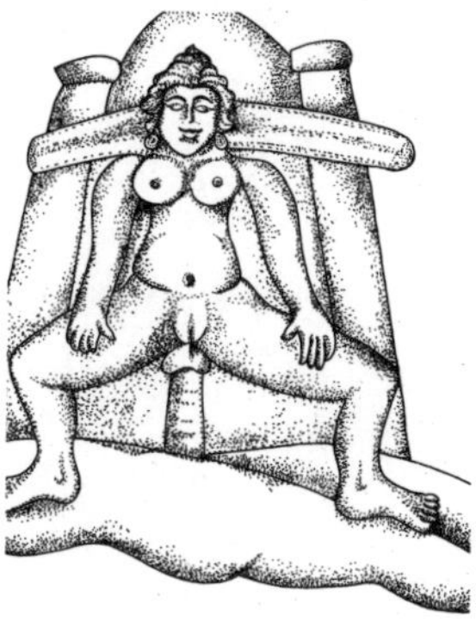

by Dirk Jan Hoens.[21] With this tāntric background, it can be claimed that the three Śaiva tāntric temples of Bauḍ, standing in a triangular shape were planned and built by advanced tāntric formulae. These temples may be assigned to the earlier period of the Somavaṁśī rule in Orissa.[22]

K.C. Panigrahi[23] also states that these three temples of Bauḍ have correlation with the Mukteśvara temple at Bhubaneswar. Mukteśvara temple has the *pañcaratha* plan with the *navagrahas* over its door jamb. Therefore, it is sure that the Kośalī style of *rekhā* temple architecture with its tāntric cult had influenced the development of *pañcaratha* plan temples of coastal Orissa, which was the matured form of Kaliṅga style. The matured *pañcaratha* planned temples, which had chronological development in their best forms in coastal Orissa, are the temples of Siṁhanātha, situated on an island in the Mahānadī river of Baramba area, the Mukteśwar temple of Bhubaneswar, the Liṅgarāja temple of Bhubaneswar, the Jagannātha temple of Purī and Sun temple of Koṇārka. This shows the influence of tāntric *kāmakalā yantra* on the temple architecture of the Mahānadī valley. Hence the Mahānadī valley which comprises Chhattisgarh and Orissa is the land of *kāmakalā*, i.e., erotic spiritual science of desire fulfilment. The highest desire of a human being is salvation or emancipation.

The study shows the development of full-fledged temple architecture in the Mahānadī river valley that took place with tāntric influence in the background.

---

21. Dirk Jan Hoens "Mantra and other Constituents of Tāntric Practices," *Handbuch der Orientalistik*, - II, *Abt.*, IV, *Band*. 2. *Abschh*, *Hindu Tantrism*, Leider/Kdn., E.J. Brill, 1979, pp. 93-95.

22. K.C. Panigrahi, *Archaeological Remains at Bhubaneswar*, Orient Longmans, New Delhi, 1961, p. 159.

23. *Ibid.*, pp. 87-93 and p. 159.

Visuals

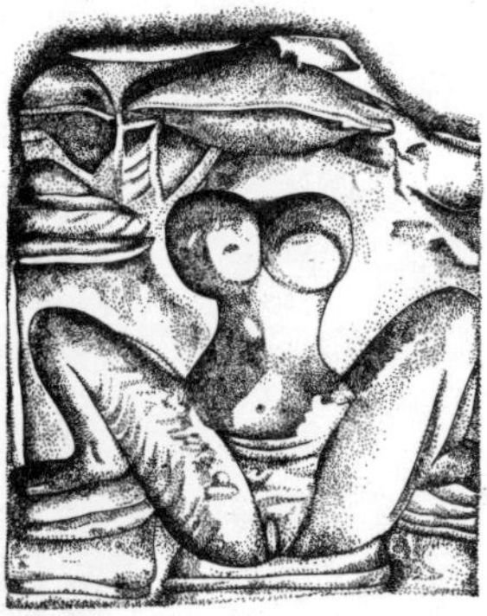

Appendix

Idealistic Translation of "Pāñcaśāyaka," Poetry into Prose

PĀÑCAŚĀYAKA, is composed by Kavi Samrāṭ Upendra Bhañja of Orissa in poetic Oriyā language. Prose translation of the required relevant portions has been done and others have been left out. Medicine (viagra), as it deals with botanical names, has been left out. Much importance is given to *candra calana*, (erogenous zones of females during different moon days) and 64 sexual *bandha*s (poses), as they are not found in the literature of any other language. It is a speciality and a gift of Orissa to the entire humanity.

Pāñcaśāyaka Prose Translation

Salutation to Ganesh.

An individual ignorant of erotic art is equal to a beast.

Types of Males

There are four types of male, viz., hare, deer, bull and horse. The hare type male is a lover of truth, religious and of normal health. His characteristic qualities are that he has well set and sharp teeth, beautiful nose and eyes, sweet voice and talks pleasant; he is cool-minded, merciful, a bit timid, uninterfering, helpful, god fearing, not poor, and satisfied with little sex indulgence. The penis of such a man is six fingers long.

The qualities of a deer man are that he talks sweetly and is pleasant, large hearted, truthful, bit timid, doubtless, amorous, fond of loneliness, not fickle-minded and the penis is eight fingers long.

A bull man is healthy, has robust body, his eyes are neat and clean, has much sexual indulgence, and has a penis of ten fingers long.

A horse man is miser, love to indulge in a sexual intercourse long duration uncourtious, spiteful, malignant, inimical, violent, and is hairy, has big teeth and a penis twelve fingers long.

Types of Females

Females are of four varieties, viz., Padminī, Citriṇī, Śaṁkhinī and Hastinī. Their distinct characteristics are being mentioned below:

Padminī: Moon like face, fare complexion, tender body, sweet voice like cuckoo, silk like hair, walks like a swan, has a charming look, a throat like conch, has big eyes, good buttocks, has proportionate teeth, nose and ears, smiling face, prefers fine clothes, eats little, shy in nature, sensitive, stable-minded and satisfied with little sex.

Citriṇī: Tint complexion, lotus faced, deer like eyes, cokoo-goose and pigeon like voice, teeth are extraordinarily beautiful, well-shaped belly with deep navel, well developed breasts, bee like hair, walks like an elephant, odour like pleasant new leaves, fond of luxury, has small diet, easily satisfied in sex, large buttocks, tender constitution and limbs are proportionate.

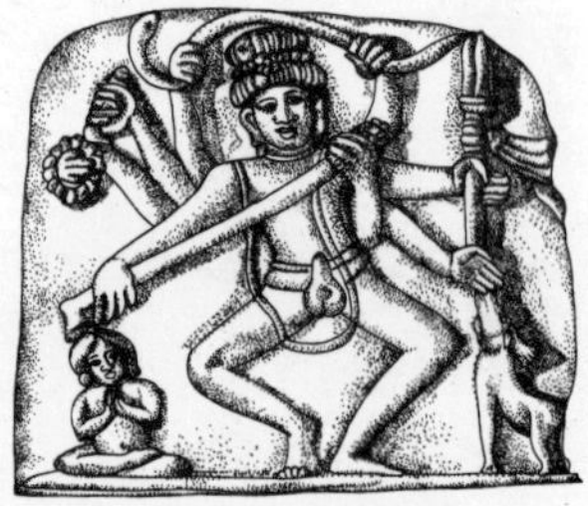

Śaṁkhinī: Long limbs, warm or cold body which is neither too thin nor not too fat, three folds on the throat which looks beautiful, voice of rattling sound, copper coloured hair, not easily satisfied in sex, fond of back biting talk, jealous, laughs loud, loves

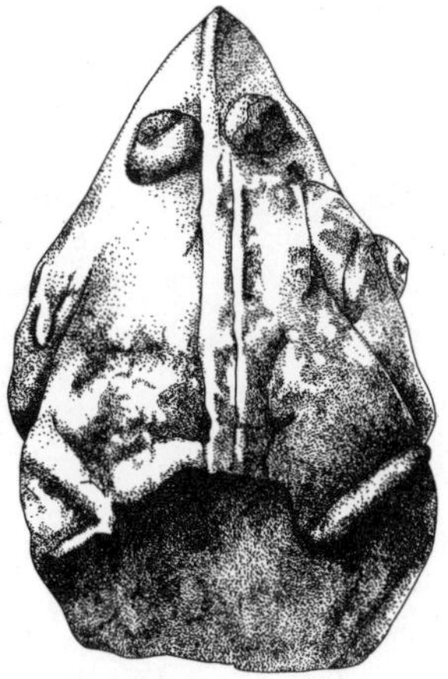

red clothes, small breast, odour like flesh, fickle-minded, loves to be embraced tightly and nail scratching.

Hastinī: Too fat body, walks like a horse, small and thin hair, rough voice, odour like wine, dark red lips, nice nose, three folds on the stomach, hairy body, very much amorous, huge thighs, thick waist, large breast, wishing sexual intercourse mostly, not fond of clothes and enjoys day time sexual intercourse.

Eroticism in Lunar days

Amorous days for *Padminī* females are first, third, fourth and fifth lunar days, for *Citriṇī* sixth, seventh, eighth and twelfth lunar days, for *Śaṁkhinī* second, ninth, eleventh and thirteenth lunar days and for *Hastinī* tenth, fourteenth and fifteenth lunar days.

Sexual Union

Women	*Men*
Padminī	Hare
Citriṇī	Deer
Śaṁkhinī	Bull
Hastinī	Horse

Variety of Penis

There are three varieties of penis: long, fat and short.

Variety of Yonis (Female Organs)

There are five varieties of *yoni* (female organ), viz, tortoise like, like the shoulder of an elephant, lotus like, *yoni* without hair and of a broad type.

*Yoni*s are cool, warm, hot and rough. The cool one is the best, warm one is better, hot one should be avoided and the rough variety is most troublesome.

Improper Union

Men	*Women*
Deer	Padminī
Hare	Citriṇī
Horse	Śaṁkhinī
Bull	Hastinī

Most Improper Union

Men	*Women*
Bull	Padminī
Horse	Citriṇī
Deer	Śaṁkhinī
Hare	Hastinī

Toilet, Dress and Ornaments suited for Amorous Encounters by Damsels

There are sixteen types of *śṛṅgāra* (toilet and dress suited for amorous encounters), viz.

1. Anointment of the body with scented paste,
2. Fresh bath,
3. Wearing of fine clothes,
4. Arrangement of hair with flowers and other ornaments,
5. Ornaments to be worn on the body,
6. *Sindūra* (vermilion) should be applied at the centre of the forehead,
7. Application of collyrium to the eyes,
8. Nose-pin to be worn,
9. Ear-rings and ear caps to be worn,
10. Necklaces to be worn,
11. Bangles to be worn,
12. Upper armlets to be worn,
13. Waste girdle to be worn,
14. *Kastūri* (musk) and sandle paste to be applied on the

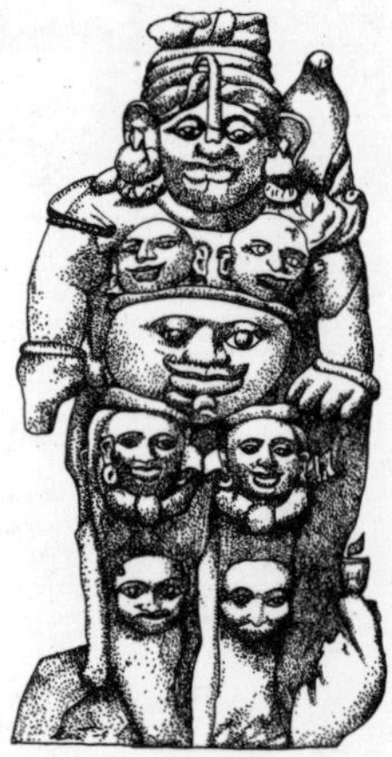

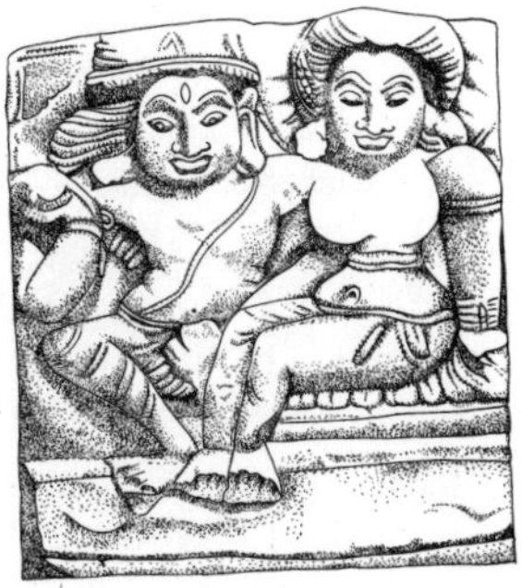

breasts, and cheeks are to be decorated with crocodile and bumble-bee designs,

15. Tinkling ring should be worn on the second finger of the legs, a ring (making sound) should be worn on the small finger of the legs, and a tinkling anklet should also be worn, and
16. Gold rings should be worn on fingers.

After these 16 *śṛṅgāra*s, the damsel should look at the mirror and be sensitive for seducing the enamoured male.

When the damsel is decorated with all these, why should Kāmadeva (Indian cupid) be not stimulated? So, it becomes natural for an individual to be aroused.

Such decorated damsels can easily seduce persons by offering beetle-nuts, cold drinks, smiles, sidelong and amorous glances which are feast to the eyes and by using a sweet language.

Sixteen Types of Amorous Encounters of the Male

The male should do 16 types of amorous encounters, viz.:

1. First embrace,
2. Kiss on the mouth,
3. Have sweet talk,
4. Do nail scratching,
5. Bite softly by teeth,
6. Have love intrigues,
7. Have sufficient love play,
8. Chest embrace and chest fondling,
9. Side feeling,
10. Navel feeling,
11. Ear feeling or biting,
12. Recite the *mantra*s (sacred mystic incantation) as given in the text,
13. By this time the lips are moistened; so derive the erotic taste,

14. Remove the under garment,
15. Indulge in penetration, and then finally, the
16. Sexual intercourse.

Amorous Feelings of Eight Types Then Follows

The amorous feelings of eight types of the females are,

1. Trembling out of excitement,
2. Bristling or thrill of joy,
3. Facilitation,
4. Tears of joy,
5. Love-quarrel,
6. Drowned in the sentiments of love (*śṛṅgāra rasa*),
7. One becomes apathetic, and
8. Finally one sleeps in the joy of orgasm after orgasm.

Acquainting Women of Different States

Southern women have beautiful faces. They put lot of flowers on their hair, which are soothing while embracing.

The women of Gauḍa state have a sensual gesture with well-shaped hips and buttocks. They are wholly beautiful, well mannered, well dressed and good in vaginal art.

The women of Mithilā have fine lips, well shaped eyes, nice *tribali* the three-fold or wrinkles of skin appearing on the belly and are desirous of frequent copulation.

Candra calana (Erogenous zones of Females during different moon days)

Erotic zones of females are those parts of the body which when stimulated arouse sexual reaction. In different moon days the erotic highs are in separate zones of the female body.

Erotic zones are situated on the right and left side of the males and females respectively. On the bright lunar fortnight (*śūkla pakṣa*) the men are stronger erotically, while on the dark lunar fortnight (*kṛṣṇa pakṣa*) the women are stronger.

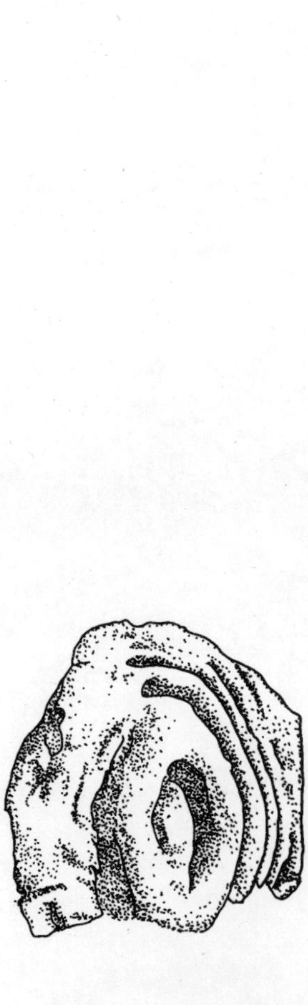

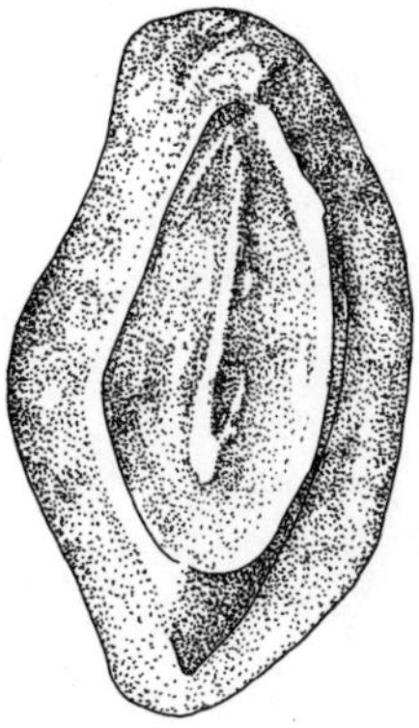

The following are the erotic zones of women:

1. lower part of the toe,
2. feet,
3. ankle joints
4. back part of the knee joints,
5. lower part of the navel and the navel itself,
6. armpits,
7. chest,
8. sides of the neck,
9. cheeks,
10. lips,
11. eyes,
12. ears,
13. forehead,
14. vulva, and
15. left arm.

According to some, the following are the erotic zones of women:

1. Sole of the feet,
2. ankle joints,
3. thighs,
4. vulva,
5. navel,
6. chests,
7. eyes,
8. armpits,
9. sides of the neck,
10. cheeks,
11. forehead,
12. ears,
13. eyes,
14. head, and
15. hair.

These series are the erotic zones during the bright lunar fortnight and it is reverse in the dark lunar fortnight.

The Method of Exciting Erotic Zones

Feet, ankle, back of the knee, breasts and armpits should be felt by the finger nail.

Vulva should be tickled by finger. Feel the breasts by palm. Bite softly at the lips and kiss on the cheeks, eyes and fore-head. Then the *mantra* (*kāma devāya rādhā mohāya svāhā* — sacred mystic incantation) should be enchanted, while exciting erotic zones of women.

Description of Copulation Time

Men of taste and wit should be skilful in the act of copulation for sexual enjoyment and should do such acts which pleases the woman partner with different poses for amorous delight.

In the fourth part of the night the Padminī women is easily pleased while in the third part the Citriṇī women gets enjoyment. Śaṁkhinī women can be pleased on the first, second and third parts of the night and Hastinī is ready to enjoy at anytime, day or night.

A lady is known as *bālā,* until her sixteenth year. Between the ages of 16 and 50 woman is fully matured. After the age of 50 a woman gets old.

Conjugation with women in *bālā,* period is enjoying as she remains much emotional. With a fully matured woman sex is enjoyed skillfully, while sex with old women is wastage of energy.

A *bālā* is seduced by presents of beetle leaves, clothes, flowers, scents, cosmetics, etc.

A women in fully matured stage is satisfied by kisses, tight embraces and intensive copulation.

For the old women, appeasement and soft words are pleasing. The seasons of eroticism for old women are autumn, spring and rainy. During summer and autumn a *bālā* is to be enjoyed.

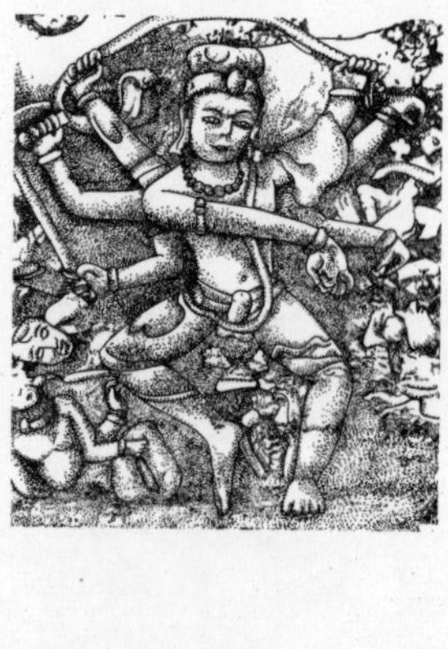

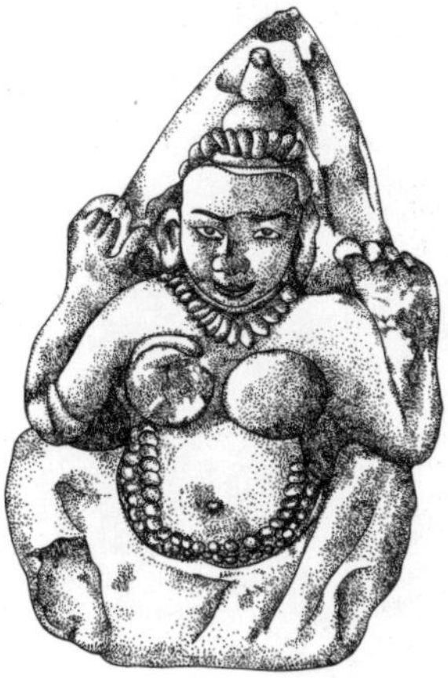

While approaching a woman for sexual act one should first please her with sweet talks, then make her sit on the lap, catch her hands and with polite love-talks make her sensuous. One should then embrace her and give delicate kisses on her lips as an enticement. Fondle her breasts tenderly. Then free kissing should be done at the erotic zones like throat, forehead, eyes, lips, breasts, cheeks, centre of the chest, ears and lips mostly. Kisses can also be given on all parts of the female body.

Then the breasts are to be felt or squeezed strongly. Nail feeling or scratching to be done at the sides of the breasts, buttocks, thighs, centre of the chest, hairs, neck, cheeks, hands and mostly at the inner side of the thighs.

After all these sensuous feelings bite her softly, wherever one likes or at the breasts, cheeks and lips. When a woman becomes aroused, lubricated and makes erotic noise, kiss her emotionally and indiscriminately wherever chance provide.

After the arousal of all these emotions the underwears are to be opened while embracing the woman tightly. The woman should not be allowed to break the aroused emotion and then the actual sexual intercourse is to be followed.

Erotic zones are always to be aroused during the action while pronouncing of the prescribed *mantra* (sacred mystic incantation). Kiss and counter-kisses are to be followed. Then the different poses are to be practised. Soft blowing should be done at the woman partner's ears. The felting on the chest and sides should not be stopped.

Bandhas (Poses)

There are 64 *bandha*s or poses and they are described below:

1. *Kāmaprada bandha*: The woman should raise her two legs, place them on the man's shoulder and place her hands on the neck of the man. The man should then have sexual penetration and kiss her on the lips.
2. *Viparīta bandha*: The woman should spread one leg on

the thigh of the male and the second foot should be placed over the shoulder. The man should catch hold of the woman's neck by one hand and should place his other hand on her breast.

3. *Nagara bandha*: The man should sit near the thigh of the woman and have sex in sitting position. The man's hands should get hold of the woman's neck.
4. *Ratipāśa bandha* : The woman should place the man locked within her thighs, and then embrace him tightly.
5. *Koyar bandha:* The woman should squeeze one thigh of the man by both of her thighs and her two hands should embrace the male.
6. *Tosaka bandha*: The man should lift the woman by catching hold of her feet. The woman should place her hands around the man's neck. The breasts of the woman are to be placed on the chest of the man.
7. *Samapāda bandha*: The woman should raise her legs towards her chest and the man should catch hold of her breasts, squeeze them and give her biting kisses.
8. *Ekapāda bandha*: The woman should place one of her legs straight, raise the other leg and catch hold of the neck of the man. Then the raised leg should be placed on the man's shoulder.
9. *Sampuṭa bandha*: The woman should lie down flat and the man should enjoy her. After this, different poses may be practised.
10. *Ardhasampuṭa bandha*: Enjoy the woman while she lies down flat by touching her breasts with one's own chest.
11. *Stanabhāra bandha*: The woman should sit on the man's lap with her legs spread apart. Then, the male should lie down and fondle the breasts of the woman extremely.
12. *Ratisundara bandha*: The woman should raise her two legs and touch them on her breasts. The man should

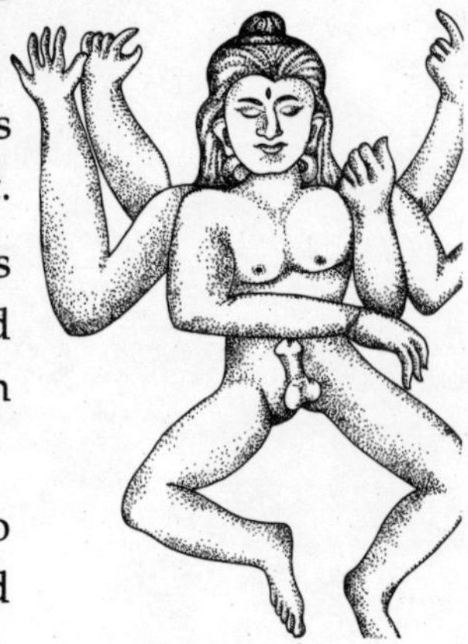

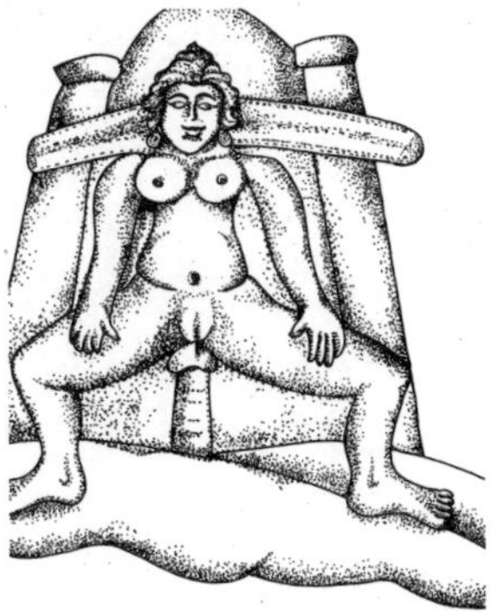

enjoy her by catching hold of her neck.

13. *Padma bandha*: Catch hold the breasts of the woman, embrace her tightly and enjoy.
14. *Ekarasa bandha*: Catch hold the waist of the woman. Then lift one of her leg and put it on the man's waist. The other leg of the woman should be straight. Then, place one hand round her neck and do movement.
15. *Cakra bandha*: Catching hold of the woman by the left hand the man should make her sit on his feet. The woman's legs should be spread apart.
16. *Second cakra bandha*: Catching hold of the two legs of the woman by the armpits the man should put his hands around her neck and touch the breasts.
17. *Bikrama bandha*: One foot of the woman should touch the man's forehead and her other leg should hold the man's waist. While kissing her the man's chest should touch the woman's breasts and thus enjoy the sexual intercourse.
18. *Vaistaka bandha*: The woman should raise her one leg and keep touching the man's chest while the other leg of her should encircle waist. This action should be done in a sitting position.
19. *Haṁsa kīlaka nīlāsana bandha*: Man lies down and the woman sitting on his thighs becomes active.
20. *Haṁsa kīlaka bandha*: Man lies down and the woman sitting on his thighs catches hold of the man's arm-pits and does movement.
21. *Nīlāsana bandha*: Man should lie down and the woman should sit over his *liṅga* (penis) and bend over the man's chest so that the woman's breasts can be caught hold by the man and in the same time the woman's breasts should touch the man's chest.
22. *Siṁha-rīti Bandha*: The two legs of the woman should be placed on the man's shoulders. The man should catch

hold of the woman's breasts and have sexual intercourse.

23. *Gaja-rati Bandha*: Making the woman sit on his thighs, the man catch hold of her. The woman's body shouldn't be allowed to touch the ground.
24. *Aśva bandha*: Making the woman bent her front the man should touch her thigh with his from the back and enjoy by having movement.
25. *Brūśa bandha*: The woman should bend her front side and rest by her hands. The man should kiss her from the side and have sexual intercourse from her back and enjoy.
26. *Mṛgamata bandha*: Make the woman bend towards her front and while resting her hands on her knee. Then, the man should have sexual intercourse from her back and enjoy.
27. *Mārjāra bandha*: The woman should lie down on her back. The man should lie on her straight. The man's hands should be spread on her hands.
28. *Raṭi bikrama bandha*: The man should raise the feet of the woman on the bed and make her spread her hands. He then has sexual intercourse and enjoys.
29. *Grāmya bandha*: The woman should lie down flat and the man should lie or sit on her so that the thighs of both should touch each other. In the meantime the woman should catch hold of the man's right hand by her left hand and should feel a fist-closed palm.
30. *Karmūka kṛti bandha* (*or bow pose*): The man should sit between the thighs of the woman and bend on her, while clasping hands.
31. *Chanda bandha*: Raising the legs of the woman on his head and sitting close to her buttocks, the man should clasp the thighs tightly and perform the sex act.
32. *Padmāsana bandha*: The man should sit in *padmāsana*

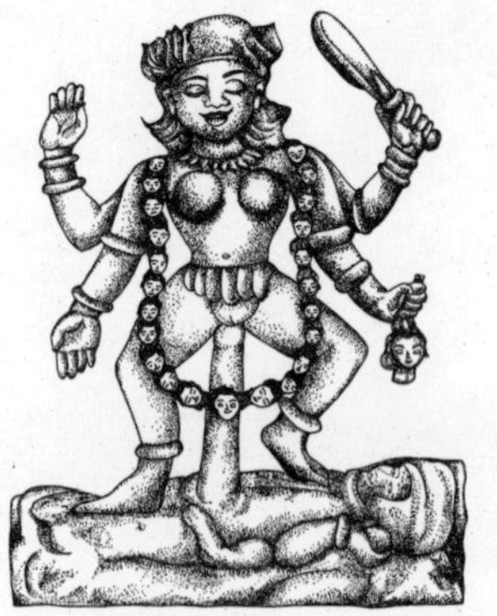

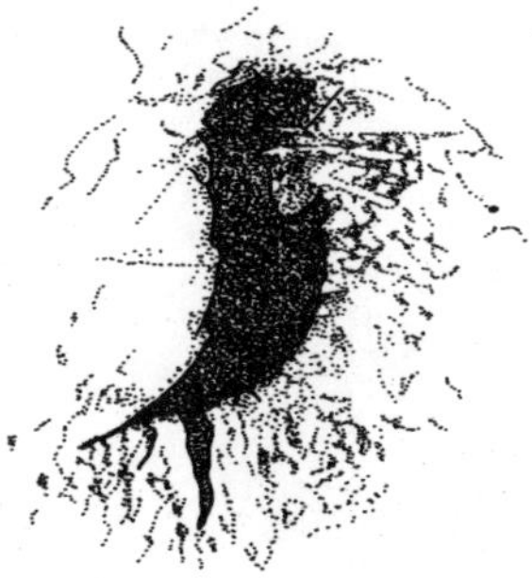

(lotus pose) and the woman should sit on his lap. Both of them should clasp their hands to form a lotus.

33. *Cakrabhava bandha*: The woman should sit on the feet of the man. The man should clasp breasts as he moves his hands through her thighs. In this pose, kissing and embracing each other should also continue.

34. *Eśa (or plough) bandha*: The woman should lie down flat and the man should rest himself on his knees and place his chest on the woman's breasts.

35. *Aśr̥ta bandha*: The woman should lie down flat and keep her one leg straight and the other leg should be placed on the thigh of the man.

36. *Sūraja-kr̥ti bandha*: Raising the legs of the woman and catching hold of her thighs, the man should place his hands on her breasts.

37. *Malla Bandha*: The man should lie down flat and raise his two legs. The woman should catch hold of the man's thighs and bend her head down like a deer. This can be done the other way also.

38. *Varuṇa bandha*: The man should raise both the legs of the woman and hold them, while the woman should hold the man's neck by her hands. The man should kiss on both breasts and perform the sex act.

39. *Gūḍharāsa bandha*: The woman should spread her legs between the legs of the man. The man should touch the cheek of the woman by one hand and catch her breast by another hand.

40. *Viparīta bandha*: The man should lie down and place one leg on the shoulder of the woman and the other leg should be straight. The woman should perform the act and the man should hold her chin.

41. *Ekapāda bandha*: The woman should lie down with one leg stretched and her other leg should be placed on the shoulder of the man.

42. *Ūrdhvapada bandha*: Let the woman lie down flat and raise her two legs up. The man should hold the woman's legs by both of his hands and do sexual intercourse energetically and tightly.
43. *Cakra bandha*: Let the woman lie down and spread her both legs and hands. The man should lie upon her and allow his chest to touch her breasts.
44. *Bhadrāsana bandha*: The man should sit in a posture of meditation and allow the woman to sit on his lap, then embrace her and kiss her proficiently.
45. *Jaṅghāsana bandha*: The man should sit over the two feet of the woman and catch hold of her body by both hands. The man's buttocks should touch the ground and enjoy the sex act.
46. *Sūsama bandha*: *Sūsama bandha* is practised very less. Place both the woman's legs on one shoulder of the man and the man should grasp the two breasts of the woman.
47. *Kūrma (or tortoise) bandha*: The man should catch hold of the woman's neck after placing her both thighs upon his.
48. *Kaṅkaṇa bandha (or bracelet pose)*: The woman and the man should embrace each other and have sexual act in standing pose.
49. *Kakarati bandha*: The man should sit down and stretch his legs. Then, the woman should sit on the lap of the man by stretching her legs, towards the back of the man.
50. *Jugala bandha*: The man and woman should stand and put one of their legs round each other's waist.
51. *Dṛḍa bandha*: The man should put his thighs on those of the woman and catch hold of her chin.
52. *Rasajita bandha*: The woman should lie down flat. The man then sits on one of her thigh and place another thigh on his own thigh.

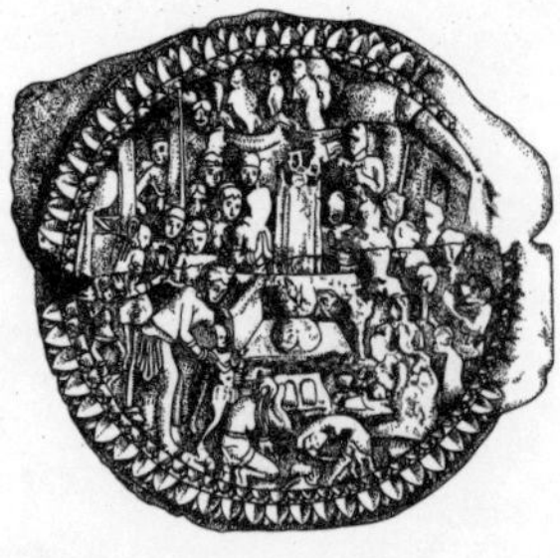

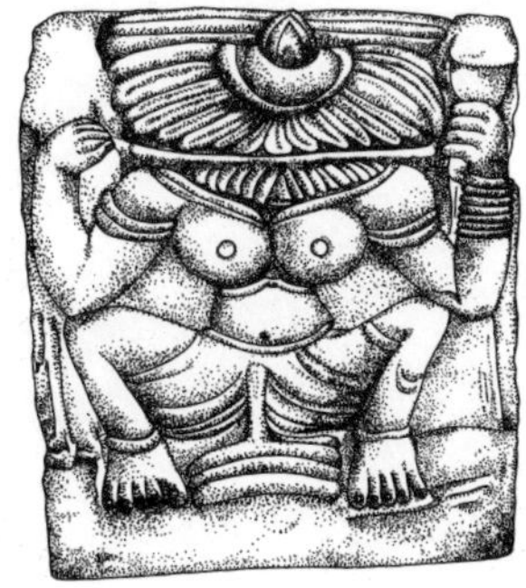

पक्षीबन्धः समुत्पन्नः दंडनाम समाचरेत्।
युगलः कंकणः प्रोक्तो सारभस्य यथाक्रमः॥

53. *Uparati bandha*: The man and the woman should lie down side by side, facing each other and perform the sex act.
54. *Saṅkaca bandha*: Make the woman lie down flat on her belly, facing the ground. The man should then lift one thigh of the woman and perform the act from her back.
55. *Trikoṇa bandha*: The man standing on the feet of the woman should stretch her hands apart by catching them.
56. *Mekhalā bandha*: The woman should place her thighs on her breasts by lifting them and hold them by her hands. The man should catch her at the waist and perform the sex act.
57. *Bikaca bandha*: The woman should sit down with crossed legs and then lie down by lifting the crossed legs. The man should penetrate his hands through the crossed legs of the woman and catch hold of her neck and perform the sex act.
58. *Ghana bandha*: The woman should cover her body with the bedsheet and stretch herself on the bed, being hidden. The man should search the proper place for the sexual intercourse.
59. *Kumuda bandha*: It is a difficult action. The woman should hold both her feet and lie down, so that she could lift them and keep on the man's shoulders. The man should enjoy sexual intercourse by placing his hands on her breasts.
60. *Bakra bandha*: Make the woman lie down flat, facing the ground. Hold her from back side. The man should bend from the waist towards her and kiss her. At the same time sexual intercourse should go on.
61. *Adhomukha bandha*: The woman should rest on her knees

and elbows. The man should penetrate from her back by kneeling and perform the sexual intercourse.

62. *Ūrdhyomukha bandha*: The man should sit down, putting his feet near the vulva of the woman, then lift her face by holding the chin and perform the sexual intercourse.

63. *Padadruta bandha*: Both the man and the woman should stand and catch hold of each others' thighs by one hand and embrace by the other. At the same time sexual intercourse should continue.

64. *Sammukha bandha*: The woman should sit on the lap of the man by stretching her legs. The man should then embrace her by the neck and kiss on her cheeks while having sexual intercourse.

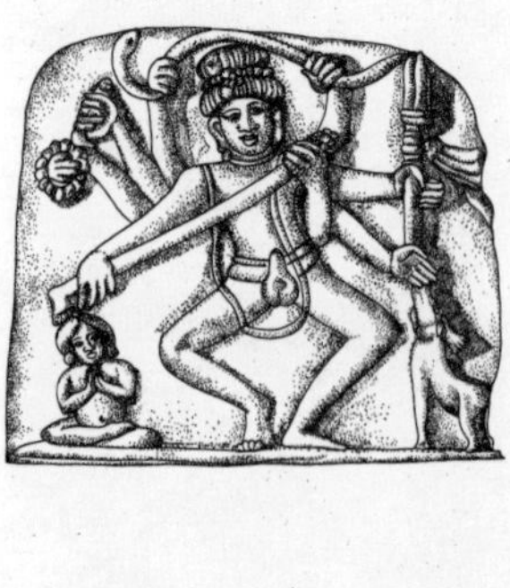

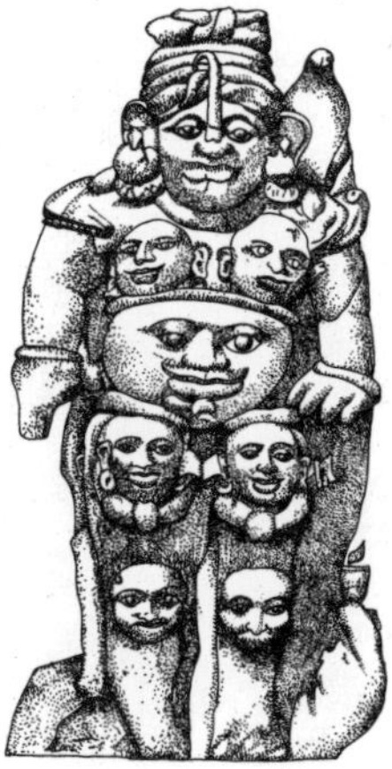

Glossary

Bindu	:	Point, point of potential energy and consciousness, nucleus. In *tantra* and *haṭha yoga*, it also represents a drop of semen.
*Bhūta*s	:	There are five subtle elements, which constitute the perceived gross world, viz. : (1) *ākāśa* (space), (2) *agni* (fire), (3) *vāyu* (air), (4) *vyāna* (water) and (5) *somāna* (earth). These *pañca* (five) *bhūta*s are found in human body, according to yogic thought.
Dakṣa	:	Prajāpati Dakṣa is father-in-law of Lord Śiva, as mentioned in the *Tantra Cūḍāmaṇi* text.
Deula	:	Temple
Kāla	:	Kāla is time and Mahākāla is the destroyer of the cosmos or the god of time.
Mantra	:	Subtle sound vibration, process of *tantra* for liberating energy and expanding consciousness from the limitations of mundane awareness.
Vaidikācāra	:	Vedic knowledge and wisdom.
*Yuga*s	:	Respective ages in Hindu calendar.
Yantra	:	A diagram which acts as a receptacle for the power of a *mantra*.
Yoga	:	State of union between two oppssite poles, viz.: Śiva and Śakti, body and mind, individual and universal awareness, process of uniting,

		opposing forces in the body and mind in order to realize the spiritual essence of being and existence.
Yogī	:	Individual who does *yoga.*
Yantra	:	Symbolic diagram utilized in *tantra*, geometrical symbol representing specific conformations of forces of Śakti and consciousness. A process of concentration upon specific forms employed in *tantra* to liberate potential energy and consciousness within an individual.

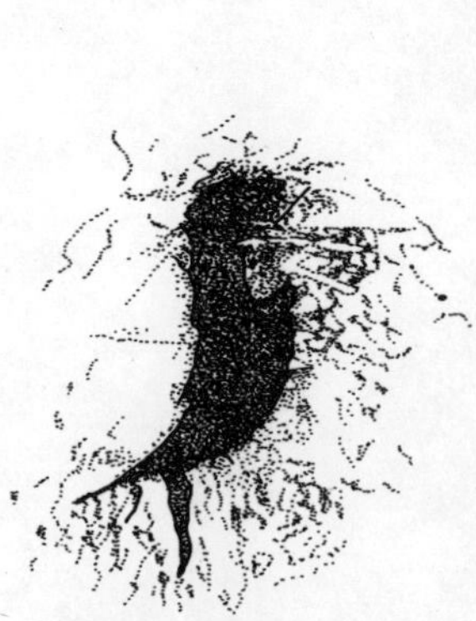

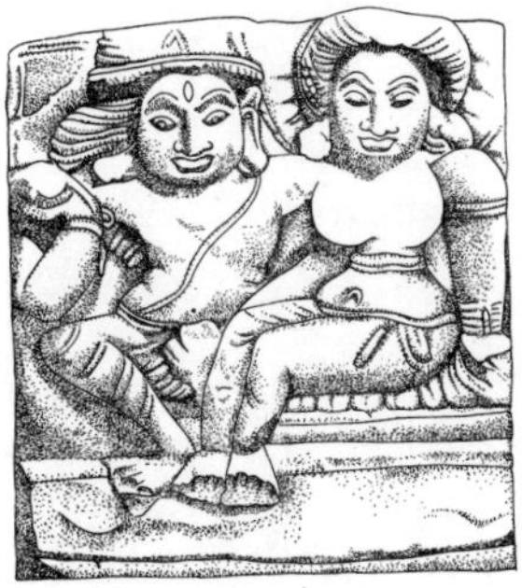

Bibliography

Antiquary, Report, Journal, Souvenir, Quarterly and Magazine

Bharati-Utkal University Journal (*Humanities*), vol. IV, July, 1971.

Cunningham, A., *Archaeological Survey of India Report*, vol. IX and vol. XIII.

Essays of History, Education & Culture (Comparative Nos. 3 & 4), Mayur Publication, Bhubaneswar, 1987.

Indian Antiquary, vol. LXII, 1933.

Indian Historical Quarterly, vol. VI.

Journal Asiatique, 1951.

Journal of Bengal Art, Dacca, vol. 4, 1999.

Journal of History, Dept. of History, Jadavpur University, vol. XIII, 1994-95, Kolkata.

Journal of Royal Asiatic Society, 1906.

Journal of the Bihar and Orissa Research Society, 1909 and 1928.

Journal of the Royal Asiatic Society of Bengal, *Letters*, vol. XIV, No. 1, 1948.

Kalahandi Utsav, *Souvenir*, 2000, Bhawanipatna.

Man 35, no. 70.

OHRJ, vols. XIV, Nos. 3 & 4, XXX, No. 1, XXX, Nos. 2, 3, & 4, XXII, No. 2, XXIV, XXV, XXVI, XXXVII, Nos. 1 to 4 & XLII, Nos. 1 to 4.

Orissa Review (*Monument Special*), A.N Tiwari (Chief ed.), January 1976, Bhubaneswar.

Prachya Pratibha, vol. V, no. 1, January 1977, Agamkala Prakashan, Delhi.

Prāgdhārā, No. 6, Journal of the Uttar Pradesh State Archaeological Organization, 1995-96.

Rupam, no. 10, April 1922.

Souvenir, District Council of Culture, 1998, Sonepur.

Souvenir, Kalahandi Utsav 1999, Bhawanipatna.

Souvenir, Kalahandi Utsav, 2002, Bhawanipatna.

Souvenir, Loka Mahosabha, 2001, Sambalpur.

Souvenir, Loka Mahosabha, 2002, Sambalpur.

The Journal of Kalinga Historical Research Society, vol. I, No. 4, March 1947 and vol. II.

The Quarterly Review of Historical Studies, Institute of Historical Studies, Kolkata, vol. XI, nos. 1 & 2, April to September 2000.

Gazetteer

Behuria, N.C. (Chief ed.), *Gazetteer of India, Orissa State*, vol. II, Cuttack, 1991.

Kuanr, D.C. (State ed.), *Gazetteer of India, Orissa, Boudh-Khondmals*, N. Senapati (Chief ed.), Cuttack, 1983.

Sahu, N.K. (State ed.), *Gazetteer of India, Orissa, Balangir*, N. Senapati, (General ed.), Cuttack, 1968.

Inscription

Inscriptions of Orissa, vol. IV, Bhubaneswar, 1966.

Shastri, Ajay Mitra, *Inscriptions of the Śarabhapuriyas, Pāṇḍuvaṁśīs and Somavaṁśīs*, Parts I & II, Motilal Banarsidass, Delhi, 1995.

———, *E.I.* vol. XXXI.

Sanskrit Text

Agni Purāṇa.

Aitareya Brāhamaṇa.

Devi Mahātmya.

Dutt, M.N., *A Prose Translation of Mahānirvāna Tantra*, Chowkhamba Sanskrit Series Office, Varanasi, 1979.

Ghosh, D. (ed.), *Ānanda-Laharī — Śaṅkarācārya*, Sanskrit Book Depot (P.), Ltd., Kolkata, 1985.

Karaṇāgama.

Mahadevan, T.M.P., *The Hymns of Śaṅkara*, Motilal Banarsidass, Delhi, 1986.

Pancham Singh (ed.), *The Haṭha-Yogta-Pradīpikā*, Munshiram Manoharlal, New Delhi, 1980.

Rukmani, T.S. (ed.), *Yogavārttika of Vijñanabhiksu*, Munshiram Manoharlal,

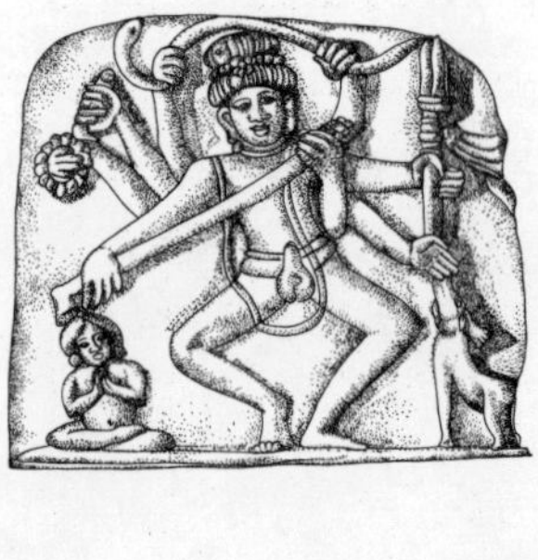

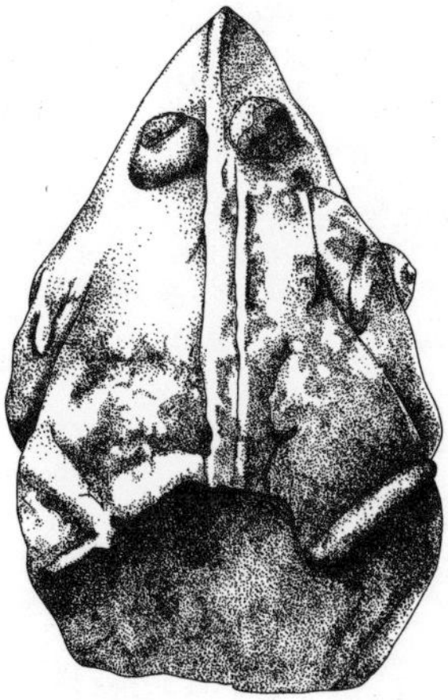

New Delhi, vol. I, 1981, vol. II, 1983, vol. III, 1998 and vol. IV 1999.

Śākta Pramoda, ed. Sri Venkatesvara Press, Bombay, 1951.

Sāṁkhyāyana Śrauta Sūtra.

Sastri, Pandit Harisadankarji (ed.), *Śyāma Rahasya Tantra*, Sanskrit Pustakalaya, Haridwar, 1911.

Śatapatha Brāhamaṇa.

Schoterman, J.A., *The Yoni Tantra*, Manohar Publications, New Delhi, 1980.

Subramanian, V.K., *Saundarya-Laharī of Śaṅkarācārya*, Motilal Banarsidass, Delhi, 1986.

Vasu, S.C. (ed.), *Śiva Saṁhitā*, Munshiram Manoharlal, New Delhi, 1970.

Vasu, S.C. (ed.), *The Gheraṇḍa Saṁhitā*, Munshiram Manoharlal, New Delhi, 1980.

Woodroffe, Sir J. (ed.), *Mahānirvāṇa Tantram*, Gita Press, (?), Gorakhpur.

Secondary Sources

Agrawal, D.P. & Chakrabarti, D.K. (eds.), *Essays in Indian Proto-history*, B.R. Publication Corporation, Delhi, 1979.

Agrawal, P.K., *Mithuna — The Male-Female Symbol in Indian Art and Thought*, Munshiram Manoharlal, New Delhi, 1983.

Alchin, F.R. & Chakrabarti, D.K. (eds.), *A Source Book of Indian Archaeology*, vol. I, Munshiram Manoharlal, New Delhi, 1979.

Anderson, Kenneth, *Secrets of Sex*, Jaico Publishing House, Bombay, 1973.

Bandyopadhyay, Pranab, *The Goddess of Tantra*, Punthi Pustak, Kolkata, 1987.

Banerjea, J.N., *Purāṇic and Tāntric Religion*, (?).

Banerjee, R.D., *History of Orissa*, vol. II, (?) Kolkata.

Basa, K.K. & Mohanty, P. (eds.), *Archaeology of Orissa*, vol. I, Pratibha Prakashan, Delhi, 2000.

Baumer, B. & Das, R.P. (eds.), *Śilparatnakośa* (*A Glossary of Orissan Temple Architecture*), by Sthāpaka Nirañjana Mahāpatra, Indira Gandhi National Centre for the Arts, New Delhi & Motilal Banarsidass, New Delhi & Delhi, 1994 (Vatsyayan, K., General editor).

Behera, K.S., *Konark The Heritage of Mankind*, vols. I & II, Aryan Books International, New Delhi, 1996.

Behera, K.S., *Temples of Orissa*, Orissa Sahitya Akademi, Bhubaneswar, 1993.

Bhargava, M.L., *The Geography of Ṛgvedic India*, The Upper India Publishing House Ltd., Lucknow, 1964.

Bhaskara Reddy, G.V., *Erotic Sculptures of Ancient India*, Inter-India Publications, New Delhi, 1991.

Bhattacharya, B., *An Introduction of Buddhist Esoterism*, (?).

Bhattacharyya, N.N., *History of Indian Erotic Literature*, Munshiram Manoharlal, New Delhi, 1975.

Bhattacharyya, N.N., *History of the Tāntric Religion*, Manohar, New Delhi, 1987.

Bolon, C.R., *Forms of the Goddess Lajjā Gaurī in Indian Art*, Motilal Banarsidass, Delhi, 1997.

Boner, A. & Sarma, S.R. (eds.), *Śilpa Prakāśa of Rāmacandra Kaulācārya*, parts I & II, Leiden, 1966.

Boner-Sarma-Baumer, *Vāstusūtra Upaniṣad* (*The Essence of Form in Sacred Art*), Motilal Banarsidass, Delhi, 1996.

Bose, D.N.-Haldar-Hiralal, *Tantras, Their Philosophy and Occult Secrets*, Oriental Publishing Co., Kolkata, 1956.

Bose, Nirmal Kumar, *Canons of Orissan Architecture*, Cosmo Publication, New Delhi, 1982.

BSOIHAC, vol. I, 1997, vol. II, 1993 and vol. XVI, 1995.

Burton, Sir R. & Arbuthnot, F.F. (trs.), *Vatsyayana's Kāmasūtra*, Orient Paperbacks, Delhi, 1982.

Cairns, G.E., *Man as Microcosm in Tāntric Hinduism*, Manohar, New Delhi, 1992.

Chakravartty, C., *Sex Life in Ancient India*, Firma K.L.M. Kolkata, 1963.

Chakravarty, K.K. & Bednari, F.G. (eds.), *Indian Rock Art and its Global Contest*, Motilal Banarsidass, (?), New Delhi.

Chakravarty, M., *Religious Life in The Kalachuri Empire*, Punthi Pustak, Kolkata, 1999.

Chawdhury, L.R., *Practicals of Yantras*, Sagar Publications, New Delhi, 1984.

Chela Buddhananda, *Moola Bandha the Master Key*, Bihar School of Yoga, Munger, Bihar, 1984.

Chidananda, Swami, *Path to Blessedness*, The Divine Life Society, Shivanandnagar, 1975.

Chinmayananda, Swami, *Vedanta The Science of Life*, Part I, Central Chinmaya Mission Trust, Bombay, 1983.

Chowdhury, A.K.R., *Bharatavarsha — An Evolutionary Synthesis of India* (*Dandakaranya & Mahakantara*), vol. I, Rupa & Co., Kolkata, 1975.

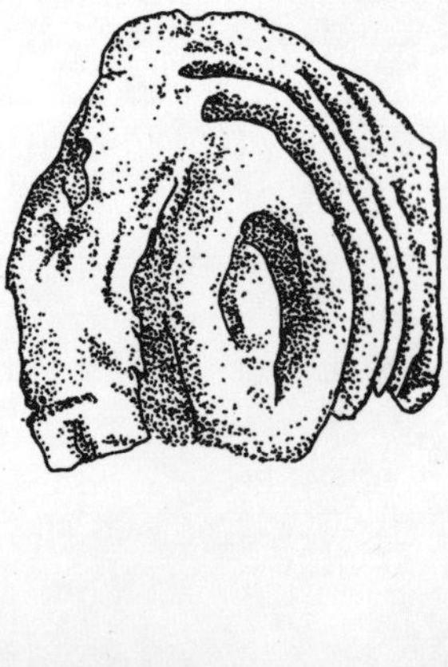

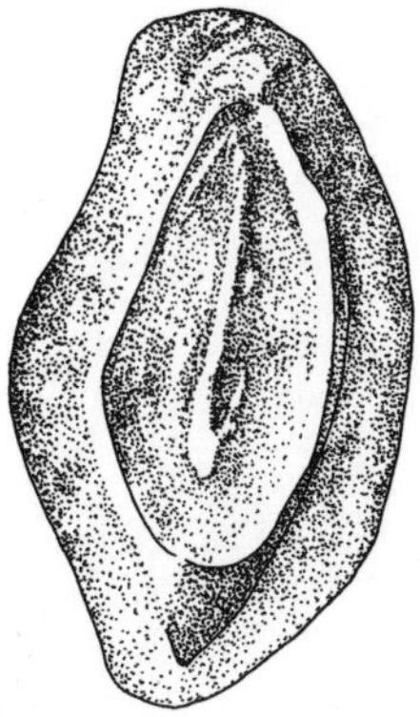

Das, Chittaranjan, *Balarama Das*, Sahitya Akademi, New Delhi, 1982.

Das, Dipakranjan, *Temples of Orissa: The Study of a Sub-Style*, Agamkala Prakashan, Delhi, 1982.

Das, H.C., *Cultural Development in Orissa*, Punthi Pustak, Kolkata, 1985.

Das, H.C., *Daśamahāvidyas* (Oriyā), S.B. Publications, Cuttack, 1983.

Das, H.C., *Iconography of Śākta Divinities*, vol. I, Pratibha Prakashan, Delhi, 1997.

Das, H.C., *Śākta Pīṭhas — A Study*, Bharati Prakashan, Bhubaneswar, 1999.

Das, H.C., *Tāntricism : A Study of Yogini Cult*, Sterling Publishers, New Delhi, 1981.

Das, M.N., (ed.), *Sidelights on History and Culture of Orissa*, Vidyapuri, Cuttack, 1977.

De, Sushil Kumar, *Ancient Indian Erotics and Erotic Literature*, Firma K.L.M. Kolkata, 1969.

Desai, Devangana, *Erotic Sculpture of India — A Socio-Cultural Study*, Tata McGraw-Hill Publishing Co., New Delhi, 1975.

Desai, Devangana, *The Religious Imagery of Khajuraho*, Project for Indian Cultural Studies Publication, IV, Mumbai, 1996.

Devaraja, N.K., *The Mind and Spirit of India*, Motilal Banarsidass, Delhi, 1967.

Dhatta, B., *The Science of Sulba*, Kolkata, 1932.

Don Mario Mazzoleni, *A Catholic Priest Meets Sai Baba*, Sri Sathya Sai Book & Publication Trust, Prashanthi Nilayam, Andhra Pradesh, 1995.

Donaldson, T.E., *Kāmadeva's Pleasure Garden: Orissa*, B.R. Publishing Corporation, Delhi, 1987.

Feuersten, G., Kal, S. & Frawley, D., *In Search of the Cradle of Civilization*, Motilal Banarsidass, Delhi, 1999.

Frawley, D., *Gods, Sages and Kings (Vedic Secrets of Ancient Civilization)*, Motilal Banarsidass, Delhi, 1995.

Frawley, David, *The Ṛgveda and The History of India*, Aditya Prakashan, New Delhi, 2001.

Garg, Ganga Ram (General ed.), *Encyclopaedia of The Hindu World*, vol. I; A-Aj., Concept Publishing Company, New Delhi, 1992.

Harding, Elizabeth U., *Kālī*, Motilal Banarsidass, Delhi, 1998.

Harshananda, Swami, *All About Hindu Temple*, Sri Ramkrishna Ashrama, Mysore, 2nd edn., 1981.

Hindu Tantrism, Hansbuch Der Orientalistek, II, ABT., IV, Band 2, ABSCH, No., Leiden/Koln, E.J. Brill, Belgium, 1979.

HYPBS, 1993.

Joanna, G.W. (ed.), *Kalādarśana* (American Studies in the Art of India), Oxford & I.B.H. Publishing Co., New Delhi, 1981.

Kara, K.K., *Ascharja Charya Chaya* (Oriyā), Odisha Sahitya Akademi, Bhubaneswar, 1969.

Khare, M.D. (ed.), *Painted Rock Shelters*, Archaeology & Museums, Madhya Pradesh, Bhopal, 1981.

Kumar, Pushpendra, *Śakti Cult in Ancient India*, Bharatiya Publishing House, Vārāṇasī, 1974.

Lal, B.B., *The Saraswati Flows on* (*The Continuity of Indian Culture*), Aryan Books International, New Delhi, 2002.

Lal, B.B., *The Earliest Civilization of South Asia*, Aryan Books International, New Delhi, 1997.

Madhu Khanna, *Yantra: The Tāntric Symbol of Cosmic Unity*, Thames & Hudson, London, 1994.

Mahārāja, Jagadguru Swami Śrī Kṛpālujī, *Philosophy of Divine Love* (*Prema Rasasiddhanta*), Sadhna Bhawan Trust, Mangarh, Uttar Pradesh, 2nd edn., 1996.

Margoliouth, D.S., *Mohammad and the Rise of Islam*, Voice of India, New Delhi, reprint 1985.

Mishra, K.C., *The Cult of Jagannātha*, Firma K.L.M., Kolkata, 1971.

Mishra, P.K. (ed.), *Culture, Tribal History and Freedom Movement*, Agamkala Prakashan, Delhi, 1989.

Mishra, R.P. (ed.), *Culture and Collections*, Punthi Pustak, Kolkata, 1996.

Mishra, R.P., *Fragments of Indian Culture* (*Ranipur-Jharial*), Punthi Pustak, Kolkata, 1995.

Mishra, R.P., *Sahajayana — A Study of Tāntric Buddhism*, Punthi Pustak, Kolkata, 1991.

Mishra, T.N., *Impact of Tantra on Religion and Art*, D.K. Printworld (P.) Ltd., New Delhi, 1997.

Misra, Shiva Sheikhar, *Fine Arts and Technical Sciences in India with Special Reference to Somesvara's Manasollasa*, Krishnadas Academy, Vārāṇasī, 1982.

Mohapatra, G.C., *The Stone Age Cultures of Orissa*, Deccan Collge, Poona, 1962.

Moharana, S.K., *Tāntric Buddhism*, Aryan Books International, New Delhi, 2001.

Nathan, R.S., *Our Heritage*, Book I, Central Chinmaya Mission Trust, Bombay, 1986.

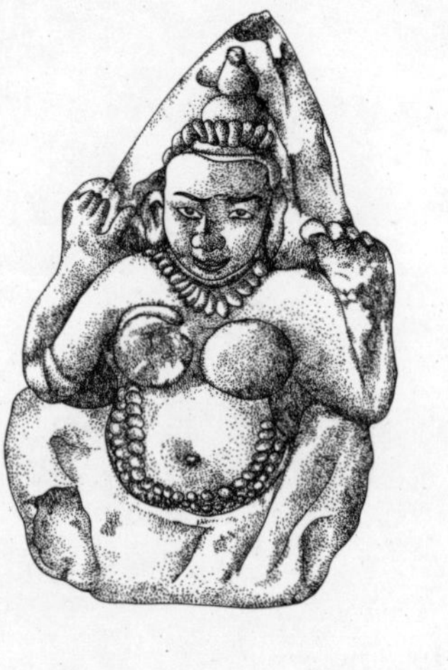

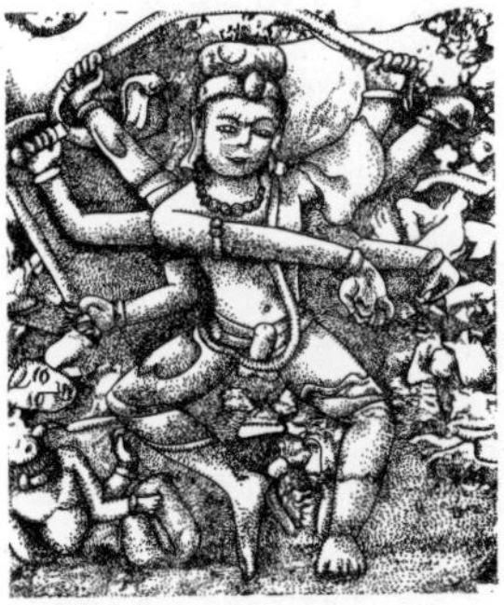

Nayak, P.M. (ed.), *Confluence*, vol. I, Registrar, Sambalpur University, Burla, 1992.

Nema, S.R., *Political History of The Somavaṁśī Kings of South Kośala and Orissa*, Oriental Publishers, New Delhi, 1978.

Neumayer, Erwin, *Lines on Stone*, Manohar, New Delhi, 1990.

NIATAL, 2nd edn., 1994.

Nigam, M.L., *Report of The Excavation of two Megalithic Burial at Hashmatpet, Hyderabad, Andhra Pradesh*, Birla Archaeological & Cultural Research Institute, Hyderabad, Andhra Pradesh, 1971.

Niranjanananda, Paramahamsa, *Yoga Darshan* (*Vision of the Yoga Upaniṣad*), Sri Panchdashnam Paramahamsa, Alakhbara, Deogarh, Bihar, 1993.

Sri Swamiji Maharaj, *Siddhānta Rahasya* (*Secrets of Spiritual living*), Śrī Pitambarapeeth Sanskrit Parishad, Datia, Madhya Pradesh, Chaitra Purnima, Samvat, 2040.

Pandey, Kanti Chandra, *Comparative Aesthetics*, vol. I, Chowkhamba Sanskrit Series, Vārāṇasī, 1959 and edition 1995.

Pandey, R. P., *Pre-historic Archaeology of Madhya Pradesh*, Sundeep Prakashan, Delhi, 1987.

Pandey, S.K., *Indian Rock Art*, Aryan Books International, New Delhi, (?).

Pandit, M.P. (Readings), *Kulārṇava Tantra*, Motilal Banarsidass, Delhi, 1994.

Panigrahi, K.C., *Archaeological Remains at Bhubaneswar*, Orient Longmans, New Delhi, 1961.

Panigrahi, K.C., *History of Orissa*, Kitab Mahal, Cuttack, 1981.

Parida, A.N., *Early Temples of Orissa*, Commonwealth Publisher, New Delhi, 1999.

Patel, C.B., *Dynastic History of Nalas*, Punthi Pustak, Kolkata, 1990.

Patel, Prof. S.R., *East and West — A Cultural Dialogue*, Bharatiya Vidya Bhavan, Bombay, 1992.

Pradhan, S. (ed.), *Orissa: History, Culture and Archaeology*, D.K. Printworld (P) Ltd., New Delhi, 1999.

Pradhan, S., *Rock Art in Orissa*, Aryan Books International, New Delhi, 2001.

Praharaj, Gopal Chandra, *Pūrna Candra Ordiā Bhāṣā Kośa*, vol. I and vol. V, Cuttack, 1931 and 1936.

Radhakrishna, B.P. & Merh, S.S. (eds.), *Vedic Sarasvati* (*Evolutionary History of a lost River of North Western India*), Geological Society of India, Bangalore, 1999.

Raghavan, V., *Yantras or Mechanical Contrivances in Ancient India*, (Transaction no. 10), The Indian Institute of Culture, Bangalore, 2nd edn., 1956.

Rai, Ram Kumar, *Kulārṇava Tantra*, Prachya Prakashan, Vārāṇasī, 1983.

Ramchandra Rao, Prof. S.K., *The Yantras*, Sri Satguru Publications, Delhi, 1988.

Rath, A.K., *Studies on Some Aspects of the History and Culture of Orissa*, Punthi Pustak, Kolkata, 1987.

Rath, C.S. "Lord Jagannātha, A Legend and a Symbol an Interpretation," in *Studies in the Cult of Jagannātha*, ed. K.C. Mishra, Institute of Orissan Culture, Bhubaneswar, 1991.

Romanis, F. De. & Techernia, A. (eds.), *Crossings: Early Mediterranean Contacts with India*, Manohar, New Delhi, 1997.

Sahu, N.K., *Buddhism in Orissa*, Utkal University, Cuttack, 1958.

Sahu, N.K., *Utkal University History of Orissa*, vol. I, Utkal University, Bhubaneswar, 1964.

Saraswati, Paramahamsa Swami Satyananda, *A Systematic Course in the Ancient Tāntric Technique of Yoga and Kriyā*, Bihar School of Yoga, Munger, 1981 and 2nd edn. 1989.

Saraswati, Paramahamsa Swami Satyananda, *Kuṇḍalinī Tantra*, Bihar School of Yoga, Munger, 1992.

Saraswati, Swami Prakashanand, *The True History and the Religion of India*, Motilal Banarsidass, Delhi, 2001

Sastri, T.V.G., Bai, K.N. & Rao, J.V.P., *Veerapuram*, Bhavani Printers, Hyderabad, 1984.

SASWITW, Delhi, 1979.

Satpathy, S., *Śakti Iconography in Tāntric Mahāvidyās*, Punthi Pustak, Kolkata, 1991.

Sengupta, S.R., *Mother Cult*, Firma K.L.M., Kolkata, 1977.

Sharma, A.K., *Archaeo-Anthropology of Chhattisgarh*, Sundeep Prakashan, New Delhi, 2000.

Sharma, R.A., *Technology and Material Life of Central India*, Agamkala Prakashan, Delhi, 1991.

Sharma, R.K. & Tripathi, K.K. (eds.), *Recent Perspectives on Pre-Historic Art in India and Allied Subjects*, Aryan Books International, New Delhi, 1996.

Shukla, L.K., *A Study of Hindu Art and Architecture, with especial Reference to Terminology*, Chowkhamba Sanskrit Series Office, Varanasi, 1972.

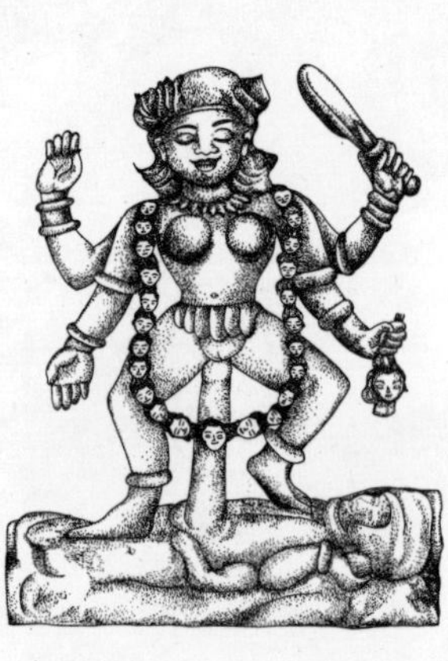

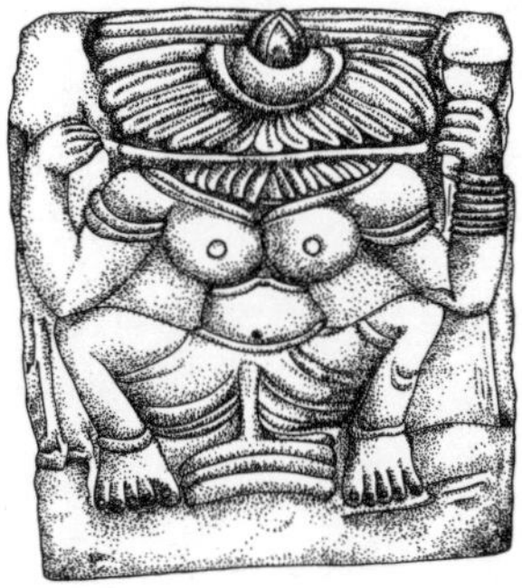

Singh Deo, J.P. *Origin of Jagannātha Deity*, Gyan Publishing House, New Delhi, 1991.

Singh Deo, J.P., *Cultural Profile of South Kośala*, Gyan Publishing House, Delhi, 1987.

Singh Deo, J.P., *Tāntric Art of Orissa*, Kalpaz Publication, Delhi, 2001.

Singh, B., *The Vedic Harappans*, Aditya Prakashan, New Delhi, 1995.

Singh, Jagabandhu, *Pracina Utkala* (Oriyā), Puri, 1929.

Singh, Ranvir, *A Study of Decorative Motifs in the Rock Art of Orissa*, M. Phil Thesis, History Dept., Sambalpur University, 1996-97, unpublished.

Singhal, J.P. *The Sphinx Speaks or the Story of the Pre-Historic Nations*, Sadgyan Sadan, New Delhi, 1963.

Sivananda, Swami, *Bliss Divine*, The Divine Life Society, Shivanandanagar, 1974.

Sivananda, Swami, *Kuṇḍalinī Yoga*, The Divine Society, Sivanandanagar, Uttar Pradesh, 1971.

Sivananda, Swami, *Lord Śiva and His Worship*, The Divine Life Society, Sivanandanagar, 1984.

Sivananda, Swami, *Mind: Its Mysteries and Control*, The Divine Life Society, Shivanandanagar, 1974.

Srivastava, Balram, *Iconography of Śakti* (*A Study based on Sritattvanidhi*), Choukhambha Orientalia, Vārāṇasī, 1978.

Stone, E.R., *The Buddhist Art of Nāgārjunakoṇḍa*, Motilal Banarsidass, Delhi, 1994.

Stutley, James & Stutley, Margaret, *Harpers' Dictionary of Hinduism*, New York, 1977.

Svoboda, R.E., *Aghora* (*At the left hand of God*), Rupa & Co., New Delhi, 1993.

Swami, Nikhilananda, *The Upaniṣads* (Abridged edition), Harper Torch Books, Harper & Row Publishers, New York & Evanston, 1963.

Talageri, S.G., *The Ṛgveda — A Historical Analysis*, Aditya Prakashan, New Delhi, 2000.

THACOTIP, vol. I, 1965, vol. II, 1968, vol. III, 1970, vol. IV, 1964 and vol. V, 1966.

The Cultural Heritage of India, vol. II, The Ramakrishna Mission Institute of Culture, Kolkata, 1969.

Tiwari, A.N. (ed.), *Reference Orissa*, Enterprising Publishers, Bhubaneswar, 1999.

Tripathy, K.C., *Lithic Industries in India (A Study of South-Western Orissa)*, Leeladevi Publications, Delhi, 1980.

TYATWG, Motilal Banarsidass, Delhi, 1996.

Upadhyaya, R.K., *The Concept of God in Śaiva Tantra*, Jnananidhi Prakashan, Muzaffarpur, 1984.

Upasak, C.S., *The History and Palaeography of Mauryan Brahmi Script*, Nalanda Publishers, (?), 1960.

Vatsyayan, K. (General ed.), *Prakṛti (The Integral Vision)*, vol. 3, Indira Gandhi National Centre for the Arts, New Delhi, D.K. Printworld (P.) Ltd., New Delhi, 1995.

Verma, V.K., *Indo-Aryan Colonization of Greece and Middle East*, vol. I & vol. II, Pratibha Prakashan, Delhi, 2000.

Waddel, L.A., *Tibetan Buddhism*, (?).

Woodroffe, Sir John (trans.), *Kāma-Kalā-Vilasa*, Ganesh & Co., Pvt., Ltd., Madras, 1971.

Woodroffe, Sir John, (ed.), *Tantra Rāja Tantra (A Short Analysis)*, Ganesh & Co. Madras, 1971.

Woodroffe, Sir John, *Śakti and Śākta (Essays & Addresses)*, Ganesh & Company, Madras, 1975.

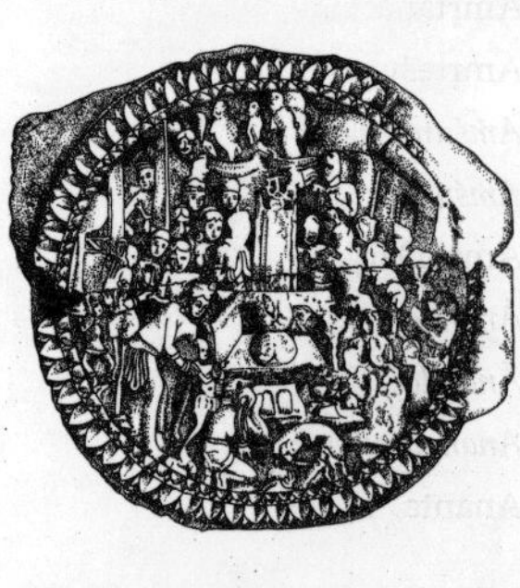

Index